Hepatitis C: From Pathophysiology to Disease Management

Hepatitis C: From Pathophysiology to Disease Management

Edited by Ned Wright

hayle
medical

New York

Hayle Medical,
750 Third Avenue, 9th Floor,
New York, NY 10017, USA

Visit us on the World Wide Web at:
www.haylemedical.com

ISBN: 978-1-63241-875-3

Cataloging-in-Publication Data

Hepatitis C : from pathophysiology to disease management / edited by Ned Wright.
    p. cm.
Includes bibliographical references and index.
ISBN 978-1-63241-875-3
1. Hepatitis C. 2. Hepatitis C--Pathophysiology. 3. Hepatitis C--Treatment.
4. Hepatitis C--Diagnosis. I. Wright, Ned.
RC848.H425 H46 2020
616.362 3--dc23

Table of Contents

Permissions

List of Contributors

Index

Preface

This book was inspired by the evolution of our times; to answer the curiosity of inquisitive minds. Many developments have occurred across the globe in the recent past which has transformed the progress in the field.

Hepatitis C is a liver disease that is caused by the hepatitis C virus. People infected by the virus do not exhibit symptoms initially but occasionally dark urine, yellow tinged skin, fever and abdominal pain may occur. The infection can potentially lead to liver disease and cirrhosis. The hepatitis C virus is spread due to the use of poorly sterilized medical equipment, transfusions, blood-to-blood contact and needlestick injuries. It may also spread when an infected mother gives birth to her baby. There is no vaccination against hepatitis C. However, hepatitis C can be prevented using a combination of harm reduction strategies, including treatment of substance abuse, provision of new syringes and needles, and screening of blood donors. Chronic infection with hepatitis C can be cured with antiviral medications such as simeprevir or sofosbuvir. This book covers in detail the clinical aspects of hepatitis C from pathophysiology to disease management. It unravels the recent studies in hepatitis C. A number of latest researches have been included to keep the readers up-to-date with the global concepts in this area of study.

This book was developed from a mere concept to drafts to chapters and finally compiled together as a complete text to benefit the readers across all nations. To ensure the quality of the content we instilled two significant steps in our procedure. The first was to appoint an editorial team that would verify the data and statistics provided in the book and also select the most appropriate and valuable contributions from the plentiful contributions we received from authors worldwide. The next step was to appoint an expert of the topic as the Editor-in-Chief, who would head the project and finally make the necessary amendments and modifications to make the text reader-friendly. I was then commissioned to examine all the material to present the topics in the most comprehensible and productive format.

I would like to take this opportunity to thank all the contributing authors who were supportive enough to contribute their time and knowledge to this project. I also wish to convey my regards to my family who have been extremely supportive during the entire project.

Editor

hepatocellular carcinoma (HCC), and coinciding lymphoproliferative disorders, remain unknown. The fate of HCV during prodromal and convalescent phases of infection is also poorly recognized. Moreover, in addition to a symptomatic infection, which is normally accompanied by circulating HCV RNA and antibodies to HCV (anti-HCV), HCV can also persist as a clinically silent (occult) infection [1–3]. This infection is accompanied by very low levels of HCV RNA in serum (usually below 100–200 virus genome copies per mL), liver, and peripheral blood mononuclear cells (PBMCs), which are detectable with a significant difficulty, if at all, by clinical assays [4, 5]. This occult HCV infection (OCI) continues for decades after either spontaneous (self-limited) or antiviral therapy-induced resolution of hepatitis [1–4, 6–10]. OCI may have epidemiologic (e.g., contamination of blood and organ donations) and pathogenic (e.g., cryptogenic liver disease and oncogenicity) consequences which are not yet well recognized. Furthermore, experimental and clinical data indicate that HCV replicates not only in the liver but also in the lymphatic system, where it can modify development, proliferation, and function of immune cells [1, 2, 4, 5, 11–18]. It is also apparent that immune cells are reservoirs of persisting HCV where virus may hide from immune surveillance and elimination, similar to that in infections with other lymphotropic viruses [19–22]. The ability of HCV to infect cells of the immune system is consistent with a significantly greater prevalence of lymphoproliferative disorders in patients chronically infected with HCV, including mixed cryoglobulinemia (MC), B-cell non-Hodgkin's lymphoma (B-cell NHL), and marginal zone lymphoma [23–26]. Regression of these diseases in considerable numbers of patients treated with anti-HCV therapies is indicative of the direct role of HCV in the pathogenesis of those diseases [27, 28].

2. Identification of lymphotropic HCV replication

The current approach to the diagnosis of HCV infection, which typically includes testing of only serum samples but not samples from liver or otherwise easily accessible PBMC, using assays detecting only HCV RNA-positive (also termed as non-replicative, genomic, or vegetative) strand and anti-HCV, is an obstacle in the precise determination of HCV clearance, that is, cure. These limitations are also a source of controversies regarding the natural history and the longevity of infection, as well as the sites of virus persistence [29–33]. Consequently, patients who are considered free of infection may produce low levels of biologically competent virus for an extended time after vanishing of symptoms and biochemical normalization of liver function achieved due to either spontaneous resolution or clinically apparent sustained virologic response (SVR) to antiviral treatment [1, 4–6, 8, 9]. Testing of serial samples of serum or plasma and, in particular, PBMC collected a few months apart increases the detection of low levels of HCV RNA during follow-up, even when clinical assays of moderate or low sensitivity are applied. This is due to the fluctuating level of circulating virus during OCI that can temporarily increase to the levels detectable by these assays [2, 4, 5].

Identification of HCV infection in immune cells is not just about the mere detection of virus RNA-positive strand, since the occurrence of this strand alone may reflect incidental cell surface attachment or cellular uptake of virus or its genomic material. A combination of a few approaches has been applied to credibly detect replicating HCV in immune cells [4]. They involve the documentation of (1) HCV RNA-negative (also termed as replicative or anti-genomic) strand [1, 6, 9, 34]; (2) viral structural and/or, preferentially, nonstructural proteins within the cytoplasm of infected cells [15, 34]; (3) distinctive HCV variants in total PBMC or their cell subsets when compared to those in plasma or in liver of infected patients, or emergence of HCV variants in cultured cells which are distinct from those occurring in inocula used to infect them [15, 34]; (4) susceptibility of infected cells to *ex vivo* treatment with interferon alpha (IFN-α) [6, 35] or direct acting antivirals (DAAs) [9, 34]; (5) transmission of infection to virus-naïve cells by cell-free supernatants from primary-cultured cells or *de novo*-infected cultures [34, 35]; (6) display of biophysical properties of virions by viral particles released during culture of infected cells [35], and (7) visualization of HCV virions released from infected cells by immunogold electron microscopy (IEM) with virus envelope-specific antibody [6, 35]. However, although the immune cells can support the complete cycle of HCV replication and production of biologically competent virion particles, the virus load per cell and the level of virus replication in either *in vivo*- or *in vitro*-infected immune cells are much lower than those seen in the HCV JFH-1 (Japanese fulminant hepatitis-1)-Huh7.5 cell infection system. Also, for comparison, the loads of HCV RNA per cell in total PBMC were found to be lower than those per hepatocyte in chronic hepatitis C (CHC), but comparable to each other during OCI [7]. Overall, investigations of HCV lymphotropism remain challenging and require highly sensitive detection techniques and meticulous approaches.

3. HCV compartmentalization in the immune system

HCV displays a remarkable genetic variability and typically exists in an infected host as a heterologous population of closely related subpopulations of viral particles carrying slightly different genomic sequences, called collectively as quasispecies. The 5′-untranslated region (5′-UTR) of virus genome contains an internal ribosome entry site (IRES) essential for viral RNA translation. This sequence is highly conserved among different HCV genomes, and arise of variants within this region is usually an indicator of a sustained virus change. HCV derived from extrahepatic locations tends to display variations in the IRES sequence when compared to the genomes from plasma and liver [5, 36]. Some of these substitutions are located at particular nucleotide positions, suggesting that they may reflect virus adaptation to replication in a non-hepatic milieu. In addition, variants within the hypervariable region-1 (HVR1) of the virus E2 protein, although much more common than those in the 5′-UTR, may also reflect the site-restricted replication of HCV variants. Overall, compartmentalization of HCV variants in immune cells is considered to be a reliable indicator of hepatocyte-independent virus replication [36].

The existence of HCV quasispecies with affinity to immune cells has been suggested shortly after HCV discovery [37–39]. Evidence for lymphotropic HCV variants was found in patients with CHC, acute hepatitis C, as well as in asymptomatic individuals with persistent OCI [4, 14, 15, 40–47]. Analyses of HCV variants residing in PBMC by clonal sequencing and single-stranded conformational polymorphism (SSCP) revealed features which argued against the possibility of carry-over of variants from plasma-derived HCV RNA or from

The studies from our laboratory showed that authentic HCV of different genotypes can infect total T cells enriched in culture from PBMC of healthy donors by their intermittent stimulation with phytohemagglutinin (PHA) in the presence of human recombinant IL-2 [6, 34, 35, 63, 64]. Replication and secretion of infectious HCV virions in this system were ascertained by the detection of (1) HCV RNA replicative strand and NS5a and/or core protein in infected cells [6, 34, 35, 63], (2) the emergence of HCV variants not existing in inocula used to infect the cells [6, 34], (3) the release of HCV RNA-reactive particles with buoyant density and ultra-structural properties of virions [34, 35], (4) virions released by infected cells via IEM [6, 34], and (5) the serial passage of HCV produced by the *de novo*-infected cells in virus-naïve primary T cells [35]. Moreover, the *de novo* HCV infection was inhibited by IFN-α- [35] and HCV-specific protease inhibitor Telaprevir [34, 63]. Furthermore, the system was adapted to include readily available Molt-4 and Jurkat T cells as infection targets, making it independent from freshly isolated human PBMC [63, 64]. In this model, the infection of essentially intact cells with unmodified, naturally occurring HCV allowed for the determination of (1) infectivity of low levels of HCV persisting in the course of OCI [6], (2) CD5 as the T-cell-specific receptor that mediates infection of the cells with patient-derived HCV [63], (3) differential expression of candidate HCV receptors in human T cells prone or resistant to infection with authentic HCV [64], and (4) an impact of infection with HCV on the suppression of CD4$^+$ T lymphocyte proliferation [72]. In the most recent study [34], the same infection system was also applied to recognize quantitative differences between CD4$^+$ and CD8$^+$ T-cell subsets in the level of HCV replication and to define properties of the virus produced by these cells. These investigations showed that although HCV replicates in both cell subtypes, the level of HCV replication in CD4$^+$ T cells was significantly higher than that in CD8$^+$ T cells. Intracellular HCV NS5a and core proteins were displayed at a similar frequency in both subtypes, that is, in 0.9 and 1.2% of CD4$^+$ and CD8$^+$ cells, respectively. Double staining for HCV NS5a protein and CD4 or CD8 T-cell differentiation markers provided conclusive evidence that virus replicated in both cell types. In addition, virus produced by CD4$^+$ and CD8$^+$ cells displayed different biophysical properties than those characterizing viral particles occurring in plasma used to infect the cells, confirming that new virus was produced, and the same virus was infectious to naïve CD4$^+$ of CD8$^+$ T cells isolated from a healthy donor. Remarkably, the data obtained from the *in vitro* infection of CD4$^+$ and CD8$^+$ T cells were comparable to those characterizing the infection of primary CD4$^+$ and CD8$^+$ T cells isolated from HCV-infected patients [15], although the level of HCV replication tended to be higher in *in vitro* than in *in vivo* conditions. Since HCV-specific T-cell effector activity is considered to be a principal factor underlying the pathogenesis of CHC as well as the resolution of hepatitis [73, 74], HCV infection of the T cells may have a direct impact on the virus-specific immune T-cell-depended responses and, in consequence, advance both virus infection and disease process.

5. Molecules mediating entry leading to HCV replication in immune cells

The HCV envelope is composed by two glycoproteins, E1 and E2. These proteins are primarily responsible for the virion attachment to the cell surface molecules serving as receptors and for the subsequent steps of viral entry [75]. The ability of HCV to infect human cells has approaches has been applied to credibly detect replicating HCV in immune cells [4]. They involve the documentation of (1) HCV RNA-negative (also termed as replicative or anti-genomic) strand [1, 6, 9, 34]; (2) viral structural and/or, preferentially, nonstructural proteins within the cytoplasm of infected cells [15, 34]; (3) distinctive HCV variants in total PBMC or their cell subsets when compared to those in plasma or in liver of infected patients, or emergence of HCV variants in cultured cells which are distinct from those occurring in inocula used to infect them [15, 34]; (4) susceptibility of infected cells to *ex vivo* treatment with interferon alpha (IFN-α) [6, 35] or direct acting antivirals (DAAs) [9, 34]; (5) transmission of infection to virus-naïve cells by cell-free supernatants from primary-cultured cells or *de novo*-infected cultures [34, 35]; (6) display of biophysical properties of virions by viral particles released during culture of infected cells [35], and (7) visualization of HCV virions released from infected cells by immunogold electron microscopy (IEM) with virus envelope-specific antibody [6, 35]. However, although the immune cells can support the complete cycle of HCV replication and production of biologically competent virion particles, the virus load per cell and the level of virus replication in either *in vivo*- or *in vitro*-infected immune cells are much lower than those seen in the HCV JFH-1 (Japanese fulminant hepatitis-1)-Huh7.5 cell infection system. Also, for comparison, the loads of HCV RNA per cell in total PBMC were found to be lower than those per hepatocyte in chronic hepatitis C (CHC), but comparable to each other during OCI [7]. Overall, investigations of HCV lymphotropism remain challenging and require highly sensitive detection techniques and meticulous approaches.

3. HCV compartmentalization in the immune system

HCV displays a remarkable genetic variability and typically exists in an infected host as a heterologous population of closely related subpopulations of viral particles carrying slightly different genomic sequences, called collectively as quasispecies. The 5′-untranslated region (5′-UTR) of virus genome contains an internal ribosome entry site (IRES) essential for viral RNA translation. This sequence is highly conserved among different HCV genomes, and arise of variants within this region is usually an indicator of a sustained virus change. HCV derived from extrahepatic locations tends to display variations in the IRES sequence when compared to the genomes from plasma and liver [5, 36]. Some of these substitutions are located at particular nucleotide positions, suggesting that they may reflect virus adaptation to replication in a non-hepatic milieu. In addition, variants within the hypervariable region-1 (HVR1) of the virus E2 protein, although much more common than those in the 5′-UTR, may also reflect the site-restricted replication of HCV variants. Overall, compartmentalization of HCV variants in immune cells is considered to be a reliable indicator of hepatocyte-independent virus replication [36].

The existence of HCV quasispecies with affinity to immune cells has been suggested shortly after HCV discovery [37–39]. Evidence for lymphotropic HCV variants was found in patients with CHC, acute hepatitis C, as well as in asymptomatic individuals with persistent OCI [4, 14, 15, 40–47]. Analyses of HCV variants residing in PBMC by clonal sequencing and single-stranded conformational polymorphism (SSCP) revealed features which argued against the possibility of carry-over of variants from plasma-derived HCV RNA or from virus nonspecifically attached to the cell surface [5–9, 13, 15, 42, 48, 49]. Furthermore, HCV variants from lymphoid cells were genetically related, but distinct from those occurring in serum or liver. In some instances, HCV quasispecies identified in lymphoid cells were detectable in serum but not in liver tissue, indicating that the majority of circulating virus could be of extrahepatic origin. In this regard, the analysis of the HVR1 from liver, PBMC, and serum showed that certain virus variants occurring in serum resided only in PBMC but not in the liver [42, 44]. Moreover, HCV quasispecies from one cell type, for example, CD8$^+$ T lymphocytes, were statistically more genetically like one another when compared to variants from other immune cell subsets, such as CD4$^+$ T cells. In one pertinent study, HCV RNA sequences carried by CD8$^+$ T lymphocytes were phylogenetically clustered close to one another, but not to those detected in CD4$^+$ T cells or CD19$^+$ B cells [48]. It has been found that certain sequence polymorphisms within the IRES of the 5'-UTR of the HCV genomes originating from lymphoid cells coincided with a different IRES translational activity which could promote HCV replication in cells carrying those variations [36, 50]. Similarly, it was demonstrated using liver-derived hepatoma Huh7 cells that HCV IRES variants originating from plasma displayed a significantly higher translational activity than those from HCV residing in B cells [51]. On the other hand, the IRES variants of virus replicating in B cells displayed a similarly low translational efficiency in Raji and Daudi B-cell lines as well as in hepatoma Huh7 cells, suggesting not only their extrahepatic origin but also a low capacity to replicate in B cells [51].

As already alluded to, the studies on HCV compartmentalization in the immune system demonstrated the existence of replicating virus in all the main subsets of circulating lymphomononuclear cells, including B cells, T lymphocytes, and monocytes [1, 13, 15, 42, 52]. There is also evidence for HCV replication in other immune cell types, such as dendritic cells (DCs) [53, 54]. In one of our studies, the virus load and the level of HCV replication were quantified in total PBMC as well as in affinity-purified cell subsets from these PBMCs, including CD4$^+$ and CD8$^+$ T lymphocytes, B cells, and monocytes from patients with CHC or OCI [15]. This investigation showed significant differences in the level of immune cell subset infection between patients with CHC and OCI with overall greater HCV loads in immune cells in CHC compared to those with OCI. In addition, monocytes carried the greatest HCV amounts in CHC, while B cells tended to contain the highest virus loads, and monocytes were the least frequently infected in OCI. Interestingly, while the total PBMCs were HCV RNA nonreactive in some individuals, the immune cell subsets isolated from these PBMCs clearly displayed virus RNA and its replicative strand, suggesting preferential or exclusive infection of the particular immune cell subset. This also indicated that the testing of total PBMC may not always identify residing virus and, thus, the analysis of individual immune cell types should be considered. In this study, HCV replication in immune cells was ascertained by the detection of (1) HCV RNA replicative (negative) strand, (2) HCV nonstructural 5a protein (NS5A), and (3) HCV variants distinct from those found in plasma of the same patients. In addition, immune cells were exposed *ex vivo* to a T-cell-stimulating mitogen in the presence of human recombinant interleukin-2 (IL-2) to augment HCV replication. We previously showed that such a treatment increases HCV replication in immune cells and improves detection of virus [15, 55]. Overall, the study identified the main immune cell types involved in HCV infection in CHC and OCI and demonstrated that the immune system supports HCV replication regardless of the clinical appearance of infection.

It should be mentioned that the identification of HCV in the lymphatic system is not limited only to PBMC. HCV genomes and its proteins were also demonstrated in lymph nodes and bone marrow [47, 56]. In regard to lymph nodes, replicating HCV genomes and virus core and NS3 proteins were detected within biopsied B-cell-rich lymphoid follicles from patients with CHC [47]. In one study, not only did B cells appear to be the primary site of HCV infection in this secondary lymphoid tissue, but clonal sequencing analyses also indicated that in certain patients, HCV residing in lymph node-derived B cells could contribute up to 40% of the total level of viremia [47]. Furthermore, it is of note that HCV RNA sequences found in cerebrospinal fluid of patients co-infected with human immunodeficiency virus type 1(HIV-1) were identified to be more similar to virus sequences in PBMC and lymph nodes than to those in plasma. This raised a possibility that cells of the monocyte/macrophage lineage may carry HCV into the brain, and that resident microglial cells maintain its replication independently of the liver [56, 57]. In addition, HCV RNA-positive and -negative strands, as well as HCV structural and nonstructural proteins, were readily detectable in CD34$^+$ hematopoietic progenitor cells in the bone marrow of patients with CHC [58], reinforcing the notion of extrahepatic HCV replication. However, there was no evidence of primary CD34$^+$ cells from healthy individuals supporting *de novo* HCV infection. The same study showed that CD34$^+$ cells from CHC patients could release HCV RNA into culture supernatant, linking the development of CD34$^+$ cells to their susceptibility to HCV.

4. Replication of HCV in primary immune cells and cultured immune cell lines

Direct support for the inherent propensity of HCV to enter and propagate in cells of the immune system stems from *in vitro* studies where HCV-susceptible stable human lymphocytic cell lines, normal human PBMC, or primary immune cell subsets isolated from PBMC were exposed to HCV. In this regard, it is important to note that only authentic, patient-derived virus, but not laboratory-constructed recombinant HCV clones, including HCV JFH-1, infect either primary immune cells or susceptible immune cell lines [59, 60]. Hence, it was reported that HCV carried in the serum or plasma of HCV-positive patients was infectious to Raji and Daudi B-cell lines [18, 61] and to T-cell lines, such as Molt-4 [62–64], HPB [65] and Jurkat (all derived from patients with acute T-lymphoblastic leukemia) [63, 64], and pre-stimulated PM1 (originated from acute cutaneous T-cell lymphoma) [63, 64]. It was also shown that HCV released from SB, a B-cell line established from the splenocytes of an HCV-positive patient with type II MC and monocytoid lymphoma [66], was infectious to human primary CD4$^+$ T cells [67], and Molt-4 and Jurkat T cells [68]. Others have demonstrated the ability of primary lymphoid cells from healthy individuals, including total PBMC [11, 43, 52], T lymphocytes [6, 15, 35], B cells [8, 15, 51, 69, 70], and monocytes/macrophages [15, 71] to support HCV infection.

The studies from our laboratory showed that authentic HCV of different genotypes can infect total T cells enriched in culture from PBMC of healthy donors by their intermittent stimulation with phytohemagglutinin (PHA) in the presence of human recombinant IL-2 [6, 34, 35, 63, 64]. Replication and secretion of infectious HCV virions in this system were ascertained by the detection of (1) HCV RNA replicative strand and NS5a and/or core protein in infected cells [6, 34, 35, 63], (2) the emergence of HCV variants not existing in inocula used to infect the cells [6, 34], (3) the release of HCV RNA-reactive particles with buoyant density and ultra-structural properties of virions [34, 35], (4) virions released by infected cells via IEM [6, 34], and (5) the serial passage of HCV produced by the *de novo*-infected cells in virus-naïve primary T cells [35]. Moreover, the *de novo* HCV infection was inhibited by IFN-α- [35] and HCV-specific protease inhibitor Telaprevir [34, 63]. Furthermore, the system was adapted to include readily available Molt-4 and Jurkat T cells as infection targets, making it independent from freshly isolated human PBMC [63, 64]. In this model, the infection of essentially intact cells with unmodified, naturally occurring HCV allowed for the determination of (1) infectivity of low levels of HCV persisting in the course of OCI [6], (2) CD5 as the T-cell-specific receptor that mediates infection of the cells with patient-derived HCV [63], (3) differential expression of candidate HCV receptors in human T cells prone or resistant to infection with authentic HCV [64], and (4) an impact of infection with HCV on the suppression of CD4$^+$ T lymphocyte proliferation [72]. In the most recent study [34], the same infection system was also applied to recognize quantitative differences between CD4$^+$ and CD8$^+$ T-cell subsets in the level of HCV replication and to define properties of the virus produced by these cells. These investigations showed that although HCV replicates in both cell subtypes, the level of HCV replication in CD4$^+$ T cells was significantly higher than that in CD8$^+$ T cells. Intracellular HCV NS5a and core proteins were displayed at a similar frequency in both subtypes, that is, in 0.9 and 1.2% of CD4$^+$ and CD8$^+$ cells, respectively. Double staining for HCV NS5a protein and CD4 or CD8 T-cell differentiation markers provided conclusive evidence that virus replicated in both cell types. In addition, virus produced by CD4$^+$ and CD8$^+$ cells displayed different biophysical properties than those characterizing viral particles occurring in plasma used to infect the cells, confirming that new virus was produced, and the same virus was infectious to naïve CD4$^+$ of CD8$^+$ T cells isolated from a healthy donor. Remarkably, the data obtained from the *in vitro* infection of CD4$^+$ and CD8$^+$ T cells were comparable to those characterizing the infection of primary CD4$^+$ and CD8$^+$ T cells isolated from HCV-infected patients [15], although the level of HCV replication tended to be higher in *in vitro* than in *in vivo* conditions. Since HCV-specific T-cell effector activity is considered to be a principal factor underlying the pathogenesis of CHC as well as the resolution of hepatitis [73, 74], HCV infection of the T cells may have a direct impact on the virus-specific immune T-cell-depended responses and, in consequence, advance both virus infection and disease process.

5. Molecules mediating entry leading to HCV replication in immune cells

The HCV envelope is composed by two glycoproteins, E1 and E2. These proteins are primarily responsible for the virion attachment to the cell surface molecules serving as receptors and for the subsequent steps of viral entry [75]. The ability of HCV to infect human cells has been interpreted almost exclusively in the context of the interactions between HCV JFH-1 strain, related strains, or pseudoparticles and hepatocyte-like Huh7 cells or their subclone Huh7.5. Based on these studies, tetraspanin CD81 [76], glycosaminoglycans [77], low-density lipoprotein receptor (LDL-R) [77], scavenger receptor class B-type 1 (SR-B1) [76, 78], the tight junction protein claudin-1 (CLDN-1) [79], occludin (OCLN) [80–82], and co-factors, such as epidermal growth factor receptor (EGFR) and ephrin receptor A2 (EphA2) [83], have been proposed to contribute either directly or indirectly to HCV entry into hepatocytes. In addition, the Niemann-Pick C1-like 1 (NPC1L1) cholesterol absorption receptor and transferrin receptor 1 (TfR1) have been implicated in HCV entry [84, 85]. However, the degree to which these individual molecules participate in HCV infection of normal human hepatocytes by naturally occurring virus requires validation, particularly since the majority of these molecules are ubiquitously displayed on many cell types. On the other hand, molecules determining HCV lymphotropism remained entirely unknown until recently.

An important finding toward the recognition of virological determinants mediating HCV lymphotropism was recently provided which showed that a distinct virus subpopulation capable of encoding particular E1E2 (envelope) epitopes might be responsible for the infection of B lymphocytes [86]. Isolated HCV E1E2 glycoproteins from patient B cells were able to confer the ability to enter and replicate in B cells to a non-lymphotropic HCV JFH-1 strain, as demonstrated by the detection of viral RNA and proteins within those cells. Interestingly, the B-cell tropism coincided with a loss of the JFH-1 strain ability to infect liver cancer-derived, hepatocyte-like Huh7 cells, implying that a lymphotropic variant constituted a separate population of viral particles displaying unique E1E2 envelope specificity. These results also supported a notion that a receptor for HCV on B cells is distinct from that on hepatocytes.

The recent finding that a co-stimulatory receptor B7.2 (CD86) is involved in the infection of human memory B cells by the abovementioned HCV SB strain [66] substantiated the involvement of a hepatocyte-distinct receptor in HCV lymphotropism [87] (**Table 1**). The study showed that the virus E1E2 envelope and 5′-UTR sequences determine lymphotropism of the SB strain and that silencing of the virus sensor retinoic acid-inducible gene I (RIGI) or overexpression of micrcoRNA-122 permitted the persistence of viral replication in B cells. Furthermore, the interaction of the SB virus E2 protein with the cell B7.2 protein reduced the surface display of B7.2 on memory B cells and inhibited their function. Interestingly, it was also found that memory B cells in HCV-infected patients expressed significantly lower levels of surface B7.2 when compared to those in HCV-negative individuals, but they carried significantly higher levels of HCV RNA than naïve B cells derived from HCV-positive patients. This comprehensive study provided important data on several aspects of HCV B-cell tropism and its potential functional and pathological consequences.

By applying the HCV-human T-cell infection system established in our laboratory [35], it was uncovered that CD5, a lymphocyte-specific 67-kDa glycoprotein belonging to the scavenger receptor cysteine-rich family, is essential for the infection of human T cells by authentic, patient-derived HCV [63] (**Table 1**). This work also demonstrated that CD81 likely contributes as a co-receptor, since both anti-CD5 and anti-CD81 monoclonal antibodies inhibited HCV infection. However, only CD5-positive T cells were susceptible to infection [63]. Thus, it appears that while CD81 contributes to the broad recognition of cells by HCV, CD5 facilitates HCV tropism toward T lymphocytes. In this context, primary human hepatocytes and hepatoma cell lines

HCV	HCV genotype	Immune cell target	Receptor molecule	Receptor properties	Receptor physiological function	Expected consequences of HCV-receptor interaction
Authentic (wild-type), patient plasma-derived (Ref. [63])	1–4	T cell	CD5	67-kDa glycoprotein, cysteine-rich scavenger receptor superfamily	Co-stimulatory molecule modulating positively or negatively intracellular signaling pathways induced by the antigen-specific T and B cell receptors	Unknown
SB variant, B-cell lymphoma-derived (Ref. [87])	2b	B cell	B7.2 (CD86)	60–100-kDa glycoprotein, immunoglobulin superfamily	Co-stimulatory molecule interacting with CD28 for T-cell activation and CTLA4 for T-cell immune regulation	Reduction of B7.2 on memory B cells and inhibition of the cells function in HCV-positive patients

Table 1. Receptor molecules mediating HCV entry and replication in human lymphocytes.

were found to express trace amounts of CD5 mRNA but not protein [63, 64], clearly indicating that HCV utilizes different receptors to enter different cell targets. This was confirmed in a subsequent study that investigated the expression of hepatocyte HCV candidate receptors on human T lymphocytes prone or resistant to HCV infection with authentic virus [64]. The expression of SR-B1, occludin, CLDN-1 and -6, CD5, and CD81 was determined by real-time polymerase chain reaction (RT-PCR), and their proteins quantified by immunoblotting in T-cell lines found to be prone or resistant to HCV infection, PBMC, primary T cells and CD4+ and CD8+ T-cell subsets, and compared to hepatoma-derived, well-differentiated Huh7.5 and HepG2 cells. SR-B1 protein was found in T and hepatoma cell lines but not on PBMC or primary T lymphocytes, while CLDN-1 was detected only in HCV-resistant (when unstimulated) PM1 cell line and hepatoma cell lines, and CLDN-6 was equally expressed across all cells investigated. OCLN protein occurred in HCV-susceptible Molt-4 and Jurkat T cells and in trace amounts in primary T cells, but not in PBMC. CD5 was expressed by HCV-prone T-cell lines, primary T cells, and PBMC, but not by non-susceptible T and hepatoma cell lines, while CD81 was detected in all cell types except HepG2. Furthermore, knocking down OCLN in a virus-prone T-cell line inhibited HCV infection, while *de novo* infection downregulated both OCLN and CD81 and upregulated CD5 without modifying SR-B1 expression. Overall, while no association between SR-B1, CLDN-1, or CLDN-6 and the susceptibility to HCV was found, CD5 and CD81 expression coincided with virus lymphotropism and that of OCLN with permissiveness of T-cell lines, but seemingly not primary T cells. This study narrowed the range of candidate entry receptors utilized by HCV to infect T lymphocytes among those already uncovered using laboratory-grown HCV and Huh7.5 cells and confirmed that authentic HCV utilizes different receptors to enter hepatocytes and lymphocytes. The use of different receptors to infect multiple cell types is not uncommon among viruses. For example, HIV-1 uses CD4 to infect T cells but predominantly CCR5 to infect macrophages [88, 89]. The measles virus utilizes SLAM to infect lymphocytes, macrophages, and DC, but also infects SLAM-negative epithelial and endothelial cells [90, 91]. Also, EBV uses CD21 to infect B cells and DC, but this virus also replicates in epithelial cells which do not transcribe CD21 [92, 93]. In summary, CD5 was the first identified cell surface receptor that governs human cell permissiveness to HCV in a cell-type-specific manner. Since CD5 is also expressed on a minor subset of human pro-B lymphocytes [94], this molecule may potentially contribute to HCV entry to these B cells. Taken together, the results from several studies imply that cell-type-specific surface molecules, rather than a combination of molecules naturally displayed on many diverse cell types, mediate HCV tropism toward lymphocytes.

6. Functional and pathological consequences of HCV lymphotropism

The replication of HCV in immune cells, even at low levels, has a potential to affect their function, proliferation kinetics, and yield pathological outcomes, similar to infections with other lymphotropic viruses. Although the data remain overall sparse, there is a meaningful progress in some aspects. In particular, the study of a lymphotropic HCV SB strain brought the recognition of various specific mechanisms by which HCV may modify immune cell proliferation and function [95]. Among others, it has been shown that the transient infection of primary CD4+ T cells and selected T-cell lines with the SB strain distorted the IFN-γ/STAT-1/T-bet signaling leading to the inhibition of IFN-γ production [67, 96]. It was also reported that infection with this strain suppressed the proliferation of primary CD4+ T cells and their differentiation toward the Th1 lineage, as well as inhibited Molt-4 T-cell proliferation while enhancing their CD95 (Fas)-mediated apoptosis [68]. A study from our group showed that naturally occurring, patient-derived HCV inhibited the proliferation of primary CD4+, but not CD8+ T cells, without augmenting cell death [72]. Interestingly, the results also suggested that just an exposure to authentic HCV in the absence of molecularly evident viral replication might be sufficient to inhibit CD4+ T-cell proliferation. It has also been shown that HCV core protein is capable of the transcriptional activation of the IL-2 promoter in T cells [97] and could modulate T-cell responses by inducing spontaneous and T-cell receptor (TCR)-mediated oscillations of calcium ions [98]. Others demonstrated that HCV core protein upregulated the expression of anergy-related genes in Jurkat T cells stably expressing this protein, and this coincided with the activation of nuclear factor of activated T cells (NFAT) and suppression of the IL-2 promoter [99]. In addition, it was reported that the direct binding of HCV core protein to complement receptor, gC1qR, on CD4+ and CD8+ T cells upregulated the expression of programmed death-1 (PD-1). This was accompanied by the dysregulation of T-cell activation, proliferation, and apoptosis [100]. These alterations were restored by blocking the engagement of the PD-1 and programmed death ligand-1 (PDL-1) pathway.

Interesting findings have been recently reported regarding the effect of exposure of primary human T cells to authentic, plasma-occurring HCV and to virus E2 protein or E2 encoding RNA on the TCR-signaling pathways [101]. It is of note that TCR signaling is critical for the normal functioning of CD4+ and CD8+ T cells, including their differentiation, activation, proliferation, and effector functions. The study showed that HCV interferes with TCR signaling and impairs T-cell activation *via* two distinct mechanisms. The first included intracellular processing of virus E2 coding RNA into a shorter, 51 nucleotide-long RNA fragment, predicted to be a dicer substrate. This virus-derived sequence targets a regulatory phosphatase involved in Src kinase signaling (abbreviated as PTPRE), subsequently inhibiting TCR signaling. In the second mechanism, the lymphocyte-specific Src kinase (Lck) phosphorylated HCV E2 protein, resulting in the inhibition of nuclear transportation of activated NFAT and in turn reducing TCR activation. It was concluded that HCV particles deliver viral RNA and E2 protein to T cells and that the highly conserved motifs of both RNA and protein inhibit TCR signaling, contributing to T-cell dysfunction and virus persistence. A second study from the same group showed that PTPRE levels are significantly reduced in liver tissue and PBMC of HCV-infected patients compared to those of uninfected controls [102]. It was demonstrated that a deficiency in PTPRE expression impaired antigen-specific TCR signaling, while antiviral therapy rescued the enzyme expression in PBMC and restored antigen-specific TCR signaling. Overall, the data indicated that HCV infection of T cells hinders TCR signaling and that short, regulatory HCV RNA sequences intracellularly derived from HCV genomic RNA are crucial in this process. The data from our studies showing that the authentic, patient-derived HCV can productively infect CD4+ and CD8+ T cells both *in vivo* [15] and *in vitro* [34] provide an indispensable link between HCV infection and the findings reported in the above studies.

The propensity of HCV to infect B cells is consistent with a significantly greater prevalence of certain B-cell proliferative disorders, particularly B-cell NHL, in HCV-infected individuals. Several lines of evidence support a link between HCV infection and B-cell NHL. These include (1) a strong epidemiological association of B-cell NHL with persistent HCV infection [25], (2) clinical data demonstrating that successful anti-HCV therapy often results in the remission of B-cell NHL [27, 28], (3) experimental data showing that transgenic mice expressing the full-length HCV genome specifically in B cells spontaneously develop B-cell NHL [103], and (4) both *in vivo* and *in vitro* data indicating that B lymphocytes are susceptible to infection and capable of supporting HCV replication [15, 18].

The mechanisms of lymphomagenesis associated with HCV infection were investigated by several groups, and a few concepts have been proposed (reviewed in [17]). However, it should be taken into consideration the fact that MC frequently precedes the development of B-cell NHL in HCV-infected individuals, indicating that MC might be a transitional step in the progression to lymphoma [104]. The proposed mechanisms of the pathogenesis of HCV-associated of lymphoma (i.e., lymphomagenesis) can be divided into two main categories. One includes the protracted stimulation of B cells by HCV antigens leading to pathologically augmented proliferation of the cells; a process that may involve different intracellular mechanisms. Another category relates to direct HCV infection and replication within B cells causing alterations in B-cell receptor (BCR) signaling or mutagenic changes in the cellular DNA

[27] Tasleem S, Sood GK. Hepatitis C associated B-cell non-Hodgkin lymphoma: clinical features and the role of antiviral therapy. Journal of Clinical and Translational Hepatology. 2015;**3**:134-139

[28] Arcaini L, Besson C, Frigeni M, Fontaine H, Goldaniga M, Casato M, Visentini M, Torres HA, Loustaud-Ratti V, Peveling-Oberhag J, Fabr_s P, Rossotti R, Zaja F, Rigacci L, Rattotti S, Bruno R, Merli M, Dorival C, Alric L, Jaccard A, Pol S, Carrat F, Ferretti VV, Visco C, Hermine O. Interferon-free antiviral treatment in B-cell lymphoproliferative disorders associated with hepatitis C virus infection. Blood. 2016;**28**:2527-2532

[29] Radkowski M, Laskus T. Persistence of hepatitis C virus after successful treatment of chronic hepatitis C: Is hepatitis C infection for life? Liver Transplantation. 2005;**11**:114-116

[30] Michalak TI, Pham TNQ, Mulrooney-Cousins PM. Molecular diagnosis of occult HCV and HBV infections. Future Virology. 2007;**2**:451-465

[31] Pham TNQ, Michalak TI. Occult persistence and lymphotropism of hepatitis C virus infection. World Journal of Gastroenterology. 2008;**14**:2789-2793

[32] Pham TNQ, Michalak TI. Hepatitis C virus in peripheral blood mononuclear cells of individuals with isolated anti-hepatitis C virus antibody reactivity. Hepatology. 2008;**48**:350-351

[33] Carreño V, Bartolomé J, Castillo I, Quiroga JA. New perspectives in occult hepatitis C virus infection. World Journal of Gastroenterology. 2012;**18**:2887-2894. DOI: 10.3748/wjg.v18.i23.2887

[34] Skardasi G, Chen AY, Michalak TI. Authentic patient-derived hepatitis C virus infects and productively replicates in primary CD4$^+$ and CD8$^+$ T lymphocytes *in vitro*. Journal of Virology. 2018;**92**:e01790-17

[35] MacParland SA, Pham TN, Gujar SA, Michalak TI. De novo infection and propagation of wild-type hepatitis C virus in human T lymphocytes in vitro. The Journal of General Virology. 2006;**87**:3577-3586

[36] Laporte J, Bain C, Maurel O, Inchauspe G, Agut H, Cahour A. Differential distribution and internal translation efficiency of hepatitis C virus quasispecies present in dendritic and liver cells. Blood. 2003;**101**:52-57

[37] Willems M, Peerlinck K, Moshage H, Deleu I, Van den Eynde C, Vermylen J, Yap SH. Hepatitis C virus-RNA in plasma and in peripheral blood mononuclear cells of haemophiliacs with chronic hepatitis C: Evidence for viral replication in peripheral blood mononuclear cells. Journal of Medical Virology. 1994;**42**:272-278

[38] Yun Z-B, Sönnerborg A, Weiland O. Hepatitis C virus replication in liver and peripheral blood mononuclear cells of interferon-treated and untreated patients with chronic hepatitis C. Scandinavian Journal of Gastroenterology. 1994;**29**:82-86

[39] Shimizu YK, Igarashi H, Kanematu T, Fujiwara K, Wong DC, Purcell RH, Yoshikura H. Sequence analysis of the hepatitis C virus genome recovered from serum, liver,

and peripheral blood mononuclear cells of infected chimpanzees. Journal of Virology. 1997;**71**:5769-5773

[40] Zignego AL, Giannini C, Monti M, Gragnani L, Hepatitis C. Virus lymphotropism: Lessons from a decade of studies. Digestive and Liver Disease. 2007;**39**(Suppl. 1):S38-S45

[41] Berthillon P, Inchauspé G, Trépo C. Evidence for lymphotropic strain of HCV. Hepatologia Clinica. 1998;**6**:71-75

[42] Navas S, Martin J, Quiroga JA, Castillo I, Carreño V. Genetic diversity and tissue compartmentalization of the hepatitis C virus genome in blood mononuclear cells, liver, and serum from chronic hepatitis C patients. Journal of Virology. 1998;**72**:1640-1646

[43] Radkowski M, Wang L-F, Vargas HE, Rakela J, Laskus T. Detection of hepatitis C virus replication in peripheral blood mononuclear cells after orthotopic liver transplantation. Transplantation. 1998;**66**:664-666

[44] Okuda M, Hino K, Korenaga M, Yamaguchi Y, Katoh Y, Okita K. Differences in hypervariable region 1 quasispecies of hepatitis C virus in human serum, peripheral blood mononuclear cells and liver. Hepatology. 1999;**29**:217-222

[45] Maggi F, Fornai C, Morrica A, Vatteroni ML, Giorgi M, Marchi S, Ciccorossi P, Bendinelli M, Pistello M. Divergent evolution of hepatitis C virus in liver and peripheral blood mononuclear cells of infected patients. Journal of Medical Virology. 1999;**57**:57-63

[46] Afonso AMR, Jiang J, Penin F, Tareau C, Samuel D, Petit MA, Bismuth H, Dussaix E, Féray C. Nonrandom distribution of hepatitis C virus quasispecies in plasma and peripheral blood mononuclear cell subsets. Journal of Virology. 1999;**73**:9213-9221

[47] Pal S, Sullivan DG, Kim S, Lai KK, Kae J, Cotler SJ, Carithers RL Jr, Wood BL, Perkins JD, Gretch DR. Productive replication of hepatitis C virus in peripheral lymph nodes in vivo: Implications of HCV lymphotropism. Gastroenterology. 2006;**130**:1107-1116

[48] Roque-Afonso AM, Ducoulombier D, Di Liberto G, Kara R, Gigou M, Dussaix E, Samuel D, Feray C. Compartmentalization of hepatitis C virus genotypes between plasma and peripheral blood mononuclear cells. Journal of Virology. 2005;**79**:6349-6357

[49] Vera-Otarola J, Barria MI, Leon U, Marsac D, Carvallo P, Soza A, Lopez-Lastra M. Hepatitis C virus quasispecies in plasma and peripheral blood mononuclear cells of treatment naive chronically infected patients. Journal of Viral Hepatitis. 2009;**16**:633-643

[50] Forton DM, Karayiannis P, Mahmud N, Taylor-Robinson SD, Thomas HC. Identification of unique hepatitis C virus quasispecies in the central nervous system and comparative analysis of internal translational efficiency of brain, liver, and serum variants. Journal of Virology. 2004;**78**:5170-5183

[51] Durand T, Di Liberto G, Colman H, Cammas A, Boni S, Marcellin P, Cahour A, Vagner S, Feray C. Occult infection of peripheral B cells by hepatitis C variants which have low translational efficiency in cultured hepatocytes. Gut. 2010;**59**:934-942

[52] Blackard JT, Smeaton L, Hiasa Y, Horiike N, Onji M, Jamieson DJ, Rodriguez I, Mayer KH, Chung RT. Detection of hepatitis C virus (HCV) in serum and peripheral-blood mononuclear cells from HCV-monoinfected and HIV/HCV-coinfected persons. The Journal of Infectious Diseases. 2005;92:258-265

[53] Navas MC, Fuchs A, Schvoerer E, Bohbot A, Aubertin AM, Stoll-Keller F. Dendritic cell susceptibility to hepatitis C virus genotype 1 infection. Journal of Medical Virology. 2002;67:152-161

[54] Goutagny N, Fatmi A, De Ledinghen V, Penin F, Couzigou P, Inchauspé G, Bain C. Evidence of viral replication in circulating dendritic cells during hepatitis C virus infection. The Journal of Infectious Diseases. 2003;187:1951-1958

[55] Pham TNQ, MacParland SA, Coffin CS, Lee SS, Bursey FR, Michalak TI. Mitogen-induced upregulation of hepatitis C virus expression in human lymphoid cells. The Journal of General Virology. 2005;86:657-666

[56] Bagaglio S, Cinque P, Racca S, Pedale R, Grasso MA, Lazzarin A, Morsica G. Hepatitis C virus populations in the plasma, peripheral blood mononuclear cells and cerebrospinal fluid of HIV/hepatitis C virus-co-infected patients. AIDS. 2005;19(Suppl 3):S151-S165

[57] Radkowski M, Wilkinson J, Nowicki M, Adair D, Vargas H, Ingui C, Rakela J, Laskus T. Search for hepatitis C virus negative-strand RNA sequences and analysis of viral sequences in the central nervous system: Evidence of replication. Journal of Virology. 2002;76:600-608

[58] Sansonno D, Lotesoriere C, Cornacchiulo V, Fanelli M, Gatti P, Iodice G, Racanelli V, Dammacco F. Hepatitis C virus infection involves CD34(+) hematopoietic progenitor cells in hepatitis C virus chronic carriers. Blood. 1998;92:3328-3337

[59] Sarhan MA, Chen AY, Russell RS, Michalak TI. Patient-derived hepatitis C virus and JFH-1 clones differ in their ability to infect human hepatoma cells and lymphocytes. The Journal of General Virology. 2012;93:2399-2407

[60] Marukian S, Jones CT, Andrus L, Evans MJ, Ritola KD, Charles ED, Rice CM, Dustin LB. Cell culture-produced hepatitis C virus does not infect peripheral blood mononuclear cells. Hepatology. 2008;48:1843-1850

[61] Quer J, Cos J, Murillo P, Esteban JI, Esteban R, Guardia J. Improved attachment of natural HCV isolate to Daudi cells upon elimination of immune complexes and close pH control. Intervirology. 2005;48:285-291

[62] Shimizu YK, Iwamoto A, Hijikata M, Purcell RH, Yoshikura H. Evidence for in vitro replication of hepatitis C virus genome in a human T-cell line. Proceedings of the National Academy of Sciences of the United States of America. 1992;89:5477-5481

[63] Sarhan MA, Pham TN, Chen AY, Michalak TI. Hepatitis C virus infection of human T lymphocytes is mediated by CD5. Journal of Virology. 2012;86:3723-3735

[64] Sarhan MA, Chen AY, Michalak TI. Differential expression of candidate virus receptors in human T lymphocytes prone or resistant to infection with patient-derived hepatitis C virus. PLoS One. 2013;**8**:e62159

[65] Shimizu YK, Purcell RH, Yoshikura H. Correlation between the infectivity of hepatitis C virus in vivo and its infectivity in vitro. Proceedings of the National Academy of Sciences of the United States of America. 1993;**90**:6037-6041

[66] Sung VM, Shimodaira S, Doughty AL, Picchio GR, Can H, Yen TS, Lindsay KL, Levine AM, Lai MM. Establishment of B-cell lymphoma cell lines persistently infected with hepatitis C virus in vivo and in vitro: The apoptotic effects of virus infection. Journal of Virology. 2003;**77**:2134-2146

[67] Kondo Y, Sung VM, Machida K, Liu M, Lai MM. Hepatitis C virus infects T cells and affects interferon-gamma signaling in T cell lines. Virology. 2007;**361**:161-173

[68] Kondo Y, Machida K, Liu HM, Ueno Y, Kobayashi K, Wakita T, Shimosegawa T, Lai MM. Hepatitis C virus infection of T cells inhibits proliferation and enhances Fas-mediated apoptosis by down-regulating the expression of CD44 splicing variant 6. The Journal of Infectious Diseases. 2009;**199**:726-736

[69] Morsica G, Tambussi G, Sitia G, Novati R, Lazzarin A, Lopalco L, Mukenge S. Replication of hepatitis C virus in B lymphocytes (CD19+). Blood. 1999;**94**:1138-1139

[70] Michalak TI. Immune cell reservoirs of persisting hepatitis C virus. Gut. 2010;**59**:867-868

[71] Laskus T, Radkowski M, Piasek A, Nowicki M, Horban A, Cianciara J, Rakela J. Hepatitis C virus in lymphoid cells of patients coinfected with human immunodeficiency virus type 1: evidence of active replication in monocytes/macrophages and lymphocytes. The Journal of Infectious Diseases. 2000;**181**:442-448

[72] MacParland SA, Chen AY, Corkum CP, Pham TN, Michalak TI. Patient-derived hepatitis C virus inhibits CD4+ but not CD8+ T lymphocyte proliferation in primary T cells. Virology Journal. 2015;**12**:93

[73] Lauer GM, Ouchi K, Chung RT, Nguyen TN, Day CL, Purkis DR, Reiser M, Kim AY, Lucas M, Klenerman P, Walker BD. Comprehensive analysis of CD8(+)-T-cell responses against hepatitis C virus reveals multiple unpredicted specificities. Journal of Virology. 2002;**76**:6104-6113

[74] Rehermann B. Hepatitis C virus versus innate and adaptive immune responses: A tale of coevolution and coexistence. The Journal of Clinical Investigation. 2009;**119**:1745-1754

[75] Ploss A, Evans MJ. Hepatitis C virus host cell entry. Current Opinion in Virology. 2012;**2**:14-19

[76] Bartosch B, Vitelli A, Granier C, Goujon C, Dubuisson J, Pascale S, Scarselli E, Cortese R, Nicosia A, Cosset FL. Cell entry of hepatitis C virus requires a set of co-receptors

that include the CD81 tetraspanin and the SR-B1 scavenger receptor. The Journal of Biological Chemistry. 2003;**278**:41624-41630

[77] Germi R, Crance J, Garin D, Guimet J, Lortat-Jacob H, Ruigrok RWH, Zarski J, Drouet E. Cellular glycosaminoglycans and low density lipoprotein receptor are involved in hepatitis C virus adsorption. Journal of Medical Virology. 2002;**68**:206-215

[78] Kapadia SB, Barth H, Baumert T, McKeating JA, Chisari FV. Initiation of hepatitis C virus infection is dependent on cholesterol and cooperativity between CD81 and scavenger receptor B type I. Journal of Virology. 2007;**81**:374-383

[79] Evans MJ, von Hahn T, Tscherne DM, Syder AJ, Panis M, Wolk B, Hatziioannou T, McKeating JA, Bieniasz PD, Rice CM. Claudin-1 is a hepatitis C virus co-receptor required for a late step in entry. Nature 2007;**446**:801-805

[80] Benedicto I, Molina-Jimenez F, Bartosch B, Cosset FL, Lavillette D, Prieto J, Moreno-Otero R, Valenzuela-Fernandez A, Aldabe R, Lopez-Cabrera M, Majano PL. The tight junction-associated protein occludin is required for a postbinding step in hepatitis C virus entry and infection. Journal of Virology. 2009;**83**:8012-8020

[81] Liu S, Yang W, Shen L, Turner JR, Coyne CB, Wang T. Tight junction proteins claudin-1 and occludin control hepatitis C virus entry and are downregulated during infection to prevent superinfection. Journal of Virology. 2009;**83**:2011-2014

[82] Ploss A, Evans MJ, Gaysinskaya VA, Panis MH, de Jong YP, Rice CM. Human occludin is a hepatitis C virus entry factor required for infection of mouse cells. Nature. 2009;**457**:882-886

[83] Lupberger J, Zeisel M, Xiao F, Thumann C, Fofana I, Zona L, Davis C, Mee CJ, Turek M, Gorke S, Royer C, Fischer B, Zahid MN, Lavillette D, Fresquet J, Cosset FL, Rothenberg SM, Pietschmann T, Patel AH, Pessaux P, Doffoël M, Raffelsberger W, Poch O, McKeating JA, Brino L, Baumert TF. EGFR and EphA2 are host factors for hepatitis C virus entry and possible targets for antiviral therapy. Nature Medicine. 2011;**17**:589-596

[84] Sainz B Jr, Barretto N, Martin DN, Hiraga N, Imamura M, Hussain S, Marsh KA, Yu X, Chayama K, Alrefai WA, Uprichard SL. Identification of the Niemann-Pick C1-like 1 cholesterol absorption receptor as a new hepatitis C virus entry factor. Nature Medicine. 2012;**18**:281-285

[85] Martin DN, Uprichard SL. Identification of transferrin receptor 1 as a hepatitis C virus entry factor. Proceedings of the National Academy of Sciences of the United States of America. 2013;**110**:10777-10782

[86] Douam F, Bobay LM, Maurin G, Fresquet J, Calland N, Maisse C, Durand T, Cosset FL, Féray C, Lavillette D. Specialization of hepatitis C virus envelope glycoproteins for B lymphocytes in chronically infected patients. Journal of Virology. 2015;**90**:992-1008

[87] Chen CL, Huang JY, Wang CH, Tahara SM, Zhou L, Kondo Y, Schechter J, Su L, Lai MM, Wakita T, Cosset FL, Jung JU, Machida K. Hepatitis C virus has a genetically determined lymphotropism through co-receptor B7.2. Nature Communications. 2017;**8**:13882

[88] Klatzmann D, Champagne E, Chamaret S, Gruest J, Guetard D, Hercend T, Gluckman JC, Montagnier L. HIV T-lymphocyte T4 molecule behaves as the receptor for human retrovirus LAV. Nature. 1984;**312**:767-768

[89] Zaitseva M, Blauvelt A, Lee S, Lapham CK, Klaus-Kovtun V, Mostowski H, Manischewitz J, Golding H. Expression and function of CCR5 and CXCR4 on human Langerhans cells and macrophages: implications for HIV primary infection. Nature Medicine. 1997;**3**:1369-1375

[90] Tatsuo H, Ono N, Tanaka K, Yanagi Y. SLAM (CDw150) is a cellular receptor for measles virus. Nature. 2000;**406**:893-897

[91] Sakaguchi M, Yoshikawa Y, Yamanouchi K. Growth of measles virus in epithelial and lymphoid tissue of cynomologous monkey. Microbiology and Immunology. 1986;**30**:883-891

[92] Nemerow GR, Siaw MF, Cooper NR. Purification of Epstein-Barr virus/C3d complement receptor of human B lymphocytes: Antigenic and functional properties of the purified protein. Journal of Virology. 1986;**58**:709-712

[93] Kasai K, Sato Y, Kameya T, Inoue H, Yoshimura H, Kon S, Kikuchi K. Incidence of latent infection of Epstein-Barr virus in lung cancers—An anlaysis of EBER1 expression in lung cancers by in situ hybridization. The Journal of Pathology. 1994;**174**:257-265

[94] Lee J, Kuchen S, Fischer R, Chang S, Lipsky PE. Identification and characterization of a human CD5+ pre-naive B cell population. Journal of Immunology. 2009;**182**:4116-4126

[95] Su WC, Machida K, Lai MMC. Extrahepatic replication of HCV. In: Muyamura T, Lemon SM, Walker CM, Wakita T, editors. Hepatitis C Virus II. Springer Japan. 2016. pp. 165-184

[96] Kondo Y, Ueno Y, Kakazu E, Kobayashi K, Shiina M, Tamai K, Machida K, Inoue J, Wakui Y, Fukushima K, Obara N, Kimura O, Shimosegawa T. Lymphotropic HCV strain can infect human primary naïve CD4$^+$ cells and affect their proliferation and IFN-γ secretion activity. Journal of Gastroenterology. 2011;**46**:232-241

[97] Bergqvist A, Rice CM. Transcriptional activation of the interleukin-2 promoter by hepatitis C virus core protein. Journal of Virology. 2001;**75**:772-781

[98] Bergqvist A, Sundström S, Dimberg LY, Gylfe E, Masucci MG. The hepatitis C virus core protein modulates T cell responses by inducing spontaneous and altering T-cell receptor-triggered Ca2+ oscillations. The Journal of Biological Chemistry. 2003;**278**:18877-18883

[99] Domínguez-Villar M, Muñoz-Suano A, Anaya-Baz B, Aguilar S, Novalbos JP, Giron JA, Rodríguez-Iglesias M, Garcia-Cozar F. Hepatitis C virus core protein up-regulates anergy-related genes and a new set of genes, which affects T cell homeostasis. Journal of Leukocyte Biology. 2007;**82**:1301-1310

[100] Yao ZQ, King E, Prayther D, Yin D, Moorman J. T cell dysfunction by hepatitis C virus core protein involves PD-1/PDL-1 signaling. Viral Immunology. 2007;**20**:276-287

[101] Bhattarai N, McLinden JH, Xiang J, Kaufman TM, Stapleton JT. Conserved motifs within hepatitis C virus envelope (E2) RNA and protein independently inhibit T cell activation. PLoS Pathogens. 2015;**11**:e1005183

[102] Bhattarai N, McLinden JH, Xiang J, Mathahs MM, Schmidt WN, Kaufman TM, Stapleton JT. Hepatitis C virus infection inhibits a Src-kinase regulatory phosphatase and reduces T cell activation in vivo. PLoS Pathogens. 2017;**13**:e1006232

[103] Kasama Y, Sekiguchi S, Saito M, Tanaka K, Satoh M, Kuwahara K, Sakaguchi N, Takeya M, Hiasa Y, Kohara M, Tsukiyama-Kohara K. Persistent expression of the full genome of hepatitis C virus in B cells induces spontaneous development of B-cell lymphomas in vivo. Blood. 2010;**116**:4926-4933

[104] Monti G, Pioltelli P, Saccardo F, Campanini M, Candela M, Cavallero G, De Vita S, Ferri C, Mazzaro C, Migliaresi S, Ossi E, Pietrogrande M, Gabrielli A, Galli M, Invernizzi F. Incidence and characteristics of non-Hodgkin lymphomas in a multicenter case file of patients with hepatitis C virus-related symptomatic mixed cryoglobulinemias. Archives of Internal Medicine. 2005;**165**:101-105

[105] Young RM, Staudt LM. Targeting pathological B cell receptor signalling in lymphoid malignancies. Nature Reviews. Drug Discovery. 2013;**12**:229-243

[106] Rosa D, Saletti G, De Gregorio E, Zorat F, Comar C, D'Oro U, Nuti S, Houghton M, Barnaba V, Pozzato G, Abrignani S. Activation of naïve B lymphocytes via CD81, a pathogenetic mechanism for hepatitis C virus-associated B lymphocyte disorders. Proceedings of the National Academy of Sciences of the United States of America. 2005;**102**:18544-18549

[107] Feldmann G, Nischalke HD, Nattermann J, Banas B, Berg T, Teschendorf C, Schmiegel W, Dührsen U, Halangk J, Iwan A, Sauerbruch T, Caselmann WH, Spengler U. Induction of interleukin-6 by hepatitis C virus core protein in hepatitis C-associated mixed cryoglobulinemia and B-cell non-Hodgkin's lymphoma. Clinical Cancer Research. 2006;**12**:4491-4498

[108] Mazan-Mamczarz K, Hagner PR, Corl S, Srikantan S, Wood WH, Becker KG, Gorospe M, Keene JD, Levenson AS, Gartenhaus RB. Post-transcriptional gene regulation by HuR promotes a more tumorigenic phenotype. Oncogene. 2008;**27**:6151-6163

[109] Machida K, Cheng KT, Sung VM, Shimodaira S, Lindsay KL, Levine AM, Lai MY, Lai MM. Hepatitis C virus induces a mutator phenotype: enhanced mutations of immuno-globulin and protooncogenes. Proceedings of the National Academy of Sciences of the United States of America. 2004;**101**:4262-4267

[110] Dammacco F, editor. HCV infection and cryoglobulinemia. Italia: Springler-Verlang; 2012

[111] Tucci F, Küppers R. Role of hepatitis C virus in B cell lymphoproliferation. Virologica Sinica. 2014;**29**:3-6

2

Neuropathological and Neuropsychiatric Determinants in HCV-Infected Patients

Vanja Vojnović

Abstract

Chronic hepatitis C virus (HCV) infection is a growing global health problem. HCV is a leading cause of chronic hepatitis, cirrhosis, and hepatocellular carcinoma (HCC) and is associated with more than 30 extrahepatic manifestations (EHMs). Although cryoglobulinemia is the main pathological cause of neurologic EHMs, HCV viral replication in the brain itself must also be taken into consideration. The most significant neurological manifestations of HCV chronic infection are stroke, leukoencephalopathy, encephalomyelitis/myelitis, and peripheral neuropathy. The most significant neuropsychological manifestations of HCV infection are fatigue, depression, anxiety, and cognitive dysfunction. Antiviral HCV treatment should be the first-line treatment for managing mild-to-moderate vascular and neurologic symptoms; most of EHMs improve or even resolve if antiviral treatment starts on time.

Keywords: hepatitis C virus, extrahepatic manifestations, cryoglobulinemia, neurological manifestations, neuropsychological manifestations, antiviral treatment

1. Introduction

Chronic hepatitis C virus (HCV) infection is a growing global health problem affecting an estimated 185 million people (a prevalence rate of 2.8%) [1]. HCV is a leading cause of chronic hepatitis, cirrhosis, and hepatocellular carcinoma (HCC) and is associated with more than 30 extrahepatic manifestations (EHMs) [2].

EHMs are immunologic and rheumatologic in their pathophysiology: they are caused by B-cell proliferation, which produce monoclonal and polyclonal autoantibodies and then activate rheumatoid factor or have cryoglobulin properties.

Cryoglobulinemia is the most frequent and best-studied EHM of HCV infection. It is detected in up to 50% of HCV-infected patients. Cryoglobulins (CGs) are cold-precipitable immunoglobulins, which make vascular deposits and then cause inflammation and occlusion of small- and medium-size blood vessels. Typical clinical manifestations of cryoglobulinemia are cutaneous purpura, arthralgias, and membranous proliferative glomerulonephritis. Also, up to 17–60% of patients with cryoglobulinemia develop peripheral neuropathy. Central nervous system (CNS) involvement occurs in approximately 6% of cases. CGs are also a risk factor for carotid plaque formation, hepatic fibrosis, and liver steatosis [3].

Although cryoglobulinemia is the main pathological cause of neurologic EHMs, special consideration must be given to HCV viral replication in brain itself. It is believed that there are specific brain HCV variants that cause neurotoxicity (induce apoptosis). So far, it has been hypothesized that microglial cells (CNS macrophages) are the main targets for HCV entry into the CNS. Detection of replicative intermediate forms of HCV RNA and viral proteins within the CNS has led to this conclusion. Furthermore, sequence analysis of HCV residing in liver and brain has suggested an evolutionary path of a virus to infect the CNS [4].

2. Neurological manifestations

HCV-related CNS complications encompass a wide spectrum of disorders ranging from cerebrovascular events to autoimmune syndromes.

1. Acute cerebrovascular events can sometimes be the initial manifestation of HCV infection.

2. Acute or subacute encephalopathic syndromes have been associated with diffuse involvement of the white matter in HCV chronically infected patients with CG and/or circulating anticardiolipin antibodies.

3. The occurrence of an immune-mediated process induced by HCV causes inflammatory disorders such as acute encephalitis, encephalomyelitis, and meningoradiculitis/polyradiculitis; there are reports of patients with rapidly evolving acute leukoencephalitis or fatal progressive acute encephalomyelitic syndromes [3].

4. HCV has been connected with the metabolic syndrome so HCV infection represents an independent risk factor for increased carotid wall thickness and plaque formation, thus contributing to significant cerebrovascular mortality [3].

Neurological manifestations are most often caused by occlusive vasculopathy (due to mixed cryoglobulinemia), ANCA-associated CNS vasculitis or anti-phospholipid associated syndrome. In addition, HCV infection may increase the risk of atherosclerosis and earlier stroke through predisposition to metabolic diseases such as type 2 diabetes [5].

3. Neuropsychological manifestations

Fatigue, cognitive dysfunction, and mood alterations display a profound effect on social and physical function of HCV-infected subjects, thus impacting health-related quality of life (HRQL).

Chronic fatigue (often called "brain fog") is perceived as a sensation of physical and mental exhaustion, and when severe, it is accompanied by deficits of attention tasks, anomia, and word-finding difficulties, in the absence of verbal memory or cognitive ability impairments [6].

It has been found that 28% of chronically HCV-infected subjects have depression [7]. The occurrence of depression has been attributed to psychological factors, or to specific determinants, including immune mechanisms, derangement of the blood–brain-barrier integrity, viral replication within the CNS, iatrogenic factors, or altered dopaminergic and serotoninergic transmission [7]. It is very important to diagnose such manifestations because in moderate-to-severe depression it is mandatory to reduce or discontinue interferon treatment.

Investigation of a large population of patients with chronic HCV infection has disclosed the occurrence of subclinical cognitive dysfunction (alterations in verbal and learning skills, concentration, attention, working memory) in 18% of subjects [8].

4. Peripheral neuropathies

In patients with HCV, the involvement of the peripheral nervous system (PNS) ranges from 26 to 86% in accordance with the disease stage [9]. Peripheral neuropathies occur mostly in the presence of circulating CG which causes ischemic nerve changes, as a consequence of small vessel vasculitis, or, less frequently, necrotizing arteritis of medium-sized vessels [9].

In patients without CG, immune complexes or HCV-induced autoimmune mechanisms may play a pathogenetic role in inducing vascular and perivascular inflammation, which may be driven by an intrinsic nerve population of immunocompetent and potentially phagocytic cells [10].

Many patients develop a symmetrical sensory or sensorimotor axonal-type polyneuropathy, with sensory loss and weakness in distal regions of limbs [11]. Others present with mononeuropathies and mononeuropathy multiplex or the asymmetrical sensory variants such as large-fiber sensory neuropathy (LFSN) and small-fiber sensory polyneuropathy (SFSN) [12]. Cranial nerves are usually spared.

One must also take into consideration that HCV-infected patients can have multiple neurological/neuropsychological manifestations.

5. Impact of HCV treatment on neurological/neuropsychiatric disorders

Antiviral HCV treatment is the first-line treatment for managing mild-to-moderate neurologic/neuropsychologic symptoms. However, patients on interferon (IFN) therapy should be monitored as IFN therapy may aggravate the symptoms of peripheral neuropathies (IFN can create the pathogenic inflammatory environment for neuropathy) [4].

Tricyclic antidepressants, local anesthetics, and opioids may be required to the standard antiviral therapy for treatment of acute pain attacks [4].

Rituximab is also useful in treating neuropathic pain, as it acts by inhibiting cryoglobulin production and its pathogenic cascade [4].

If EHMs do not improve after antiviral treatment, the use of immunosuppressants is also a treatment possibility, but only as a last resort in patients not responding to antiviral treatment or with refractory disease (because of possible worsening of viral infection) [4].

Also, when discussing neuropathological and neuropsychiatric manifestations in HCV-infected patients, it is very important to distinguish between neuropsychiatric diseases caused by the virus itself and those caused by the treatment.

There are many neurological side effects of HCV treatment: up to 70% of HCV patients treated with IFN may develop depression [13]. Neurovegetative symptoms like loss of appetite, fatigue, sexual impairment, and psychosomatic symptoms start to occur within 4 weeks of IFN treatment [13]. The confusional state induced by IFN is associated with psychomotor retardation, disorientation, Parkinsonism, psychosis, and manic disorder [14]. As mentioned above, IFN therapy can also aggravate the symptoms of peripheral neuropathies.

6. Conclusions

Sometimes EHMs can be the first clinical manifestation of HCV infection. This is why in the diagnostic work-up of a patient with the above reported neurological/psychiatric disorders without more obvious causes, clinicians should always consider screening for HCV infection.

Antiviral HCV treatment should be the first-line treatment for managing mild-to-moderate vascular and neurologic symptoms. Persistence or relapse of neurologic symptoms despite viral clearance suggest the presence of other diseases, so further diagnostic work-up should be undertaken.

Author details

Vanja Vojnović[1,2]*

*Address all correspondence to: vanja_vojnovic@yahoo.com

1 Faculty of Medicine, Josip Juraj Strossmayer University, Osijek, Croatia

2 Department of Neurology, University Hospital Dubrava, Zagreb, Croatia

References

[1] Mohd Hanafiah K, Groeger J, Flaxman AD, Wiersma ST. Global epidemiology of hepatitis C virus infection: New estimates of age-specific antibody to HCV seroprevalence. Hepatology. 2013;57:1333-1342. DOI: 10.1002/hep.26141 23172780

[2]   Jacobson IM, Cacoub P, Dal Maso L, Harrison SA, Younossi ZM. Manifestations of chronic hepatitis C virus infection beyond the liver. Clinical Gastroenterology and Hepatology. 2010;**8**(12):1017-1029

[3]   Monaco S, Ferrari (S), Gajofatto A, Zanusso G, Mariotto S. HCV-Related Nervous System Disorders. Clinical and Developmental Immunology, vol. 2012, Article ID 236148, 9 pages, 2012. doi:10.1155/2012/236148

[4]   Mathew S, Faheem M, Ibrahim SM, Iqbal W, Rauff B, Fatima K, Qadri I. Hepatitis C virus and neurological damage. World Journal of Hepatology. 2016;**8**(12):545-556. DOI: 10.4254/wjh.v8.i12.545

[5]   Adinolfi LE, Nevola R, Lus G, Restivo L, Guerrera B, Romano C, Zampino R, Rinaldi L, Sellitto A, Giordano M, Marrone A. Chronic hepatitis C virus infection and neurological and psychiatric disorders: An overview. World Journal of Gastroenterology. 2015;**21**(8):2269-2280. DOI: 10.3748/wjg.v21.i8.2269

[6]   Goh J, Coughlan B, Quinn J, O'Keane JC, Crowe J. Fatigue does not correlate with the degree of hepatitis or the presence of autoimmune disorders in chronic hepatitis C infection. European Journal of Gastroenterology and Hepatology. 1999;**11**(8):833-838

[7]   Carta MG, Angst J, Moro MF, et al. Association of chronic hepatitis C with recurrent brief depression. Journal of Affective Disorders. 2012;**141**:361-366

[8]   Kramer L, Bauer E, Funk G, et al. Subclinical impairment of brain function in chronic hepatitis C infection. Journal of Hepatology. 2002;**37**(3):349-354

[9]   Vital C, Vital A, Canron MH, et al. Combined nerve and muscle biopsy in the diagnosis of vasculitic neuropathy. A 16-year retrospective study of 202 cases. Journal of the Peripheral Nervous System. 2006;**11**(1):20-29

[10] Bonetti B, Monaco S, Giannini C, Ferrari S, Zanusso GL, Rizzuto N. Human peripheral nerve macrophages in normal and pathological conditions. Journal of the Neurological Sciences. 1993;**118**(2):158-168

[11] Authier FJ, Bassez G, Payan C, et al. Detection of genomic viral RNA in nerve and muscle of patients with HCV neuropathy. Neurology. 2003;**60**(5):808-812

[12] Bant A, Hurowitz B, Hassan N, Van Thiel DU, Nadir A. Complex regional pain syndrome (Reflex sympathetic dystrophy) in a patient with essential mixed cryoglobulinemia and chronic hepatitis C. Journal of the Pakistan Medical Association. 2007;**57**(2):96-98

[13] Mariotto S, Ferrari S, Monaco S. HCV-related central and peripheral nervous system demyelinating disorders. Inflammation & Allergy: Drug Targets. 2014;**13**:299-304 [PMID: 25198705. DOI: 10.2174/1871528113666140908113841]

[14] Rifai MA, Gleason OC, Sabouni D. Psychiatric Care of the Patient With Hepatitis C: A Review of the Literature. Primary Care Companion to The Journal of Clinical Psychiatry. 2010;**12**(6):PCC.09r00877. doi:10.4088/PCC.09r00877whi

3

Hepatitis C Viral Dynamics using a Combination Therapy of Interferon, Ribavirin, and Telaprevir: Mathematical Modeling and Model Validation

Philip Aston, Katie Cranfield, Haley O'Farrell,
Alex Cassenote, Cassia J. Mendes-Correa,
Aluisio Segurado, Phuong Hoang,
George Lankford and Hien Tran

Abstract

Groundbreaking new drugs called direct acting antivirals have been introduced recently for the treatment of chronic Hepatitis C virus infection. We introduce a mathematical model for Hepatitis C dynamics treated with the direct acting antiviral drug, telaprevir, alongside traditional interferon and ribavirin treatments to understand how this combination therapy affects the viral load of patients exhibiting different types of response. We use sensitivity and identifiability techniques to determine which model parameters can be best estimated from viral load data. Parameter estimation with these best estimable parameters is then performed to give patient-specific fits of the model to partial virologic response, sustained virologic response and breakthrough patients.

Keywords: hepatitis C dynamics, inverse problem, subset selection, sensitivity analysis, identifiability analysis, automatic differentiation

1. Introduction

Over 200–300 million people worldwide are infected with a virus called Hepatitis C (HCV) that affects the liver, which was discovered in 1989 [1]. It is usually spread by blood-to-blood contact via intravenous drug use, poorly sterilized medical equipment and transfusions.

Scarring of the liver and ultimately cirrhosis are just a few of the more severe complications associated with HCV [2].

Six different genotypes of HCV exist due to the highly error prone RNA polymerase with the most common being genotype 1 that has the lowest levels of response to standard treatment [3, 4]. Genotype 1 patients have about a 50% chance for sustained virologic response (SVR), while non-genotype 1 patients have about an 80% chance for SVR [5]. The clinical data used for this study were provided by the University of Sao Paulo, School of Medicine in Sao Paulo, Brazil and consist of genotype 1 patients.

One of the first treatments for HCV was 6–12 months monotherapy with interferon glyco-proteins. Interferon is naturally secreted from our bodies to fight off infection and monotherapy treatment with them is associated with around 10% SVR [6]. The addition of ribavirin (RBV), a drug believed to render some of the virus non-infectious, increased SVR to around 30% [6]. RBV monotherapy is not recommended because it does not give a significant benefit to SVR [7]. Until recently, the most common therapy was a combination of pegylated Interferon (IFN) and RBV for 24–48 weeks that yielded about a 45% SVR [5, 6]. One of the major differences between IFN and standard inteferon glycoproteins is that the pegylation allows the drugs to stay in the body longer [8]. There have also been clinical trials with RBV monotherapy before and after IFN + RBV therapy as described in [9]. Recently, new drugs called direct-acting antiviral agents (DAAs) have raised the chance for SVR for HCV patients.

DAAs give an increase to about an 80% chance for SVR for genotype 1 [10]. According to the FDA, DAAs are drugs that interfere with specific steps in the HCV replication cycle by taking advantage of the biological makeup of HCV [11]. HCV is a single-stranded RNA molecule that is several nucleotides in length. During HCV's life cycle, it is translated into a polyprotein that is composed into structural and nonstructural proteins that aid in replication. During post-translational processing, DAAs called protease inhibitors block a key protease from the repli-cation process and hinders further infection [10, 12]. Among the protease inhibitors available are boceprevir, telaprevir and simeprevir. Simeprevir is recommended over telaprevir and boceprevir because of both improved efficacy and less side effects, but telaprevir continues to be used because of its cost efficiency [13, 14].

Integration of mathematical modeling of viral dynamics with clinical data has led to further understanding of how different treatment strategies dictate viral load dynamics. One of the first mathematical models was given by Neumann et al. which attempted to describe HCV dynamics with interferon monotherapy [4]. Improvements were made to the Neumann's model to better describe different mechanisms in the liver during treatment including the regeneration of liver cells. Adjustments were also made to include the standard of care, IFN, and RBV. Some of these modifications can be found in [5, 15]. In particular, Snoeck et al. [5] had data after the end of the treatment phase so that the model can give a more accurate representation of its prediction of SVR. The introduction of DAAs has ushered in more mathematical models that include this type of therapy [16]. For example, mathemat-ical models have been proposed using telaprevir monotherapy [17–20] and in combination

with IFN and RBV [18] that uses Bayesian feedback to estimate the parameters in the model. The challenges that come with modeling DAAs is that since they are relatively new, there is not as much data available [17]. It can be difficult to predict SVR because of a lack of data after the treatment phase ends due to how recent the drugs have been approved.

This chapter introduces a novel approach for the development of a mathematical model describing HCV dynamics given the triple-drug combination treatment of IFN, RBV, and the DAA telaprevir. In Section 2, we describe how we adapted a previously known HCV model to include telaprevir and the available clinical data. Section 3 describes the a priori analysis of sensitivity and identifiability and its incorporation into the parameter estimation problem. Section 4 gives the parameter estimation results using several patient specific clinical data including partial virologic response, sustained virologic response and breakthrough. Finally, concluding remarks are provided in Section 5.

2. Mathematical models of HCV dynamics

The original model for HCV dynamics in Neumann et al. [4] was frequently used to assess viral-load profiles after short-term treatment and is given by

$$\frac{dT}{dt} = s - dT - (1 - \eta)\beta VT,$$
$$\frac{dI}{dt} = (1 - \eta)\beta VT - \delta I, \qquad (1)$$
$$\frac{dV}{dt} = (1 - \varepsilon)pI - cV,$$

where T and I denote the concentrations of healthy and infected hepatocytes, and V represents viral concentration in the liver fluid. One of the key contributions of the model was the understanding of the mechanism of IFN. It was unknown whether it acted through $\eta > 0$ (i.e., inhibiting the infection of healthy liver cells) or $\varepsilon > 0$ (i.e., reducing virion production in infected cells). In [4], it is determined that it is through ε which inhibits production of the virus. The drawback to (1) is that it cannot describe patients exhibiting breakthrough, relapse, and most importantly SVR. These responses are reasons that early viral response does not uniformly predict responses in the long term. Another important aspect is the handling of viral load measurements below the lower limit of quantification (LLOQ). Previous analysis omitted the data below LLOQ, but it can contain critical information regarding long-term treatment outcome. Snoeck et al. [5] present a mathematical model for the dynamics of HCV with the drug treatment combination of IFN and RBV that attempts to address both the long-term responses and the use of the LLOQ. The model described in [5] is given by the following system of nonlinear differential equations

$$\frac{dT}{dt} = s + rT\left(1 - \frac{T+I}{T_{max}}\right) - dT - \beta V_I T, b$$

$$\frac{dI}{dt} = \beta V_I T + rI\left(1 - \frac{T+I}{T_{max}}\right) - \delta I,$$

$$\frac{dV_I}{dt} = (1 - \bar{\rho})(1 - \bar{\varepsilon})pI - cV_I,$$

$$\frac{dV_{NI}}{dt} = \bar{\rho}(1 - \bar{\varepsilon})pI - cV_{NI}, \tag{2}$$

where T (uninfected hepatocytes), I (infected hepatocytes), V_I (infectious virions) and V_{NI} (noninfectious virions) are natural states (international units IU/mL). This model was adapted from a standard model of viral infection [4]. The number of uninfected hepatocytes increases each day with reproduction rate s and regeneration rate r. That number decreases each day as those hepatocytes die naturally at a rate d or infected at a rate β. The maximum number of hepatocytes per mL is T_{max}. The number of infected hepatocytes increases when the healthy liver cells are infected and when the infected cells regenerate themselves. That number decreases when they die off naturally at a rate δ. Infected hepatocytes produce both infectious and noninfectious virions at a rate p. Virions are naturally cleared at a rate c. IFN inhibits virus production while RBV renders some of the virus noninfectious. The drug efficacies of IFN and RBV are represented by ε and ρ, respectively. The bounds for IFN and RBV are $0 < \varepsilon \leq 1$ and $0 < \rho \leq 1$ where the more effective the drug is, the closer the efficacy of the drug will be to 1. Snoeck uses data that extend beyond treatment for patients so the terms $\bar{\varepsilon}$ and $\bar{\rho}$ in (2) account for the exponential decays of the efficacies of the drugs after treatment has ceased. The exponential decay of the drug efficacies is given by

$$\bar{\varepsilon} = \varepsilon e^{-k(t-t_{end})_+}, \tag{3}$$

and

$$\bar{\rho} = \rho e^{-k(t-t_{end})_+}, \tag{4}$$

where k is the efficacy decay rate, t_{end} marks the end of treatment, and

$$(a)_+ = \begin{cases} a & \text{if } a \geq 0, \\ 0 & \text{otherwise.} \end{cases}$$

The drug efficacies ε and ρ are related to the drug dosage levels by the following expressions

$$\varepsilon = \frac{\text{Dose}_{\text{PEG}}}{\text{ED50}_{\text{PEG}} + \text{Dose}_{\text{PEG}}}, \tag{5}$$

and

$$\rho = \frac{\text{Dose}_{\text{RBV}}}{\text{ED50}_{\text{RBV}} + \text{Dose}_{\text{RBV}}}, \tag{6}$$

where Dose $_{\text{PEG}}$ is the weekly subcutaneous dose of IFN and ED50$_{\text{PEG}}$ is the estimated weekly dose that causes 50% inhibition of virion production. Dose$_{\text{RBV}}$ represents the daily dose of

Parameter	Value
s	$6.17 \times 10^4 \; \frac{\text{hepatocyte}}{\text{mL} \cdot \text{day}}$
r	$.00562 \; \text{day}^{-1}$
β	$8.7 \times 10^{-9} \; \frac{\text{mL}}{\text{virion} \cdot \text{day}}$
δ	$.139 \; \text{day}^{-1}$
c	$4.53 \; \text{day}^{-1}$
$T_{\max}$	$1.85 \times 10^7 \; \frac{\text{hepatocytes}}{\text{mL}}$
d	$.003 \; \text{day}^{-1}$
p	$25.1 \; \frac{\text{virions}}{\text{hepatocyte} \cdot \text{day}}$
ε	$.896$
ρ	$.4$–$.6$
k	$.0238 \; \text{day}^{-1}$

Table 1. Typical values from [5].

RBV/kg body weight, and $\text{ED}_{50_{\text{RBV}}}$ represents the estimated daily dose in mg/kg that makes 50% of the virions noninfectious. Biologically, all state variables and parameters are non-negative. Typical values for model parameters used by Snoek et al. [5] are given in **Table 1**.

2.1. HCV model with DAA

Snoeck's model is adapted to incorporate the DAA, telaprevir. Recall that a DAA targets specific parts of the genome of the virus to inhibit both replication and infection. The hindrance of replication of the virus in the infected hepatocytes results in the virus not being produced by those cells. This means that the DAA should be implemented as part of the infection term, $\beta T V_I$, for inhibiting infection and viral production terms, pV_I and pV_{NI}, for inhibiting replication of the virus in (2). However, after simulations and analysis, it is concluded in this study that the obstruction of the infection and replication of the virus by telaprevir can be described solely as an amplifier for mitigating the production of virions alongside IFN. With this assumption, the model in [5] is modified to include the triple drug combination of IFN, RBV and telaprevir as follows:

$$\dot{T} = s + rT\left(1 - \frac{T+I}{T_{\max}}\right) - dT - \beta V_I T$$

$$\dot{I} = \beta V_I T + rI\left(1 - \frac{T+I}{T_{\max}}\right) - \delta I \tag{7}$$

$$\dot{V}_I = (1 - \bar{\rho})(1 - \bar{\varepsilon})(1 - \bar{\gamma})pI - cV_I$$

$$\dot{V}_{NI} = \bar{\rho}(1 - \bar{\varepsilon})(1 - \bar{\gamma})pI - cV_{NI},$$

where $\bar{\gamma}$ represents the exponential decay of the telaprevir efficacy and is defined similarly as for $\bar{\varepsilon}$ and $\bar{\rho}$ (see (3) and (4)). In [21], existence and uniqueness of solutions to this updated

HCV dynamical model were established, and a steady-state stability analysis was also performed.

2.2. Treatment schedule

The data in this research uses the treatment schedule timeline as follows (also summarized in **Figure 1**).

1. The patient is treated with the triple drug combination of IFN + RBV + te1aprevir for the first 12 weeks.

2. If at 12 weeks, viral load > 1000 IU/mL, then discontinue treatment. Otherwise, continue 12-week treatment of IFN + RBV.

3. If at 24 weeks, viral load > LLOQ (12–15 IU/mL), then discontinue treatment. Otherwise, continue 12-week treatment of IFN + RBV.

4. If at 36 weeks, viral load > LLOQ, then discontinue treatment. Otherwise, continue 12-week treatment of IFN + RBV.

5. End of treatment at 48 weeks.

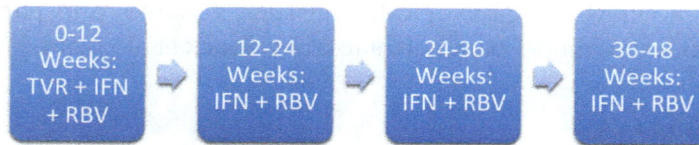

Figure 1. Treatment schedule for patients used for data received from patients treated at University of Sao Paulo, School of Medicine in Sao Paulo, Brazil.

3. Subset selection

The *forward problem* refers to using a model to predict the future behavior of a system given a set of parameters. The *inverse problem*, on the other hand, is the parameterization of a model from empirical data [22–24]. There have been extensive studies about parameter selection while solving the inverse problem for biological models and other applications that can be found in [3, 22, 25–27] and references therein. In this study, we use a simple algorithm to choose a subset of parameters to be estimated from clinical data based on both sensitivity and identifiability as follows:

1. Start with the full parameter set Q.

2. Remove parameters that are not locally sensitive to attain $Q_S \subset Q$.

3. Remove parameters that are not locally identifiable from Q_S to obtain sensitive and identifiable parameter set Q_{SI}

Since these are local analyses, this procedure is repeated over a large number of parameter sets and the parameters that appear most often in Q_{SI} are the parameters that are estimated. All other parameter values are fixed to values from the literature. A biological and structural explanation for some of the fixed parameters is given in the next section.

3.1. Fixed parameters

The assumptions for fixed parameters are the same as in [5]. Since the maximum number of hepatocytes in the liver is 2.50×10^{11} and HCV RNA is distributed in plasma and extracellular fluids with a volume of $\sim 1.35 \times 10^4$ ml, then $T_{max} = \frac{2.50 \times 10^{11}}{1.35 \times 10^4} = 1.85 \times 10^7$. d is obtained from hepatocyte turnover being every 300 days and $s = T_{max} \cdot d$ can be deduced in the absence of liver disease. p is always fixed because $p(1 - \varepsilon)$ appears in $\dot{V}$ and $\dot{V}_{NI}$ making p and ε, impossible to estimate uniquely. The rest of the parameters will be considered in the sensitivity analysis.

3.2. Sensitivity analysis

A sensitivity analysis is the process of understanding how the model output is affected by changes in the parameters. Sensitivity analyses are used in many branches of mathematics such as statistics, partial differential equations (PDEs), and control design [28, 29]. The parameters that give the most change in the output are said to be sensitive parameters. This is important in the *forward problem* because it allows an understanding of which parameters will give useful information. Once the parameters have been identified, a sensitivity analysis for the *inverse problem* is usually performed to determine the sensitive parameters. Parameters with minimal impact are fixed from the literature. There are two different types of sensitivity analysis: global and local. A global sensitivity analysis heavily depends on the structure of the model and quantifies how uncertainties in outputs can be apportioned to uncertainties in inputs. We refer the reader to [30] for a more comprehensive discussion. Our study uses a local sensitivity analysis that depends on the prescribed values of the parameters.

3.2.1. Sensitivity equations

The sensitivity analysis presented in this section uses a derivative-based approach. Consider the general form of an ODE model and a function z of its output

$$\frac{dy}{dt} = f(t, y; q),$$
$$z = g(t, y; q),$$

(8)

whereby the vectors y and q contain the variables and parameters of the model, respectively. Since we are concerned with how our model output, z, is influenced by changes to our parameters, q, then we consider the partial derivative of z, $\frac{\partial z}{\partial q}$, with respect to q. One approach to computing this partial derivative is by solving the associated sensitivity equations. Differentiating both sides of the output Eq. (8) with respect to the parameter q yields

$$\frac{\partial z}{\partial q} = \frac{\partial g}{\partial t}\frac{\partial t}{\partial q} + \frac{\partial g}{\partial y}\frac{\partial y}{\partial q} + \frac{\partial g}{\partial q}\frac{\partial q}{\partial q}$$

$$= \frac{\partial g}{\partial y}\frac{\partial y}{\partial q} + \frac{\partial g}{\partial q} \qquad (9)$$

since $\frac{\partial t}{\partial q} = 0$ and $\frac{\partial q}{\partial q} = 1$. The two components $\frac{\partial g}{\partial y}$ and $\frac{\partial g}{\partial q}$ can be directly calculated from g, but can be cumbersome to do by hand depending on the complexity of the function g. Thus, one can employ automatic differentiation to evaluate these derivatives. Since any mathematical function can be decomposed into elementary functions, automatic differentiation numerically implements the chain rule and basic arithmetic equations repeatedly to compute the total derivative of a function with accuracy to working machine precision [31]. This is achieved with table lookups and tabulating all the functional compositions [32, 33]. An automatic differentiation (AD) code developed by Martin Fink in MATLAB was employed [34]. Finally, to calculate $\frac{\partial y}{\partial q}$, it is noted that y is continuous in t and q. Since $\frac{\partial y}{\partial q}$ exists, by taking the partial derivative with respect to q of the state equations and reversing the order of differentiation [35], we obtain

$$\frac{\partial}{\partial q}\left(\frac{dy}{dt}\right) = \frac{d}{dt}\left(\frac{\partial y}{\partial q}\right) = \frac{\partial f}{\partial t}\frac{\partial t}{\partial q} + \frac{\partial f}{\partial y}\frac{\partial y}{\partial q} + \frac{\partial f}{\partial q}\frac{\partial q}{\partial q}$$

$$= \frac{\partial f}{\partial y}\frac{\partial y}{\partial q} + \frac{\partial f}{\partial q}. \qquad (10)$$

Similar to $\frac{\partial g}{\partial y}$ and $\frac{\partial g}{\partial q}$, $\frac{\partial f}{\partial y}$ and $\frac{\partial f}{\partial q}$ are calculated using automatic differentiation. From (10), the sensitivity equations are given by the following coupled system of differential equations

$$\frac{dy}{dt} = f(t, y; q),$$

$$\frac{d}{dt}\left(\frac{\partial y}{\partial q}\right) = \frac{\partial f}{\partial q}\frac{\partial y}{\partial q} + \frac{\partial f}{\partial q}. \qquad (11)$$

Solving the sensitivity equations yields $\frac{\partial y}{\partial q}$, which, in turn, gives $\frac{\partial z}{\partial q}$ from (9).

3.2.2. Model considerations and sensitivity results

The sensitivities of each parameter are ranked to obtain which parameters are most sensitive. Since there is a large range of parameter and viral load values, each parameter, q_j, is log scaled in association with the state variable, y, that is,

$$\frac{d \log_{10}(y)}{d \log_{10}\left(q_j\right)} = \frac{q_j}{y}\frac{dy}{dq_j}$$

is considered instead of $\frac{dy}{dq_j}$. This allows a comparison of the sensitivities of each parameter using similar magnitudes. The l_2- norm is used to nondimensionalize the sensitivities over time so the following sensitivity coefficient is considered for each parameter

$$S_{ij} = \left\| \frac{\partial y_i}{\partial q_j} \right\|_2 = \left[\frac{1}{t_f - t_0} \int_{t_0}^{t_f} \frac{\partial y_i}{\partial q_j} \left(\frac{q_j}{\max y_i} \right)^2 dt \right]^{\frac{1}{2}} . \tag{12}$$

Eq. (12) is defined to be the relative ranking sensitivity of each variable y_i in y with respect to each individual parameter q_j.

Since the local sensitivity analysis depends on values in q, independent sets of parameters that have a log-normal distribution are created from the population-based model fit in Snoeck et al. [5]. That is, a sequence of independent parameter sets $\{q_k\}$ is generated from this distribution using the typical values from [5] as the mean. To determine pseudo-global sensitivities, a sensitivity coefficient, S_{ij}^k, is computed for each parameter in the k th parameter set. Then, if B parameter sets are to be analyzed, then an average for all the parameter sets is computed by

$$\overline{S}_{ij} = \frac{1}{B} \sum_{k=1}^{B} S_{ij}^k . \tag{13}$$

A cutoff is determined based on the ranking of the averages attained in (13). Those parameters above the cutoff are further examined in the identifiability analysis. This method is a version of what is referred to as Morris Screening in [30]. Similar to the work done here, the Morris algorithm [36] averages local derivative approximations to provide more global sensitivity measures. The difference being that the variance in the parameter sets is also considered. Here that variance would be given by

$$\sigma_{ij}^2 = \frac{1}{B-1} \sum_{k=1}^{B} \left(S_{ij}^k - \overline{S}_{ij} \right)^2 . \tag{14}$$

As explained in [30], while the mean (13) quantifies the individual effect of the input on the output, the variance (14) estimates the combined effects of the input due to nonlinearities or interactions with other inputs. The reader is referred to [30, 36] and references therein for a more detailed analysis of Morris Screening. It is noted that only the marginal distributions are given in [5], so computations are ignorant of any covariances between parameters. The data that were used contain only the viral load observations. So the sensitivities of $V = V_I + V_{NI}$ are of interest. Therefore, (8) is considered where

$$y = [T \ I \ V_I \ V_{NI}]^T,$$

with output

$$z = V = V_I + V_{NI}.$$

Two different sets of time points are used during this analysis. The first and second set of time points come from the partial virologic response (PVR) case and Breakthrough case, respectively. This will provide a better illustration of sensitivities given that treatment decays in the Breakthrough case, but does not in PVR. The sensitivity rankings are given in **Figure 2** for over

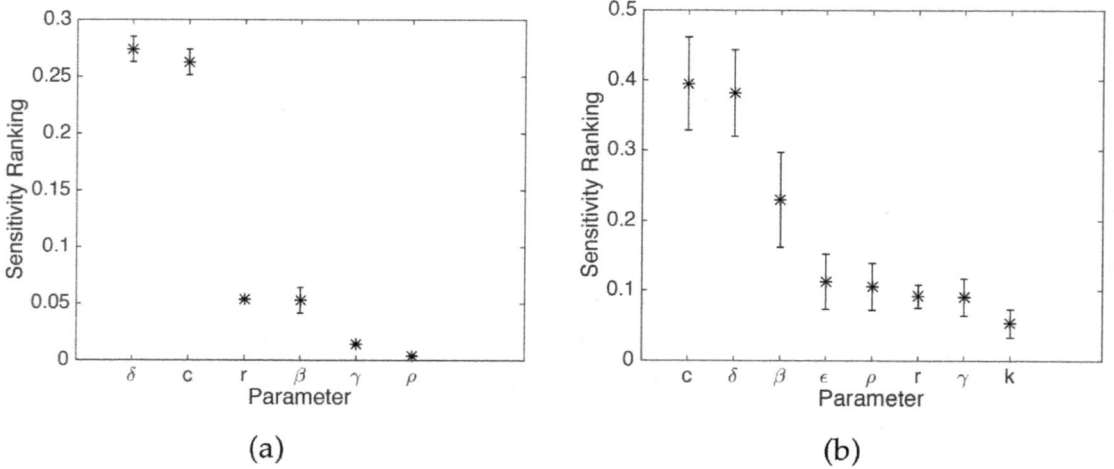

Figure 2. Sensitivity rankings using PVR (a) and Breakthrough time points (b).

2000 (a) and 400 (b) parameter sets, respectively. Error bars that are two standard deviations from the mean are included. The sensitive parameters for the PVR and Breakthrough time points are $Q_{PVR} = \{\delta, c, \beta, r, \gamma\}$ and $Q_{Brk} = \{\delta, c, \beta, r, \rho, \gamma, \varepsilon\}$, respectively. These parameters are considered in the identifiability analysis. Note that γ is always considered in the identifiability analysis due to there not being a value from the literature to fix it to for this model. It is used to determine whether it affects the identifiability of other parameters.

3.3. Identifiability analysis

After deciding which parameters are sensitive, consideration is given to understanding which sensitive parameters can uniquely be identified from the data. In this study, we employed a sensitive-based approach for local identifiability analysis. To this end, we consider the parameters contained in q which minimize the cost function

$$J(q) = \frac{1}{N} \sum_{i=1}^{N} \left(V_d^i - V(t_i; q)\right)^2,$$

with $V(t_i; q)$ denoting the model output and V_d^i denoting the corresponding data value at time point t_i for $i = 1, \ldots N$, where N is the number of data values. Similar to [37], let us assume that q^* is the minimum of this cost function. Then by using a Taylor series expansion around q^*, we obtain

$$V(t_i, q) = V(t_i; q^*) + \frac{dV(t_i; q^*)}{dq}(q - q^*) + \ldots$$

If we only consider the first two elements of $V(t_i, q)$ under the assumption that $q \approx q^*$ and substitute this expression into the cost function we find that

$$J(q) = \frac{1}{N} \sum_{i=1}^{N} \left(V_d^i - V(t_i; q^*) - \frac{dV(t_i; q^*)}{dq} (q - q^*) \right)^2,$$

$$= \frac{1}{N} \sum_{i=1}^{N} \left(\frac{dV(t_i; q^*)}{dq} (q - q^*) \right)^2, \tag{15}$$

where we used the fact that q^* is the minimum of the cost function so that $V_d^i \approx V(t_i; q^*)$. Let

$$S = \frac{dV}{dq} = \begin{bmatrix} \frac{dV}{dq_1}(t_1) & \frac{dV}{dq_2}(t_1) & \cdots & \frac{dV}{dq_l}(t_1) \\ \frac{dV}{dq_1}(t_2) & \frac{dV}{dq_2}(t_2) & \cdots & \frac{dV}{dq_l}(t_2) \\ \vdots & \vdots & \vdots & \vdots \\ \frac{dV}{dq_1}(t_N) & \frac{dV}{dq_2}(t_N) & \cdots & \frac{dV}{dq_l}(t_N) \end{bmatrix}, \tag{16}$$

be an $(N \times l)$ sensitivity matrix relating to the sensitivities $\frac{dV}{dq_j}(t_i)$ of the output with $i = 1, ..., N$ and $j = 1, ..., l$, where l denotes the number of parameters. The cost function of (15) is rewritten in terms of this sensitivity matrix

$$J(q) = \frac{1}{N} (S(q - q^*))^T (S(q - q^*)),$$

$$= \frac{1}{N} (S\Delta q)^T (S\Delta q),$$

where $\Delta q = q - q^*$. Rearranging $\Delta q = q - q^*$, we formulate the cost function in terms of $q^* + \Delta q$:

$$J(q^* + \Delta q) = \frac{1}{N} \Delta q^T S^T S \Delta q. \tag{17}$$

If we suppose that Δq is an eigenvector of $S^T S$ with $S^T S \Delta q = \lambda \Delta q$, then we have

$$J(q^* + \Delta q) = \frac{1}{N} \Delta q^T (\lambda \Delta q),$$

$$= \frac{1}{N} \lambda \|\Delta q\|_2^2.$$

We note that if Δq is an eigenvector with eigenvalue $\lambda = 0$, then the cost function to second-order approximation is $J(q^* + h\Delta q) = 0$. The least squares cost function does not change values when moving from q^* to $q^* + h\Delta q$, with h arbitrary. Thus, the parameters are locally unidentifiable at q^*. If $S^T S$ has very small eigenvalues, this can also be a problem for parameter identification. There have been studies about how the Fisher Information Matrix ($S^T S$) can be used for parameter identification [38, 39]. For example, in [38], they search all possible parameter combinations and choose them based on the rank of the sensitivity matrix, S, and asymptotic standard error uncertainty. We use the following algorithm as described in [39] to determine which of the parameters in our model will be unidentifiable.

1. Create the matrix $S^T S$, compute its eigenvalues, and order them such that

$$|\lambda_1| \le |\lambda_2| \le \cdots \le |\lambda_n|.$$

2. If $|\lambda_1|$ is less than some threshold ε (typically taken to be 10^{-4}), we say that there is a parameter that is unidentifiable.

3. The largest magnitude component of the eigenvector Δq_1 associated with the eigenvalue λ_1 corresponds to the least identifiable parameter. Remove the corresponding column from S and repeat step 1.

After performing this procedure, we now have a set of sensitive and locally identifiable parameters to estimate. The rest of the parameters are set to "typical values" found in the literature. The identifiability algorithm is applied to all the parameter sets of sensitive parameters, Q_{PVR} and Q_{Brk}, obtained in the previous section. It is observed from **Figure 3** that the parameters in $Q_{PVR} = \{\delta, c, \beta, \gamma\}$ are identifiable at least 50% of the time and the parameters in $Q_{Brk} = \{\delta, c, \beta, \gamma, \varepsilon\}$ are identifiable at least 50% of the time. The parameters contained in Q_{PVR} and Q_{Brk} are those that will be estimated from the clinical data.

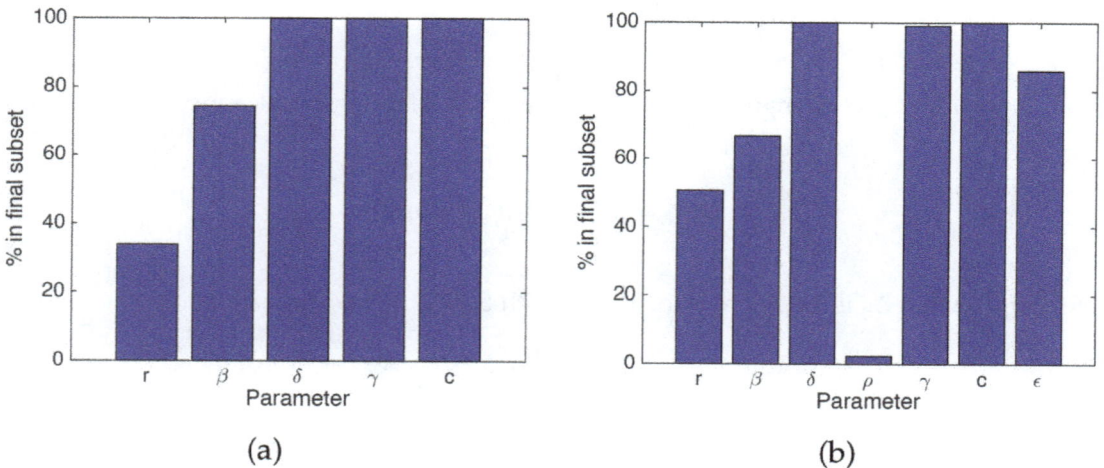

(a)   (b)

Figure 3. Final subset percentages using PVR (a) and Breakthrough time points (b).

4. Parameter estimation

The parameters in Q_{PVR} and Q_{Brk} are estimated using the weighted sum of squares of errors (WSSE) given by

$$J(q) = \sum_{i=1}^{N} w_i \left[\log\left(V_d^i\right) - \log\left(V(t_i; q)\right) \right]^2, \tag{18}$$

where w_i is the weight for the error term $\left[\log\left(V_d^i\right) - \log\left(V(t_i; q)\right) \right]$ at time t_i, V_d^i is data measurement of viral load at the i th time point and $V(t_i; q)$ is the model output with parameters q. We used both sampling and gradient based methods to minimize this function implemented in MATLAB. The model was fit to three data sets; namely, PVR, ETR (end-of-treatment response) and Breakthrough. PVR represents when the patient has an initial positive reaction to the therapy, but then the viral load rebounds during treatment and never goes below detection. ETR represents when the viral load drops below detection and does not rebound. Breakthrough represents when the patient's viral load drops below detection, but rebounds. In our data, the LLOQ is 15 IU/ml. When the data drop below the LLOQ, least squared estimation does not suffice as a statistically rigorous methodology. Instead, we employ the expectation maximization (EM) [40] to compute maximum likelihood estimates of our patient specific parameters. For a detailed description of the EM algorithm, we refer the reader to [41]. The RBV dosage depends on the patient's body weight and was sometimes modified during treatment due to different symptoms of the patients such as blood thinning. The patients experiencing PVR and Breakthrough had constant RBV dosage for the entire treatment while the patient exhibiting ETR had modified dosage. The RBV efficacy is fixed to $\rho = .1222$ from [22] for the PVR and Breakthrough patients. The efficacies for the ETR patient were modified based on time, t, in days since initial treatment and are presented in **Table 2**.

The parameters not in Q_{PVR} or Q_{Brk} are fixed to the values in **Table 3** from [5, 22]. As in [5], the infected steady state is used for the initial conditions for (7) because the patients considered had chronic infection. The values in **Table 4** are obtained after estimating the parameters in Q_{PVR} and Q_{Brk}. These estimates produce the model fits (graphs on the left) and residuals (graphs on the right) in **Figures 4–6**. It is noted that in **Figure 6**, the ETR patient's viral load goes to zero, and the residuals for censored data are set to zero.

In practice, the mathematical model is never exact (model misspecification), and the data contain noise (human errors, instrument errors). Hence, confidence and prediction intervals are used to understand the extent of uncertainty involved in estimating our parameters. In

Parameter	$t \leq 27$	$27 < t \leq 83$	$t > 83$
ρ	.5127	.3185	.219

Table 2. Patient ETR's RBV efficacies based on modified dosage.

Parameters	s	r	T_{max}	d	p	ε
Values	6.17×10^4	.00562	1.85×10^7	.003	25.1	.6138

Table 3. Fixed parameter values from [5, 22].

Patient	PVR	ETR	Breakthrough
δ	$.1883 \pm .0462$	$.7211$	$.3293$
c	2.717 ± 2.724	11.67	2.089
γ	$.9987 \pm .0015$	$.9999$	$.6575$
β	$1.875 \times 10^{-5} \pm 1.688 \times 10^{-5}$	8.684×10^{-8}	2.259×10^{-6}
ε	$.6138$	$.9829$	$.9875$

Table 4. Values from parameter estimation for (7).

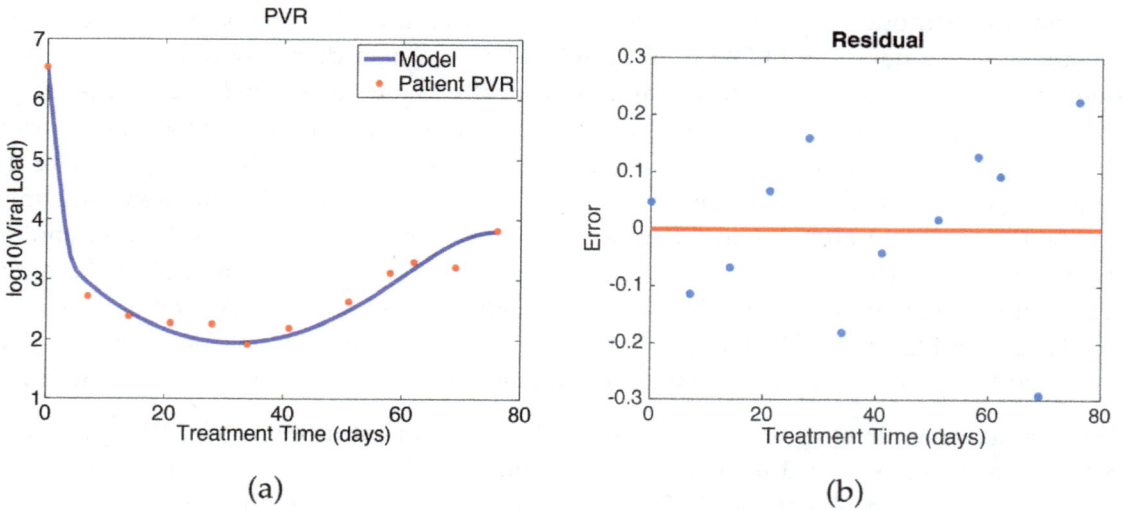

(a)   (b)

Figure 4. Viral load model fit (a) and residual plot (b) for PVR patient data.

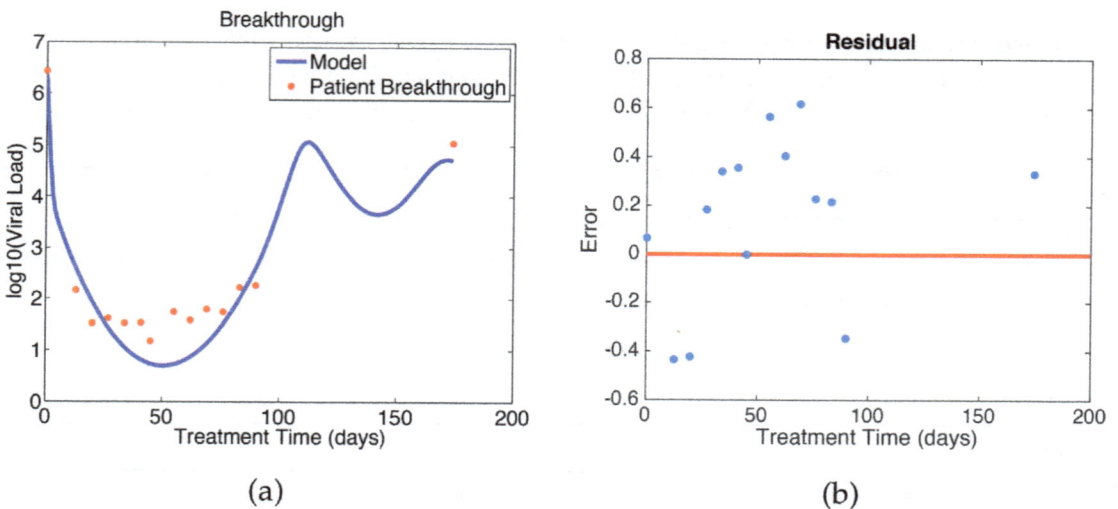

(a)   (b)

Figure 5. Viral load model fit (a) and residual plot (b) for Breakthrough patient data.

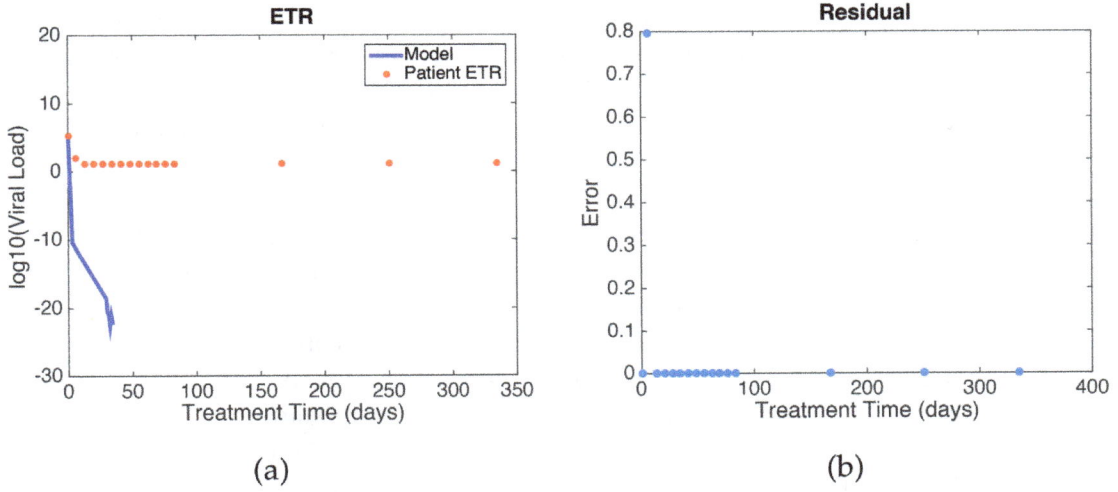

Figure 6. Viral load model fit (a) and residual plot (b) for ETR patient data.

calculating these intervals, standard errors are computed from the model predictions using the parameters that have been estimated. Moreover, 95% parameter and predictive confidence intervals and prediction intervals for the PVR parameters (attached as half-widths in **Table 4**) and predictions are calculated using the asymptotic theory outlined in [22, 27, 30, 41, 42]. The predictive confidence intervals and prediction intervals are shown in **Figure 7**.

5.1. Discussion

The higher values in c and δ in the ETR patient lead us to believe that the immune response along with the drugs has a stronger impact on the mutation and clearance of the virus. It is known that the immune response is strongly correlated with the clearance

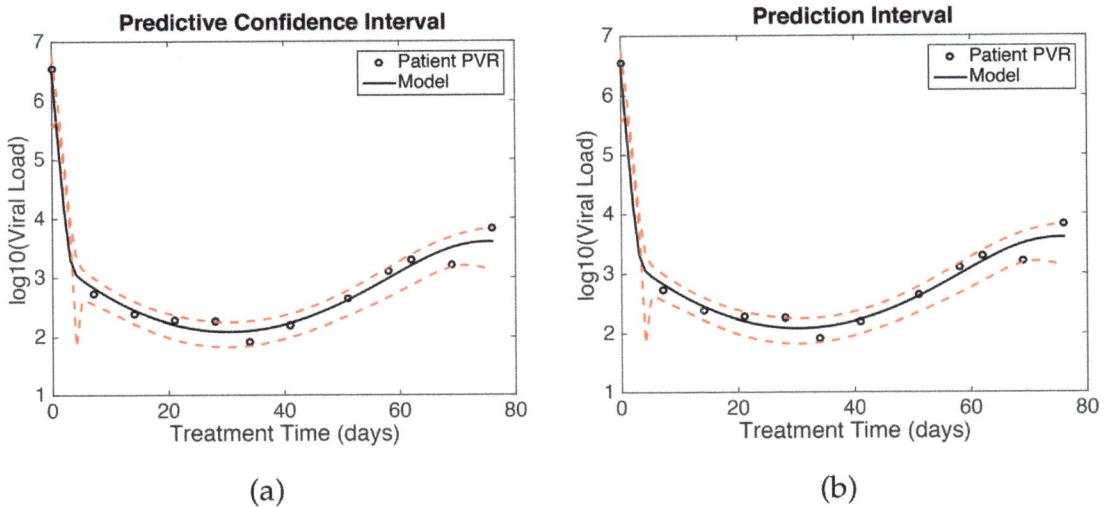

Figure 7. Predictive confidence intervals (a) and prediction intervals (b).

of the virus. Since the initial conditions of (7) are at the infected steady state, introduction of the drugs could be a mechanism to jump start the immune response. We note that even when the virus is not cleared, telaprevir still has a strong impact on viral load decay. This behavior corresponds with how powerful DAAs can be in reducing viral load even when it rebounds. The rebound could be because of mutations which are neglected in this model as stated earlier. There is a dip at around the 150th day in the Breakthrough response that is unquantifiable due to lack of information regarding the other three states or a dynamic immune response. However, this type of dip is observed in [5, 27] where data are available around this time. We conjecture that this dip is due to the immune response being stimulated by the spike in viral load and infection. The residuals in the PVR fit in **Figure 4** seem to be i.i.d. because the errors seem to be randomly distributed and are on both sides of the zero axis. This is unlike the Breakthrough fit in **Figure 5** which have most of the residuals above the zero axis. The predictive confidence intervals and prediction intervals look almost the same because the variance is very small, and the model fits the data very well. The reader is referred to [30] for further details on differences between the predictive confidence intervals and prediction intervals.

6. Conclusion

The missing data between weeks 12–24, 24–36 and 36–48 for the ETR and Breakthrough patients make parameter estimation challenging. The predictions would also be more robust if information concerning states T, I, and V_{NI} were available. These issues should be considered when making remarks about the estimations and confidence measures. DAAs were introduced in 2011, so there is not as much data available, but in the future, we hope for a larger quantity of data to make more precise estimations.

This chapter describes a model for patients with HCV who are treated with IFN, RBV, and telaprevir combination therapy. The development of this model was motivated by the desire for a model that can be validated and calibrated using sensitivity and identifiability techniques while simultaneously incorporating the new DAA, telaprevir. The model can be used to accurately describe patients exhibiting PVR, ETR, and Breakthrough.

Author details

Philip Aston[1], Katie Cranfield[1], Haley O'Farrell[1], Alex Cassenote[2], Cassia J. Mendes-Correa[2], Aluisio Segurado[2], Phuong Hoang[3], George Lankford[3] and Hien Tran[3]*

*Address all correspondence to: tran@ncsu.edu

1 University of Surrey, Guildford, United Kingdom

2 University of Sao Paulo, Sao Paulo, Brazil

3 North Carolina State University, Raleigh, United States

References

[1] Strader DB, Wright T, Thomas DL, Seeff LB. Diagnosis, management, and treatment of hepatitis c. Hepatology. 2004;**39**:1147-1171

[2] Rehermann B. Hepatitis c virus versus innate and adaptive immune responses: A tale of coevolution and coexistence. The Jounal of Clinical Investigation. 2009;**119**:1745-1754

[3] Baraldi R, Cross K, McChesney C, Poag L, Thorpe E, Flores K, Banks H. Mathematical modeling of HCV viral kinetics, Tech. Rep. Raleigh, NC: Center for Research in Scientific Computation; July 2013

[4] Neumann A, Lam N, Dahari H. Hepatitis c viral dynamics in vivo and the antiviral efficacy of interferon-alpha therapy. Science. 1998;**282**:103-107

[5] Snoeck E, Chanu P, Lavielle M, Jacqmin P, Jonsson E, Jorga K, Goggin T, Grippo J. A comprehensive hepatitis c viral kinetic model explaining cure. Clinical Pharmacology & Therapeutics. 2010;**87**:706-713

[6] Kim AI, Saab S. Treatment of hepatitis c. The American Journal of Medicine. 2005;**118**:808-815

[7] Brok J, Gluud LL, Gluud C. Ribavirin monotherapy for chronic hepatitis c. The Cochrane Database of Systematic Reviews. 2009;(4):CD005527

[8] Veronese FM, Mero A. The impact of pegylation on biological therapies. BioDrugs. 2008;**22**:315-329

[9] Quiles-Perez R, de Rueda PM, Maldonado AM-L, Martin-Alvarez A, Quer J, Salmeron J. Effects of ribavirin monotherapy on the viral population in patients with chronic hepatitis c genotype 1: Direct sequencing and pyrosequencing of the hcv regions. Journal of Medical Virology. 2014;**86**:1886-1897

[10] Takayama K, Furusyo N, Ogawa E, Shimizu M, Hiramine S, Mitsumoto F, Ura K, Toyoda K, Murata M, Hayashi J. A case of successful treatment with telaprevir-based triple therapy for hepatitis c infection after treatment failure with vaniprevir-based triple therapy. Journal of Infection and Chemotherapy. 2014;**20**:577-581

[11] Food and D. Administration, Guidance for Industry Chronic Hepatitis C Virus Infection: Developing Direct-Acting Antiviral Drugs For Treatment. Silver Spring, MD, USA: Center for Drug Evaluation and Research; 2013

[12] Kiser JJ, Flexner C. Direct-acting antiviral agents for hepatitis c virus infection. Annual Review of Pharmacology and Toxicology. 2013;**53**:427-449

[13] Bichoupan K, Martel-Laferriere V, Sachs D, Ng M, Schonfeld EA, Pappas A, Crismale J, Stivala A, Khaitova V, Gardenier D, Linderman M, Perumalswami PV, Schiano TD, Odin JA, Liu L, Moskowitz AJ, Dieterich DT, Branch AD. Costs of telaprevir-based triple therapy for hepatitis c: $189,000 per sustained virological response. Hepatology. 2014;**60**: 1187-1195

[14] Hill A, Khoo S, Fortunak J, Simmons B, Ford N. Minimum costs for producing hepatitis c direct-acting antivirals for use in large-scale treatment access programs in developing countries. Clinical Infectious Diseases Advance Access. 2014

[15] Dahari H, Ribeiro RM, Rice CM, Perelson AS. Mathematical modeling of subgenomic hepatitis c virus replication in huh-7 cells. Journal of Virology. 2007;**81**:750-760

[16] Chatterjee A, Guedj J, Perelson AS. Mathematical modelling of HCV infection: What can it teach us in the era of direct-acting antiviral agents. Antiviral Therapy. 2012;**17**:1171-1182

[17] Adiwijaya BS, Herrmann E, Hare B, Kieffer T, Lin C, Kwong AD, Garg V, Randle JCR, Sarrazin C, Zeuzem S, Caron PR. A multi-variant, viral dynamic model of genotype 1 HCV to assess the in vivo evolution of protease-inhibitor resistant variants. PLOS Computatioal Biology. 2010;**6**:e1000745

[18] Adiwijaya BS, Kieffer TL, Henshaw J, Eisenhauer K, Kimko H, Alam JJ, Kauffman RS, Garg V. A viral dynamic model for treatment regimens with direct-acting antivirals for chronic hepatitis c infection. PLOS Computatioal Biology. 2012;**8**:e1002339

[19] Guedj J, Perelson AS. Telaprevir-based therapy increases with drug effectiveness: Implications for treatment duration. Hepatology. 2011;**53**:1801-1808

[20] Rong L, Ribeiro RM, Perelson AS. Modeling quasispecies and drug resistance in hepatitis c patients treated with a protease inhibitor. Bulletin of Mathematical Biology. 2012;**74**: 1789-1817

[21] Lankford G. Optimization, Modeling, and Control: Applications to Klystron Designing and Hepatitis C Virus Dynamics, Phd Thesis. Raleigh, North Carolina: North Carolina State University; 2016

[22] Arthur JG, Tran H, Aston P. Feasibility of parameter estimation in hepatitis c viral dynamics models. Journal of Inverse and Ill-Posed Problems. 2016

[23] Clermont G, Zenker S. The inverse problem in mathematical biology. Mathematical Biosciences. 2014;**260**:11-15

[24] Zenker S, Rubin J, Clermont G. From inverse problems in mathematical physiology to quantitative differential diagnoses. PLOS Computatioal Biology. 2007;**3**:2072-2086

[25] Banks H, Baraldi R, Cross K, Flores K, McChesney C, Poag L, Thorpe E. Uncertainty quantification in modeling HIV viral mechanics, Technical Report 16. Raleigh, NC, USA: Center for Research in Scientific Computation; December 2013

[26] Banks H, Cintron-Arias A, Kappel F. Parameter selection methods in inverse problem formulation, Technical Report 03. Raleigh, NC, USA: Center for Research in Scientific Computation; November 2010

[27] Banks H, Tran H. Mathematical and Experimental Modeling of Physical and Biological Processes. Boca Raton, FL, USA: Chapman and Hall/CRC; January 2009

[28] Banks H, Bekele-Maxwell K, Bociu L, Noorman M, Tillman K. The complex-step method for sensitivity analysis of non-smooth problems arising in biology, Technical Report 11. Center for Research in Scientific Computation; October 2015

[29] Wentworth MT, Smith RC, Banks H. Parameter selection and verification techniques based on global sensitivity analysis illustrated for an hiv model. SIAM/ASA Journal on Uncertainty Quantification. 2016;**4**:266-297

[30] Smith RC. Uncertainty Quantification: Theory, Implementation, and Applications. Philadelphia, PA, USA: SIAM; 2014

[31] Carmichael GR, Sandu A, Potra FA. Sensitivity analysis for atmospheric chemistry models via automatic differentiation. Atmospheric Environment. 1997;**31**:475-489

[32] Griewank A. On Automatic Differentiation, Mathematical Programming: Recent Developments and Applications1989. pp. 83-108

[33] Neidinger RD. Introduction to automatic differentiation and matlab object-oriented programming. SIAM Review. 2010;**52**:545-563

[34] Fink M. Automatic differentiation for Matlab: Version 1.0, June 2006. http://www.mathworks.com/matlabcentral/fileexchange/15235-automatic-differentiation-for-matlab

[35] Trench WF. Advanced Calculus. New York, NY, USA: Harper & Row Publishers; 1978

[36] Morris M. Factorial sampling plans for preliminary computational experiments. Technometrics. 1991:161-174

[37] Miao H, Xia X, Perelson AS, Wu H. On identifiability of nonlinear ode models and applications in viral dynamics. SIAM Review. Society for Industrial and Applied Mathematics. 2011;**53**:3-39

[38] Cintron-Arias A, Banks H, Capaldi A, Lloyd AL. A sensitivity matrix based methodology for inverse problem formulation, Technical Report 09. Raleigh, NC, USA: Center for Research in Scientific Computation; April 2009

[39] Quaiser T, Monnigmann M. Systematic identifiability testing for unambiguous mechanistic modeling - application to jak-stat, map kinase, and nf-kb signaling pathway models. BMC Systems Biology. 2009;**3**. Article number 50

[40] Dempster A, Rubin NLD. Maximum likelihood from incomplete data via the em algorithm. Journal of the Royal Statistical Society. 1977;**39**:1-38

[41] Attarian AR. Patient Specific Subset Selection, Estimation and Validation of an HIV-1 Model with Censored Observations under and Optimal Treatment Schedule, PhD thesis. North Carolina State University; 2012

[42] Seber GAF, Wild CJ. Nonlinear Regression, Vol. 585 of Wiley Series in Probability and Statistics. Hoboken, NJ: Wiley; 2003

4

Hepatitis C Treatment in Elderly Patients

Takashi Honda, Masatoshi Ishigami,
Kazuhiko Hayashi, Teiji Kuzuya, Yoji Ishizu,
Yoshiki Hirooka and Hidemi Goto

Abstract

The patients with chronic hepatitis C (CHC) are getting older and the demands for treatment to those patients are increasing due to the high risk of development of hepatocellular carcinoma. Elderly patients were previously defined as 60 years and over, however definition of the elderly patients shifted to be older year to year. Interferon (IFN) and ribavirin combination therapy was significantly improved efficacy of treatment, however ribavirin induces anemia, resulted in lower efficacy due to reduction of ribavirin for the elderly patients. And efficacy of over 60 years old was comparable to the patients under 60 years. In the CHC patients with genotype 1, the efficacy of elderly patient was significantly lower than that of younger patients, especially in female. Direct-acting antivirals (DAAs) therapy makes treatment efficacy improved to over 90% and side effect of treatment was dramatically reduced compared to IFN-based therapy. The efficacy of dual oral therapy by using asunaprevir (ASV) and daclatasvir (DCA) for elderly patients with hepatitis C virus (HCV) genotype 1b has not been fully clarified. In this article we would like to show the efficacy of elderly patients with CHC, especially patients infected with genotype 1b, from the era of IFN monotherapy to the era of new DAAs.

Keywords: hepatitis C virus, peginterferon, ribavirin, direct-acting antivirals, elderly patient

1. Introduction

The first in the world, the demand for treatment to the elderly patients with chronic hepatitis C (CHC) has increased in Japan. The prevalence of anti-hepatitis C virus (HCV) shows the peak is in the older generation and the rate of anti-HCV increases with the increase in age in Japan. In other country, the peak of prevalence differs from country to country. These differences

- Interferon-α2b/ribavirin
- Genotype 1 ,2
- n=220, aged 60 years or older; n=66 (30.0%)

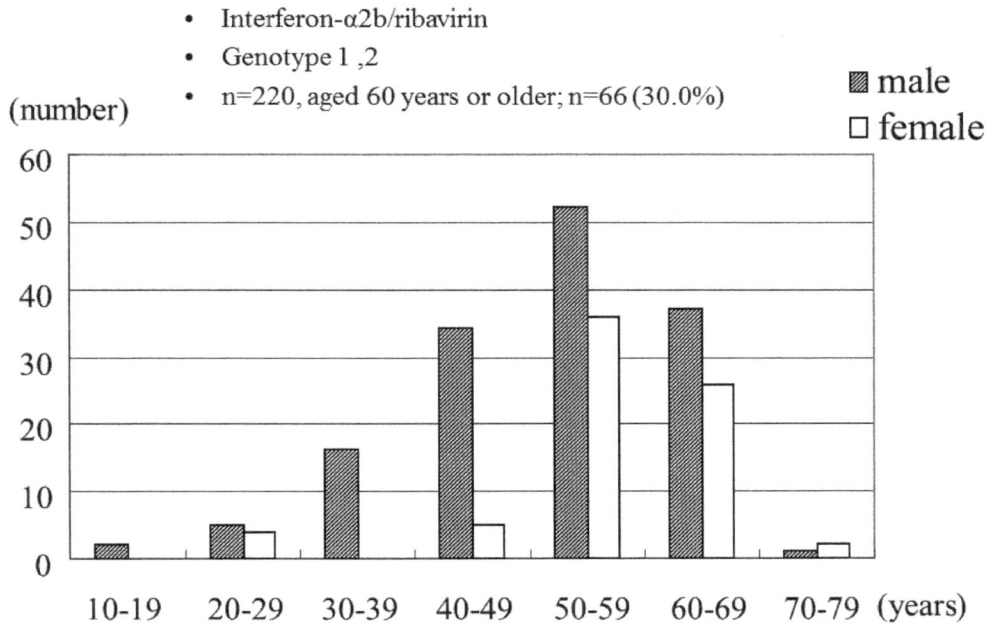

Figure 1. Patient age distribution by decade.

come from one of the reasons when the war was held in each country. During the war, HCV infection spread among drug users, blood donors and the wounded. Thereafter medical treatment with intravenous injection using contaminated needles and syringes during that time easily transmitted HCV. Therefore in Japan the peak of prevalence of anti-HCV was shifted to the older comparing to other country [1]. Previously, we compared SVR rate of ribavirin plus interferon (IFN)-α2b in CHC patients aged ≥60 years with patients aged <60 years [2]. Our study showed age distribution of the CHC patients treated by IFN-α plus ribavirin was peaked around 50 generation in 2002 (**Figure 1**). At that time we defined over 60 years as elderly patients.

2. Ribavirin and IFN-based treatment

The sustained virological response (SVR) rates of treatment in the patients with genotype 1 and a high viral load aged 60 years and older was below 10% by IFN monotherapy. However, SVR rate of IFN and ribavirin combination therapy was significantly improved by over 20%. And efficacy of over 60 years old was comparable to the patients under 60 years (**Figure 2**) [2]. In this study adding of ribavirin increased SVR rate, but ribavirin induces anemia, resulted in lower SVR rate due to reduction of ribavirin in the elderly patients. During combination of IFN-α2b plus ribavirin therapy, over 50 generation and 60 generation had high dose reduction and cessation of treatment (**Figure 3**) [2].

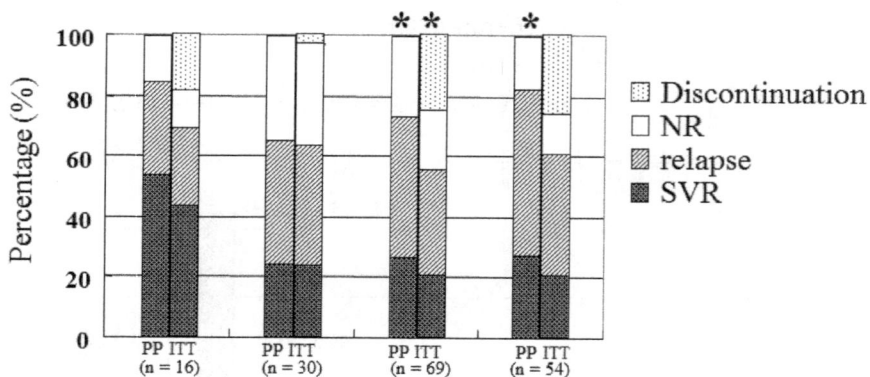

Figure 2. Virologic response to combination therapy and interferon monotherapy. * Indicate significant differences vs the respective IFN monotherapy (*P < 0.05).

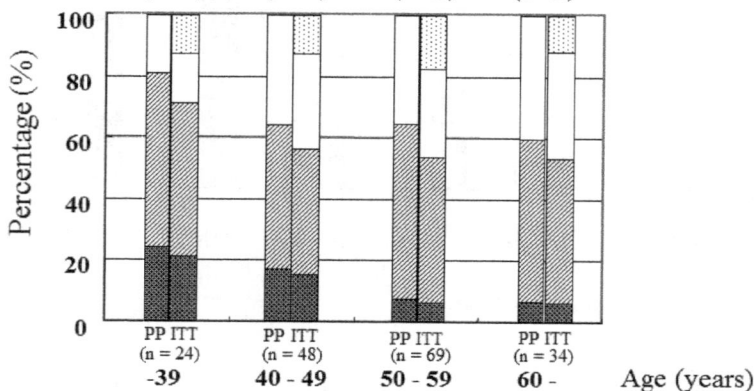

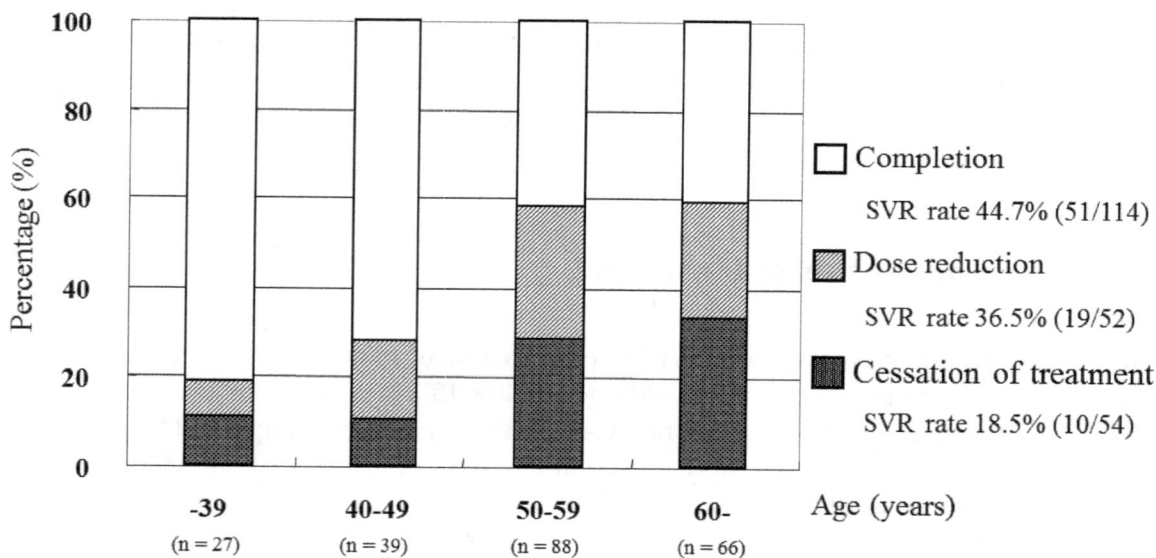

Figure 3. Ribavirin dose reduction and discontinuation rates according age of patients.

3. Ribavirin and PegIFN-based treatment

Peginterferon (PegIFN) plus ribavirin therapy improved the SVR rate of HCV treatment. We conducted the study of efficacy of PegIFN-α2b plus ribavirin and the number of the CHC patients in that study was 591. The distribution of elderly patients was around 20% in 2007. At that time elderly patients were defined as aged 65 years or older [3]. In the CHC patients with genotype 1, the SVR rate of elderly patient was significantly lower than that of younger patients, especially in female (**Figure 4**) [3]. On the other hand, patients with genotype 2 had comparable SVR rate of elderly patients to the younger patients (**Figure 5**) [3].

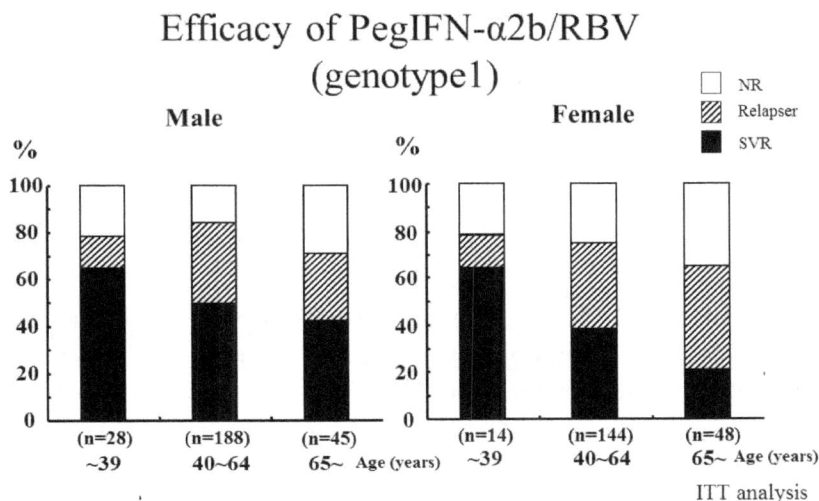

Figure 4. A virological response to combination therapy according to the age and gender of patients with genotype 1.

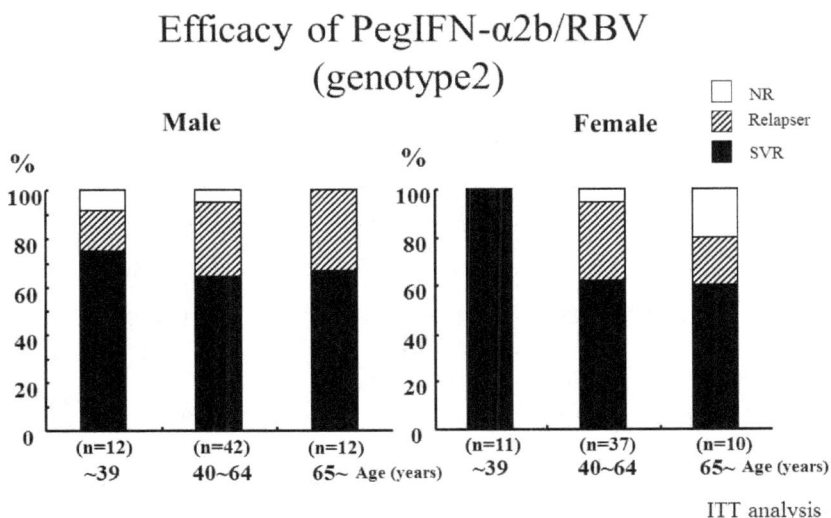

Figure 5. A virological response to combination therapy according to the age and gender of patients with genotype 2.

4. DAA-based treatment

Emerge of direct-acting antiviral's (DAA's) therapy makes SVR rate improved to over 90% and side effect of treatment was dramatically reduced compared to IFN-based therapy. Ribavirin free regimen also has benefit for the elderly patients due to avoidance of ribavirin-induced anemia. Akuta et al. reported that high SVR rate was achieved by daclatasvir (NS5A replication complex inhibitor) (DCA) and asunaprevir (NS3 protease inhibitor) (ASV) even in the elderly patients infected with HCV genotype 1b aged 70 and older [4]. They showed predictive factors associated with SVR12 in elderly patients was NS5A-Y93H mutation under 20%, non-treated by triple therapy with simeprevir, lower level of viremia under 6 logIU/mL, hemoglobin under 13.0 g/dl.

We also conducted the study of efficacy of DAA's therapy for the genotype 1-infected patients with CHC. Here we show the results of the patients with DCA and ASV therapy, 287 patients were analyzed and the patient's background shows that patients were getting older and we defined elderly patients as aged 70 older. The study protocol was approved by the ethics committee of our hospital and affiliated hospital. The inclusion criteria included positive anti-HCV and positive HCV RNA and having findings of active hepatitis. Exclusion criteria included positive for serum hepatitis B surface antigen, alcohol abuse, autoimmune hepatitis, primary biliary cirrhosis, coexisting serious psychiatric or medical illness.

Elderly patients account for 57.8% (166/287) of total treated patients (**Table 1**). Baseline ALT, γ-glutamyl transpeptidase (GGT) hemoglobin and eGFR in elderly patients were significantly lower than that of younger patients. Renal function in elderly patients was worse comparing

	Total patients (n = 287)	Patients aged <70 years (n = 121)	Patients aged ≥70 years (n = 166)	P value
Sex ratio (male/female)	123/164	55/66	68/98	0.448
Age (years)	72.0 (65.0–77.0)	63.0 (58.0–66.0)	76.0 (73.0–79.0)	<0.001
AST (IU/L)	46.0 (35.0–68.0)	48.0 (35.0–75.0)	44.0 (34.0–60.3)	0.124
ALT (IU/L)	39.0 (27.0–63.0)	48.0 (30.5–74.0)	37.0 (23.8–52.3)	<0.001
GGT (IU/L)	32.0 (22.0–53.0)	35.0 (22.0–69.0)	29.5 (21.0–46.0)	0.021
Hemoglobin (g/dl)	13.2 (12.0–14.2)	13.5 (12.3–14.4)	13.0 (11.8–14.0)	0.010
Platelets (×10^4/μL)	12.8 (8.8–17.1)	13.6 (9.2–18.1)	12.4 (8.5–16.8)	0.302
eGFR	71.7 (60.2–84.5)	80.6 (67.8–91.3)	68.2 (56.6–77.0)	<0.001
HCV RNA (KIU/mL)	6.1 (5.6–6.5)	6.1 (5.7–6.5)	6.1 (5.6–6.5)	0.556
Previous therapy (naive/ ineligible/intolerant/NVR/ relapse)	146/5/26/75/25	54/3/14/31/14	92/2/12/44/11	0.276
NS5A Y93H, n (%)	9 (3.1)	6 (5.0)	3 (1.8)	0.122
NS5A L31M, n (%)	4 (1.4)	3 (2.5)	1 (0.6)	0.230

ALT, alanine aminotransferase; GGT, γ-glutamyl transpeptidase; eGFR, estimated glomerular filtration rate; HCV RNA, hepatitis C virus RNA; KIU, kilo international units; NVR, null virological response.

Table 1. Baseline clinical characteristics of patients treated with DAA's therapy.

to the younger patients as expected. There was no patient with dose reduction due to renal insufficiency. The results of DAA's therapy showed that the SVR24 rate in elderly patients was high even in younger patients (92.2 vs. 85.1%). The factors associated with an SVR24 in DAA's therapy were determined by multivariate analysis. Gender [P = 0.014, odds ratio 0.301 (0.115–0.785)], GGT [P = 0.032, odds ratio 0.992 (0.985–0.999)] and absence of NS5A Y93H [P < 0.001, odds ratio 16.50 (3.801–71.66)] were significantly associated with an SVR24 while patient age did not affect SVR24. In elderly patients, the factors associated with an SVR24 in DAA's therapy were determined by multivariate analysis. Gender [P = 0.025, odds ratio 0.071(0.007–0.716)], GGT [P = 0.006, odds ratio 0.982 (0.970–0.995)] and absence of NS5A Y93H [P = 0.018, odds ratio 58.47 (2.024–1689.3)] were significantly associated with an SVR24.

5. Prevention of HCC

Aging is one of the factors associated with development of HCC in the CHC patients [5]. IFN therapy was reported to have reduction in development of HCC among virological or biochemical responders [6, 7]. We previously researched how benefit of reduction of HCC after eradication of HCV by PegIFN plus ribavirin. As shown in the **Figure 6** cumulative incidence of HCC in the elderly patients was higher than that in the younger patients [8]. However, if the elderly patients achieved a SVR, patients have marked reduction of cumulative incidence of HCC [8]. From the multivariate analysis in all patients age, advanced fibrosis, treatment efficacy and gender was associated with development of HCC. In elderly patients, GGT and treatment efficacy were factors associated with development of HCC. Receiver operating characteristic

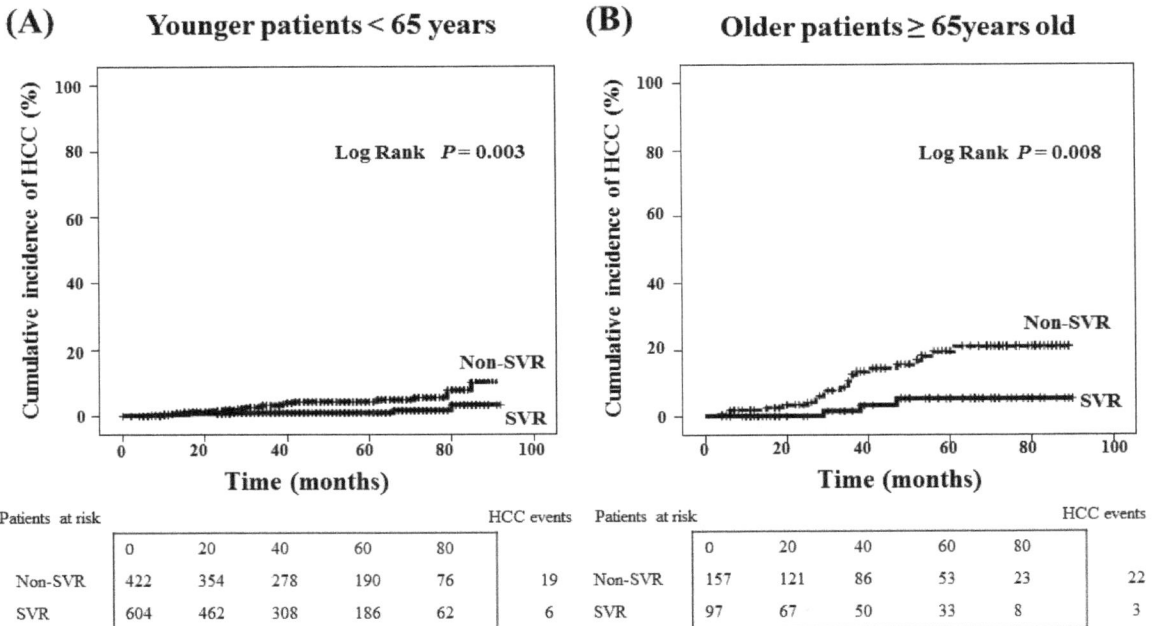

Figure 6. Cumulative incidence of HCC after peginterferon alfa-2b and ribavirin in patients who achieved SVR (solid line) or did not achieve SVR(dashed line) in younger patients < 65 years old (A) and older patients ≥ 65years old (B).

(A)   **Patients with GGT < 44 IU/L**   **(B)**   **Patients with GGT ≥ 44 IU/L**

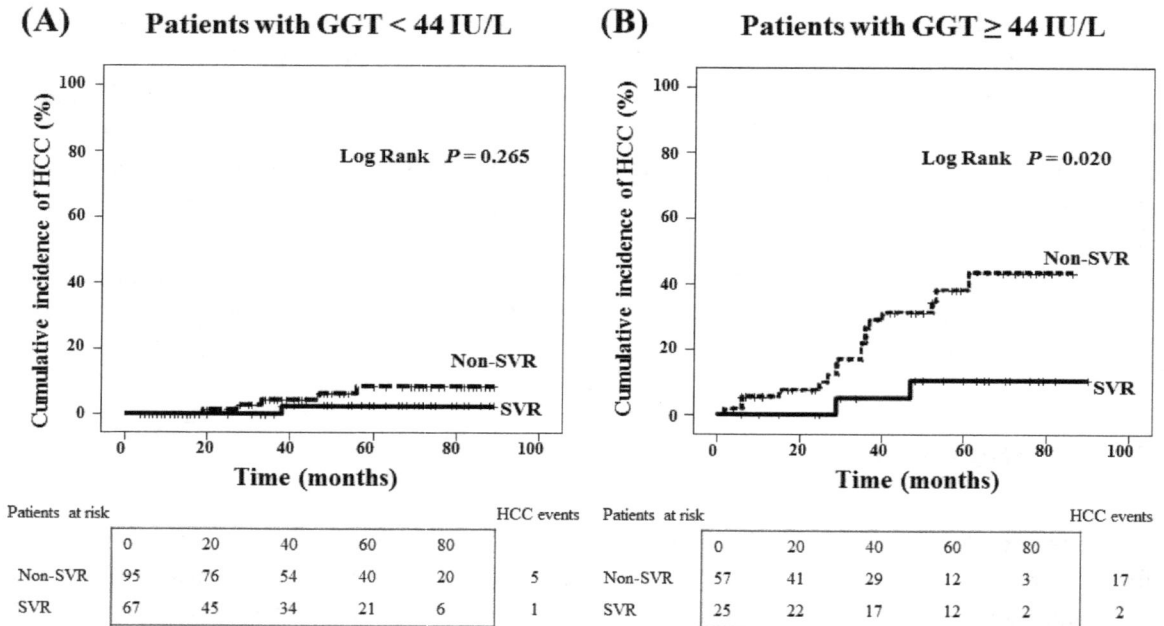

Patients at risk

Non-SVR	0	20	40	60	80	HCC events
Non-SVR	95	76	54	40	20	5
SVR	67	45	34	21	6	1

Patients at risk

Non-SVR	0	20	40	60	80	HCC events
Non-SVR	57	41	29	12	3	17
SVR	25	22	17	12	2	2

Figure 7. Cumulative incidence of HCC after peginterferon alfa-2b and ribavirin in older patients who achieved SVR (solid line) or did not achieve SVR(dashed line), among those with GGT < 44 IU/L (A) and GGT ≥ 44 IU/L (B). HCC, hepatocellular carcinoma; GGT, gamma-glutamyltranspeptidase; SVR,sustained virological response.

(ROC) curve indicated the cut off vale was 44 IU/L to predict for HCC. Among elderly patients with GGT < 44 IU/L, the cumulative incidence of HCC in patients with non-SVR was higher than patients with SVR, but this difference was not significant (**Figure 7A**). However, in elderly patients with SVR and GGT ≥ 44 IU/L, there was a marked reduction in the development of HCC compared with the elderly patients with SVR and GGT ≥ 44 IU/L (elderly patients with GGT < 44 IU/L, $P = 0.265$; elderly patients with GGT ≥ 44 IU/L, $P = 0.020$, log-rank test) (**Figure 7B**).

6. Discussion

Elderly patients with CHC are getting older and definition of elderly patients shifted from 60 to 70 years in our study during 13 years. In these days, the change of physical function according to age is seen 10 years older than that was seen in 10–20 years ago. Therefore, The Japan Geriatrics Society proposed elderly patients are defines as 75 years and over due to these rejuvenation phenomenon and the extension of the average life expectancy in 2017. If this phenomenon would be seen in all over the world, it will be globally accepted in the future.

DCV/ASV therapy for Japanese elderly patients with CHC had high SVR rate and is comparable to younger patients [4]. Our result indicated there is a possible to be higher SVR rate in elderly patients treated by DCV/ASV therapy than that in younger patients. For another type of DAA's therapy Ledipasvir/Sofosbuvir (LDV/SOF) therapy for the older CHC patients with genotype 1 from the Phase III had high SVR rate as well as younger patients [9]. They defined patients aged 65 years or older as elderly patients and those are still small population of CHC patients in the United States (12%). In other study CHC patients aged ≥65 years who were treated with different combinations of DAAs had high efficacy and took significantly more concomitant medications [10]. Therefore, they indicated assessment of concomitant medications and drug-drug interactions would be needed before DAAs therapy especially for the elderly patients. As well as PegIFN plus ribavirin therapy, DAA's therapy including ribavirin regimen needs close monitoring of anemia in the elderly patients. Elderly patients with GGT > 44 IU/L and advanced fibrosis have high risk of development of HCC when we treated older CHC patients by PegIFN plus ribavirin. These patients would be high priority to be treated with DAA, because patients who achieved SVR had a marked reduction in the development of HCC compared with elderly patients who did not achieve SVR. Compared to the RBV and IFN or PegIFN-based treatment, DAA-based treatment improved efficacy of treatment even in non-elderly patients. Therefore, indication for the elderly patients will expand. However, due to the high costs of current DAA's therapy at the moment, it is better to evaluate life expectancy. Higher age, HCV-related liver disease (advanced fibrosis, HCC) and other concomitant disease affect life expectancy. Elderly patients took many other medications, therefore evaluation of drug-drug interaction between DAA and other medication is necessary. If HCV-related liver diseases are likely to affect survival and quality of life (QOL) and there are no economic restrictions in country where patients will be treated, the patients are better to be treated. If HCV-related liver diseases are not likely to affect survival and QOL or there are economic restrictions in that country, the patients should be closely monitored and be regularly reevaluated. Therefore, physician needs more knowledge of interaction of other diseases and to have a long-term of view on the CHC patients.

Author details

Takashi Honda, Masatoshi Ishigami*, Kazuhiko Hayashi, Teiji Kuzuya, Yoji Ishizu, Yoshiki Hirooka and Hidemi Goto

*Address all correspondence to: masaishi@med.nagoya-u.ac.jp

Department of Gastroenterology and Hepatology, Nagoya University Graduate School of Medicine, Nagoya, Japan

References

[1] Yoshizawa H. Hepatocellular carcinoma associated with hepatitis C virus infection in Japan: Projection to other countries in the foreseeable future. Oncology. 2002;**62** Suppl 1: 8-17

[2] Honda T, Katano Y, Urano F, et al. Efficacy of ribavirin plus interferon-alpha in patients aged >or=60 years with chronic hepatitis C. Journal of Gastroenterology and Hepatology. 2007;**22**:989-995

[3] Honda T, Katano Y, Shimizu J, et al. Efficacy of peginterferon-alpha-2b plus ribavi-
     rin in patients aged 65 years and older with chronic hepatitis C. Liver International.
     2010;**30**:527-537

[4] Akuta N, Sezaki H, Suzuki F, et al. Favorable efficacy of daclatasvir plus asunaprevir
     in treatment of elderly Japanese patients infected with HCV genotype 1b aged 70 and
     older. Journal of Medical Virology. 2017;**89**:91-98

[5] Asahina Y, Tsuchiya K, Tamaki N, et al. Effect of aging on risk for hepatocellular carci-
     noma in chronic hepatitis C virus infection. Hepatology. 2010;**52**:518-527

[6] Imai Y, Kawata S, Tamura S, et al. Relation of interferon therapy and hepatocellular carci-
     noma in patients with chronic hepatitis C. Osaka Hepatocellular Carcinoma Prevention
     Study Group. Annals of Internal Medicine. 1998;**129**:94-99

[7] Ikeda K, Saitoh S, Arase Y, et al. Effect of interferon therapy on hepatocellular carcino-
     genesis in patients with chronic hepatitis type C: A long-term observation study of 1,643
     patients using statistical bias correction with proportional hazard analysis. Hepatology.
     1999;**29**:1124-1130

[8] Honda T, Ishigami M, Masuda H, et al. Effect of peginterferon alfa-2b and ribavirin on
     hepatocellular carcinoma prevention in older patients with chronic hepatitis C. Journal
     of Gastroenterology and Hepatology. 2015;**30**:321-328

[9] Saab S, Park SH, Mizokami M, et al. Safety and efficacy of ledipasvir/sofosbuvir for
     the treatment of genotype 1 hepatitis C in subjects aged 65 years or older. Hepatology.
     2016;**63**:1112-1119

[10] Vermehren J, Peiffer KH, Welsch C, et al. The efficacy and safety of direct acting anti-
     viral treatment and clinical significance of drug-drug interactions in elderly patients
     with chronic hepatitis C virus infection. Alimentary Pharmacology & Therapeutics.
     2016;**44**:856-865

5

Hepatitis C Virus and Inflammation

Binod Kumar, Akshaya Ramachandran and
Gulam Waris

Abstract

Inflammation is often a rapid coordinated response generated in the host against evading microbial infections or tissue injury. Microorganisms like bacteria and viruses instigate inflammation mediated by pro-inflammatory cytokines and activate cascade of signaling events leading to the recruitment of inflammatory cells (neutrophils and macrophages). Although the main function of inflammation is the resolution of infection, several viruses, including the hepatitis C viruses (HCV) have evolved to utilize this host response and make the cellular environments conducive to infection. In majority of infected individuals, HCV causes persistent chronic liver inflammation leading to development of liver cirrhosis and hepatocellular carcinoma. HCV induces reactive oxygen species (ROS) and activates nuclear factor-κB (NF-κB) leading to the activation of cyclooxygenase-2 (Cox-2) that ultimately produces prostaglandin-E2 (PGE2), thus enhancing inflammatory process. Interestingly, HCV further activates NACHT, LRR, and PYD domains-containing protein 3 (NLRP3) inflammasome (a multiprotein complex) by recruiting adaptor protein apoptosis-associated speck-like protein containing a carboxy-terminal CARD (ASC) which are involved in activation of caspase-1 leading to production of interleukin-1beta (IL-1β) and interleukin-18 (IL-18). In this chapter we have highlighted the recent advancements in HCV-induced inflammatory responses and discussed potential future directions to understand the role of inflammation during HCV infection.

Keywords: PAMP, DAMP, TLR, NLRP3, AIM2, RIG-I, IFI16, inflammation, inflammasome, IL-Iβ, Caspase-1, HCV, HBV, herpesvirus

1. Introduction

Inflammation, often triggered by harmful stimuli such as tissue injury and pathogenic infections, is an adaptive response that underlies a wide variety of both physiological and pathological processes [1]. Inflammation can be acute or chronic. Acute inflammation is generally induced by tissue injury, noxious compounds or invasion of pathogens with general clinical signs like swelling, redness, pain and heat at the site of the insult. Acute inflammation is the initial response of body during which, the small immune-mediating molecules called anaphylatoxins are recruited to site where it stimulates mast cells to release histamine, serotonin and prostaglandins. This event is followed by vasodilation to allow immune cells such as the neutrophils to rush to the site to respond to the causative agent. During the acute stage, the inflammation remains a beneficial process to heal and provide relief within few days. Chronic inflammation, however, lasts for weeks, months or even years and cause tissue damage. At the chronic stage, the inflammation becomes a problem rather than solution to infection or disease. In contrast to acute inflammation, the chronic inflammation is generally seen in viral infections and other hypersensitive disorders where the inflammation is persistent for a longer duration. During chronic inflammation, the primary immune cells are macrophages and T lymphocytes which play crucial roles by producing cytokines and other enzymes that are detrimental to cells. Several studies have focused on the chronic inflammation that occurs during type-2 diabetes, cardiovascular and autoimmune diseases and during localized chronic inflammation that occurs due to chronic infections. In spite of so much advancements made in inflammation biology, the causes and mechanistic details are still partly understood and need an in-depth analysis to completely unravel the mystery.

During pathogenic invasion, the host immune system initiates an immediate defense mechanism. The pathogens are recognized by the pattern-recognition receptors (PRR) [2] that identify pathogen-associated molecular patterns (PAMPs) [3] and danger-associated molecular patterns (DAMPs) to rapidly activate the innate arm of the host immune system, including the secretion of chemokines and cytokines [4]. The PRRs, like the Toll-like receptors (TLRs) [5] are present on the plasma membrane and in the endosomes while the RIG-I-like receptors (RLRs) [6], NOD-like receptors (NLRs) [7] and AIM2-like receptors (ALRs) [8] reside in the cytoplasm. During viral infections, the viral RNA is sensed by TLR3, TLR7 and TLR8, and viral DNA is sensed by TLR9. Similarly, viruses are also recognized by soluble sensors such as the RNA-sensing RIG-like helicases (RIG-I and MDA5) or the DNA-sensing PRRs (DAI and AIM2). The viral RNA in cytoplasm is detected by the helicase domain of either RIG-I or MDA5 followed by the exposure of the caspase recruitment domain (CARD) to interact with the N-terminal of mitochondrial adaptor protein (MAVS). This CARD-CARD interaction leads to dimerization of MAVS in the mitochondria to form the MAVS signalosome which further activates the NF-κB, production of type I interferons (IFNs) and the secretion of proinflammatory cytokines (IL-1β and IL-18) and chemokines [9, 10]. The maturation of IL-1β and IL-18 depends on the proteolytic cleavage of the pro-form of caspase-1 to release the active forms of IL-1β and IL-18 [11]. The formation of the active caspase-1 (p10/p20) is often regulated by multi-protein complexes called the inflammasomes [12].

Several distinct inflammasomes including the NLRP3 inflammasome, the absent in melanoma 2 (AIM2) inflammasome, the γ-interferon-inducible protein 16 (IFI16) inflammasome and the RIG-I inflammasomes have been identified to be activated during specific viral and bacterial infections [13]. Several viruses such as vaccinia virus (VACV) [14], HCV [15], hepatitis B virus (HBV) [16], human papillomavirus [17], mouse cytomegaloviruses (mCMV) [14, 16], influenza virus [9, 18] and Vesicular stomatitis viruses (VSV) [19] have been reported to activate inflammasomes. In this book chapter, we have reviewed the role of inflammation and discussed the detailed mechanism of activation, following viral invasions, specifically during HCV infection.

2. Overview of inflammatory response to viral infections

2.1. Virus-induced inflammatory response

Inflammation is very crucial in maintaining the homeostasis that's altered during any exogenous stimuli such as the tissue injury or a pathogenic infection. Several viruses are known to induce inflammatory response. The virus is sensed by TLRs (TLR3/7, TLR8/9), RLRs (RIG-I and MDA5) and RNA-dependent protein kinases (PKR), to induce the production of inflammatory mediators and IFNs. The dsRNA is usually sensed through RIG-I and/or TLR3 in the monocytes, macrophages and non-immune cells (endothelial cells, epithelial cells and hepatocytes) whereas in plasmacytoid dendritic cells, TLR7 is highly expressed and acts as the major ssRNA sensor [20–23]. The activation of RLRs and TLRs then promote the secretion of IFNs and proinflammatory cytokines. The inflammation is further amplified when the proinflammatory cytokines and chemokines, such as IL-6, IL-8, tumor necrosis factor alpha (TNF-α) and Rantes starts recruiting other cell types to the infected tissue. These events not only contribute in the control of virus replication but also significantly enhance the inflammatory responses and disease severity.

The endoplasmic reticulum is the major site for protein synthesis including viral protein synthesis that disturbs the ER homeostasis and causes ER stress [24]. The main stress response pathway in the ER is the unfolded protein response (UPR) which has been linked to enhanced cytokine (TNF-α and IL-6) production due to activation of NF-κB and pro-inflammatory transcription factors [25, 26]. Thus the UPR pathway serves as the internal danger signal and compliments the cellular viral sensors to boost subsequent antiviral response [27]. Since the ER stress in the absence of any viral infection also leads to production of IL-1β secretion and cell death, it would be interesting to investigate further if there is a crosstalk between the UPR pathway and inflammasome activation during viral infection. The mitochondrial stress has also been associated with formation of ROS that can result in the activation of NF-κB, Cox-2, PGE2, IL-6 and activating protein-1 (AP-1), that subsequently up-regulate antioxidants and inflammatory pathways, including the ISGs [28].

Several viruses such as influenza viruses (human H1N1 and avian H5N1) have been shown to infect the microglia, astrocytes and neuronal cell lines and produce pro-inflammatory cytokines, ultimately leading to cell apoptosis [29]. A recent study also showed that influenza virus infection of mouse primary cortical neurons enhanced the mRNA levels of inflammatory cytokines, chemokines, and type I IFNs [30]. The Epstein–Barr virus (EBV) also triggers the TNF-α signaling by its LMP1 protein, activating NF-κB and resulting in production of IL-6 and subsequently a number of pro-inflammatory and immune stimulatory cytokines [31–33]. Similarly, the KSHV encodes several genes specially the viral Fas-associated death domain-like IL-1-converting enzyme inhibitory protein (vFLIP) that induce NF-κB activation that subsequently upregulates the chemokine CCL20 and its receptor CCL6. The CCL20 then recruits dendritic cell and lymphocyte and thus contributes to the inflammatory infiltrate in the Kaposi's sarcoma lesions [34, 35]. In case of hepatitis B and C viruses, the liver cancer develops due to years of inflammation, oxidative stress (OS) and cell death leading to chronic liver damage. The liver infiltrating lymphocytes contributes majorly in the production of pro-inflammatory cytokines such as TNF-α, IL-6 and IL-1β during chronic HBV/HCV infection [36, 37].

2.2. Virus-induced inflammasomes

Several viruses like the influenza viruses, Respiratory syncytial virus (RSV), hepatitis B and C viruses, Dengue virus and herpesviruses have been reported to induce inflammation and activate the inflammasomes (**Table 1**). Few viruses are cleared, while a majority of viruses that cause chronic infection and cancer tend to utilize the inflammasome complex and the cellular milieu for their survival and have successful infection. The various inflammasomes that gets activated during different viral invasions are shown in **Table 1** and **Figure 1**.

The inflammasomes further contribute in secretion of inflammatory cytokines during viral infections. The following inflammasomes have been widely discussed during viral infections:

2.2.1. NLRP3 inflammasome

The NLRP3 inflammasome is the best-studied inflammasome and is known to be activated by viruses belonging to different families, suggesting a common pathway for detection of viruses and appropriate response by the host cells. NLRP3 is a multi-domain protein comprising of the N-terminal caspase recruitment domain (CARD), a PYD, a central nucleotide-binding and oligomerization domain (NACHT) (also termed NOD) and the C-terminal leucine-rich repeats (LRRs) [50]. The N-terminal domain helps in signal transduction by interacting with other CARD or PYD-containing proteins. The central NACHT domain serves as the scaffold protein and helps in oligomerization, thus activating the inflammasome. The LRRs are believed to act as ligand sensors. The formation of NLRP3 inflammasome induces the activation of caspase-1 and production of mature IL-1β and IL-18 [11]. NLRP3 inflammasome has been shown to be activated by ATP mediated efflux of PAMPs [51], lysosome/cathepsin B [52] and Ca^{2+}/ROS [53]. Viruses from different families are known to activate and modulate NLRP3 inflammasomes.

PRR	Pathogens	PAMPs recognized	Cytokines expression modulated	Refs
NLRP3	Influenza virus, Sendai virus, Vaccinia virus, HCV, RSV, VSV and Rabies virus	RNA	IL-1β and IL-18	[15, 18, 38–43]
AIM2	VACV, HBV, HPV and mCMV	Cytoplasmic DNA	IL-1β and IL-18	[14, 16, 17, 44]
RIG-I	Influenza virus, HCV, Rabies virus, JEV, RSV	RNA	Type I IFNs, IL-1β and IL-18	[6, 9, 45, 46]
IFI16	KSHV, EBV, HSV-1	Nuclear DNA	Type I IFNs, IL-1β	[47–49]

Table 1. Virus-induced inflammasome activation and modulation of cytokines.

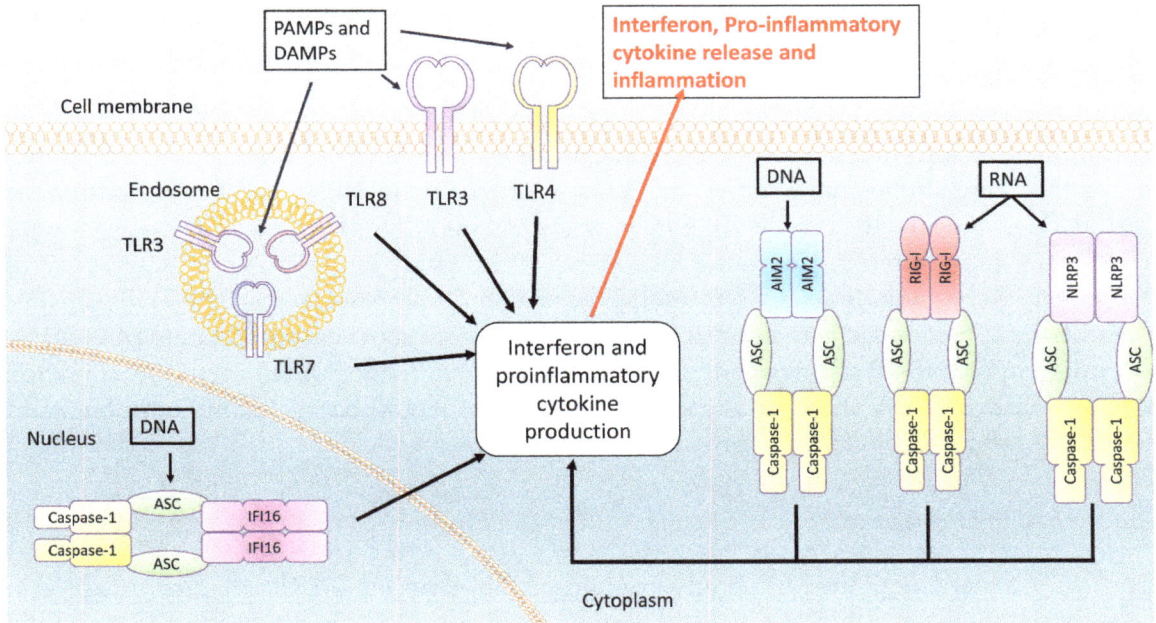

Figure 1. Inflammasome activation during viral infection. Infection with viruses leads to inflammasome activation. Depending on the type of nucleic acid composition of the invading pathogen different types of inflammasomes are activated. TLRs do not form inflammasome but do sense PAMPs and DAMPs associated with pathogens and its associated products. TLRs are located on either the cell membrane (TLR3 and TLR4) or endosome (TLR7 and TLR8). Sensing of PAMPs and DAMPs by TLRs activates cellular pathways which leads to the production of IFNs and proinflammatory cytokines. IFI16 detects DNA in the nucleus and is activated through formation of a complex formed with ASC and caspase-1. Similarly, AIM2 also detects pathogen DNA in the cytoplasm and forms an inflammasome with ASC and caspase-1. Whereas, RIG-I and NLRP3 both sense RNA PAMPs from pathogens, and similar to IFI16 and AIM2, form an inflammasome complex with adaptor ASC and effector caspase-1. Formation of inflammasome complex leads to its activation and release of IFN and proinflammatory cytokines which ultimately causes inflammation.

Influenza viruses are the most common activators of NLRP3 inflammasome [38]. Studies have further shown that the influenza virus proton-specific ion channel M2 protein activates NLRP3 inflammasome in the acidic trans-Golgi network [54]. The hepatitis C virus (JFH-1) also activates the NLRP3 inflammasome in Huh7.5 cells and THP-1 macrophages and leads to the production of IL-1β [15, 43]. The ROS inhibitor diphenyleneiodonium (DPI) has been shown to inhibit the HCV-induced IL-1β production [43]. Thus HCV has been shown to activate the NLRP3 inflammasomes both through the HCV genomic RNA and ROS model. Others viruses like the Rabies virus [42], modified vaccinia virus [14], Japanese encephalitis virus [55] and Rift Valley fever viruses [56] are also shown to induces IL-1β production and NLRP3 inflammasome activation.

Apart from RNA viruses, the DNA viruses are also reported to activate NLRP3 inflammasome. The Herpes simplex virus 1 (HSV-1) infection triggers the association of ASC with NLRP3 along with the production of mature caspase-1 and IL-1β in the human foreskin fibroblasts [49]. Adenovirus activates IL-1β secretion in monocytic cells. The transfected adenoviral DNA was known to activate the inflammasome which was NLRP3 independent, however later in a study, it was observed that adenoviral infection could activate the NLRP3 inflammasome, thus suggesting that NLRP3 inflammasome activation could be dependent on the route of viral DNA. The study further showed that NLRP3 knockout mice showed decreased IL-1β induction in response to adenoviral infection thus indicating the possibility of other sensors identifying transfected adenoviral DNA in previous studies [57]. In another study, the Varicella-Zoster Virus (VZV) was also demonstrated to activate the NLRP3 followed by recruitment of ASC and caspase-1 in monocytic and melanoma cell lines and in skin xeno-grafts [58]. Few studies have shown the relation of NLRP3 in HBV infections, however the results does not directly correlate the increased expression of NLRP3 in CHB patients with HBV-DNA copy number. Hence the increase in NLRP3 may be due to an indirect effect of HBV such as the liver damage [59]. Another recent study has shown that HBV-HBeAg sup-pressed the LPS-induced activation of the NLRP3 inflammasome and production of IL-1β by suppressing the NF-κB pathway and ROS production [60]. Since studies about the activation of NLRP3 during HBV infection are still progressing, it would be interesting to understand how HBV modulates inflammasomes for its propagation.

2.2.2. RIG-I inflammasome

The RIG-I, a member of the RLR family, contains two N-terminal CARDs that recruits several adaptor proteins, a central RNA helicase domain that has an ATPase activity and a C-terminal regulatory domain (CTD) that binds to the dsRNA to collectively induce the type I IFN pro-duction [61]. The RIG-I has been shown to recognize the dsRNA replication intermediates of several RNA viruses [62]. Influenza virus, HCV, Sendai virus, New castle disease virus, rabies virus and RSV showed defective IFN production in the absence of RIG-I [6]. The role of RIG-I as inflammasome activator has been shown in a study that was conducted with rhab-dovirus VSV infection in murine dendritic cells in which there was RIG-I dependent produc-tion of IL-1β and IL-18 via NF-κB, caspase-1, and caspase-3 activation. The knockdown of RIG-I in mice inhibited the secretion of IL-1β [19]. Another study however showed conflicting results in which the infection with VSV was shown to be activated by NLRP3 and not by RIG-I [41]. These contrary results highlight the possible dual role of RIG-I in the inflammasome and type 1 IFN pathways. A study conducted with influenza virus infection in the primary human bronchial epithelial cells demonstrated both RIG-I-dependent priming of the NLRP3 inflammasome as well as direct RIG-I-mediated inflammasome activation [9]. Thus extensive research is still needed to analyze the roles of RIG-I during viral infections.

2.2.3. AIM2 inflammasome

The AIM2 is a member of the interferon (IFN)-inducible protein with a 200 amino acid repeat family (also known as the HIN200 family of IFI200 family) containing an N-terminal PYD and a C-terminal HIN200 domain. The family includes at least six members in mice (IFI202, IFI203, IFI204, IFI205, PYHIN1 and AIM2) and four members in humans (IFI16, MNDA, IFIX and AIM2). Studies have demonstrated that AIM2 senses the cytoplasmic bacterial, viral, or even the host double-stranded DNA (dsDNA) [8, 16]. The AIM2 utilizes its PYD domain to interact with ASC and recruit caspase-1 for the AIM2 inflammasome formation and IL-1β and IL-18 secretion [16]. AIM2 has been shown to be required for activation of caspase-1 during the VACV and MCMV infection in cell culture system but not during the HSV-1 infection [14, 63]. The sensing of VACV and MCMV but not HSV-1 indicates that few viruses have evolved to block the AIM2 mediated recognition of their genome and downstream signaling. It has been further shown that AIM2$^{-/-}$ mice infected with MCMV were defective in IL-18 and IFN-γ production as compared to their control littermates [14]. The human hepatocytes have also been shown to express AIM2. An *in vitro* study has shown that the AIM2 senses the hepatitis B virus in hepatocytes and increases the production of IL-18. Further, the study showed that the expression of AIM2 in chronic hepatitis B (CHB) patients was higher than that of controls and which positively correlated to the severity of liver inflammation [64]. In another study conducted on peripheral blood mononuclear cells (PBMCs) from patients with acute hepatitis B (AHB) and CHB during different clinical phases, the expression of AIM2, IL-1β, and IL-18 was observed to be significantly high in AHB compared with expression in CHB patient samples [44]. The low expression in CHB patients also suggests that AIM2 may be associated with the chronic development of hepatitis [44]. It would be interesting to study if all the family of DNA viruses is sensed by the AIM2 inflammasomes.

2.2.4. IFI16 inflammasome

Similar to AIM2, the IFI16 belongs to the ALR family however they differ in their cellular localization. The former is strictly cytosolic while the latter is mainly localized in the nucleus due to its nuclear localizing sequence (NLS). Since both AIM2 and IFI16 recognizes DNA, these sensors are also reported to get activated by self-DNA, potentially leading to various autoimmune and auto inflammatory diseases such as lupus pathogenesis [65], Sjögren's syndrome [66] and systemic sclerosis [67]. The IFI16 is also known to sense viral DNA during infection. A study conducted on KSHV has shown that IFI16 recognized the viral DNA in the nucleus and later translocated to cytoplasm only in infected cells [68]. Upon recognition of the KSHV genome, the IFI16 is acetylated in the nucleus and later redistributed to the cytoplasm with the help of BRCA1 [48, 69]. Among others, the herpes simplex virus 1 (HSV-1), Epstein–Barr virus (EBV), and bovine herpesvirus 1 (BoHV-1) are also reported to activate the IFI16-ASC inflammasomes and produce inflammatory cytokine IL-1β [47, 49, 70].

3. Hepatitis C virus and liver inflammation

Hepatitis C virus is a hepatotropic virus, belongs to the *Flaviviridae* family. It is a positive sense single-stranded RNA virus. The RNA genome is present in an icosahedral structure made up of core proteins, which is further encapsulated in lipid bilayer which contains E1/E2 glycoproteins in a heterodimer on the membrane [71]. The RNA genome contains a 5'UTR which has an internal ribosomal entry site (IRES) and is required for cap–independent translation [72, 73]. On the other hand, the 3'UTR consists of mainly a poly (U/UC) tract and X-tail which have been shown to be required for replication of viral RNA [74, 75]. In between the two UTRs exists the genomic region which translates into a 3000aa polyprotein which is cleaved by host peptidases and viral proteins to form structural (core, E1 and E2) proteins, p7 and non-structural (NS2, NS3, NS4A, NS4B, NS5A, and NS5B) proteins. The virus is known to cause chronic infections in liver and eventually cancer (**Figure 2**). HCV causes chronic inflammation leading to liver fibrosis, steatosis, cirrhosis and finally hepatocellular carcinoma (HCC).

Inflammation is a crucial physiological event that occurs during chronic HCV infection. Chronic inflammation is defined by the persistence of inflammatory cells and destruction of liver cells. The liver cells have a unique regenerative capacity and can replace a significant loss of liver cells by compensatory proliferation. However, the chronic liver damage and regeneration results in scarring of liver called liver fibrosis. The fibrotic stage is characterized by the activation of HSCs and extracellular matrix (ECM) secretion. The liver fibrosis is also enhanced due to promotion of activated hepatic stellate cells (HSCs) survival in a NF-κB dependent manner by the KCs and recruited macrophages [76]. The ROS released by KCs and NADPH oxidase stimulated ROS production in HSCs and hepatocytes, result in robust induction of OS leading to DNA damage, enhanced expression of proinflammatory genes, fibrogenesis and malignancy [77]. The fibrotic stage gradually progresses to late stage of fibrosis called cirrhosis, which is the hallmark of an irreversible advanced stage liver injury. At this stage the dense bands of fibrotic scar develops into abnormal nodules of hepatocytes, resulting mainly from regenerative hyperplasia, separated by fibrous tissues. The disease progression eventually leads to the loss of normal functionality of liver such as xenobiotic metabolism and the metabolism of carbohydrates, proteins and other crucial molecules. In case of HCV infection, the complication progresses as a mild liver disease for 15–20 years after which a substantial number of individuals develop liver cirrhosis with clinical complications such as ascites, variceal hemorrhage and hepatic encephalopathy [78]. The ultimate complication of cirrhosis is the development of hepatocellular carcinoma.

In HCV infected individuals, besides a local inflammation in the liver, a mild systemic inflammation is also observed due to increased pro-inflammatory cytokine serum levels and

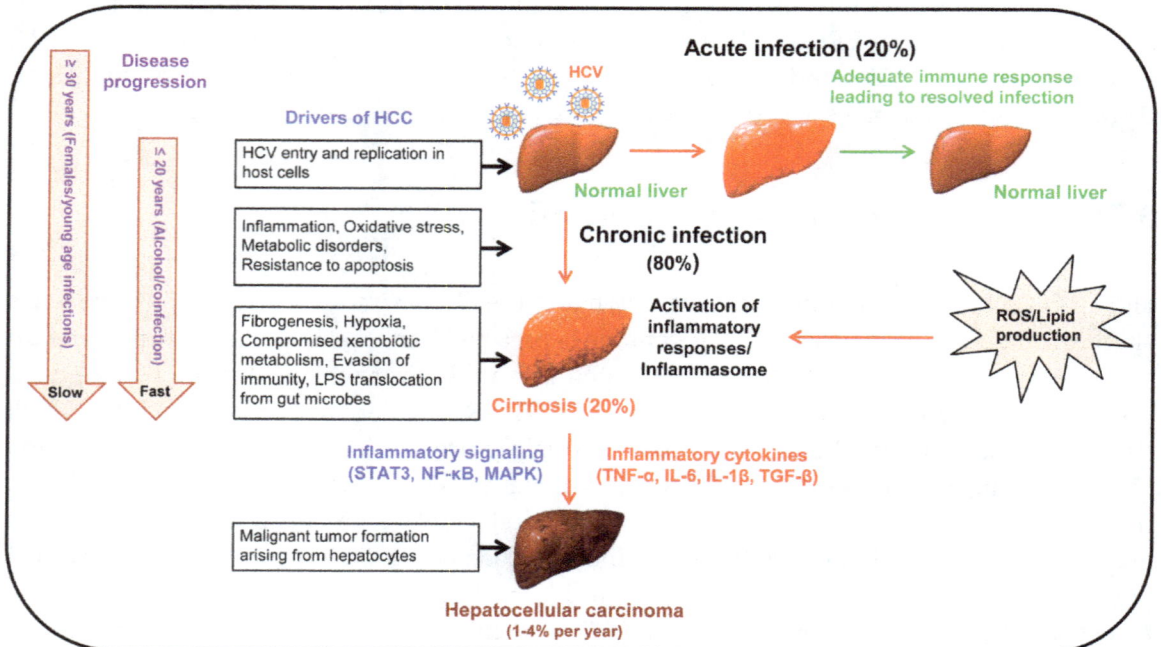

Figure 2. Schematic diagram representing different stages of HCV-induced liver disease progression.

activation of blood monocytes. The OS generated during chronic infection also plays key roles in the development of local and systemic inflammation. HCV proteins activate several pathways responsible for increased inflammatory response. The NS5A, for example, promotes upregulation of Cox-2 which contributes to chronic inflammation and fibrosis through production of various prostaglandins [79]. The chronic liver damage due to continuous inflammatory response (various inflammatory cytokines) and OS for several years ultimately leads to liver cancer [36]. Similarly, HCV infection also leads to an enrichment of proinflammatory cytokines in the liver cells ultimately leading to increased secretion of TNF-α, IL-6 and IL-1β [80]. These inflammatory events make the HSCs highly responsive to the transforming growth factor β (TGF-β) [81] that promotes hepatic fibrogenesis and eventually the progression and prognosis of HCC [82, 83]. HCV also induces the ER stress that increases the intracellular ROS levels which ultimately leads to increase in inflammatory gene expression by activation of NF-κB, AP-1 and STAT3 [84, 85]. A study has shown that the HCV core induces lipid accumulation leading to increased ROS production and inflammation ultimately promoting the HCC in transgenic mice [86, 87]. Osteopontin (OPN) is a cytokine that either remain intracellular or is secreted to allow both autocrine and paracrine signaling. Studies have shown the correlation of hepatic inflammation with increased expression of OPN [88, 89]. Recent studies have also shown that OPN is a crucial player during HCV infection and plays roles in epithelial to mesenchymal transition of hepatocytes [90, 91].

3.1. Role of various cytokines in HCV-induced inflammation

Cytokines belong to a large group of proteins that are secreted from specific cells of the immune system and perform a wide range of biological functions including innate and acquired immunity, hematopoiesis and inflammation. They mainly include the interleukins, chemokines, IFNs, TNF etc. Viral proteins and dsRNA from HCV triggers the induction of proinflammatory cytokines and chemokines. HCV core protein has been shown to induce inflammatory cytokines through the STAT3 signaling pathway [92]. A study further showed that a cross-talk existed between the HSCs and HCV-infected hepatocytes. The IL-1β secreted by HSCs co-cultured with the hepatocytes, ignited the production of several pro-inflammatory cytokines and chemokines, such as IL-6, IL-8, MIP-1α and MIP-1β, by the hepatocytes [93]. The HCV proteins (NS3, NS4 and NS5) are also reported to induce the human Kupffer cells (KCs) to synthesize inflammatory cytokines such as TNF-α and IL-1β [94]. The HCV-NS5A protein has been shown to induce high levels of pro-inflammatory chemokine IL-8 to inhibit IFN-α thus facilitating the viral replication despite IFN α/β induction [95]. *In vitro* studies have shown that IL-10 production is regulated by HCV structural proteins to inhibit IL-12 production in myeloid cells. This also correlated with reduced IL-12 levels observed in chronic hepatitis C patients [96]. Serum cytokine levels were evaluated in HCV patients, and it was observed that both T helper (Th) 1 and Th2 lymphocytes were highly associated with chronic HCV infection [97]. This lead to the increased production of IL-2, IL-4, and IL-6 cytokines in all chronic active hepatitis patients [97]. Liver fibrosis has been shown to progress due to the persistent inflammation activating the HSCs, myofibroblasts, and fibroblasts which are regulated by pro-inflammatory cytokines such as TGF-β, IL-6, TNF-α, CCL21, and platelet-derived growth factor (PDGF) [98]. The HCV related mixed cryoglobulinemia

(MC) (MC + HCV) is an extrahepatic disease associated with HCV infection. In a study, the MC + HCV was shown to express significantly higher mean IL-1β, IL-6, and TNF-α levels than the controls or the HCV patients [99]. A recent study has shown the importance of Th17/IL-17 axis in HCV-induced chronic hepatitis and progression to cirrhosis. It promotes the recruitment of inflammatory cells and cytokines IL-6 and IL-23. A similar observation was also made in HCV patients with orthotopic liver transplantation (OLT). The recipients with HCV-induced allograft fibrosis or cirrhosis presented with higher levels of HCV-specific Th17 cells along with proinflammatory mediators (IL-17, IL-1β, IL-6, IL-8, and MCP-1) [100]. In a study conducted to analyze the expression of cytokines in HCV infected patients, it was observed that TNF-α expression was localized mainly in liver sinusoidal cells (macrophages, endothelial cells) and a high proportion of hepatocytes demonstrated expression of TNF-α, IL-1α, and IL-2 [101]. IL-32 has also been shown to be expressed by human hepatocytes and hepatoma cells and is involved in HCV-associated liver inflammation [102]. In addition, IL-32 was found to be constitutively expressed in the human hepatoma cells and was observed to be upregulated by IL-1β and TNF-α [102].

3.2. HCV-induced oxidative stress adds to inflammatory response

Oxidative stress plays a significant role in HCV-induced liver damage. HCV infection has also been reported to activate the liver-residing macrophages- Kupffer cells (KC) and result in ROS production. The activated KCs enhance the production of TNF-α and ROS as a mechanism to cope with HCV infection by killing hepatocytes [103]. HCV has also been shown to induce OS through calcium signaling [84, 104, 105]. The HCV infection also induces ROS that stimulates the NF-κB to activate Cox-2. This event ultimately leads to overexpression of Cox-2 thereby increasing the levels of pro-inflammatory molecules, PGE_2 (**Figure 3**) [104]. The ROS also activates a transcription factor, STAT-3, that controls important cellular processes required for cell survival, proliferation, differentiation and oncogenesis [106] and constitutive activation of NF-κB and STAT-3 by HCV has been shown to be involved in acute and chronic liver disease associated with HCV infection [107]. ROS has also been shown to increase the proliferation of HSCs as well as TGF-β and collagen synthesis to promote fibrogenesis [108]. Hepatic steatosis, reported in more than 50% of HCV-infected patients, has also been linked to OS in CHC patients infected with HCV genotype non-3 [109]. The HCV-infected human hepatoma cells enhance the expression of TGF-β1 by induction of transcription factors AP-1, Sp1, NF-κB and STAT-3 via OS [110].

3.3. Role of inflammasomes in HCV-induced inflammatory response

HCV infection in liver cells stimulates host responses which triggers PRRs to recognize HCV components. Recognition usually occurs through TLR3 and TLR7 on either the cell surface or the endosomal compartments during HCV infection (**Figure 3**) [111]. TLR expression and recognition of HCV associated PAMPs has led to production of IFN as well as activation of NF-κB mediated inflammatory molecules which ultimately cause inflammation. TLR3 signaling pathway is led by TIR-domain-containing adaptor-inducing interferon-B (TRIF) which activates IRF-3 and NF-κB which produces pro-inflammatory cytokines, chemokines and type I IFN. Even though TLR3 expression was observed in HCV infected cells it was identified that the downstream signaling is impaired by HCV non-structural proteins NS3/4A, NS5A

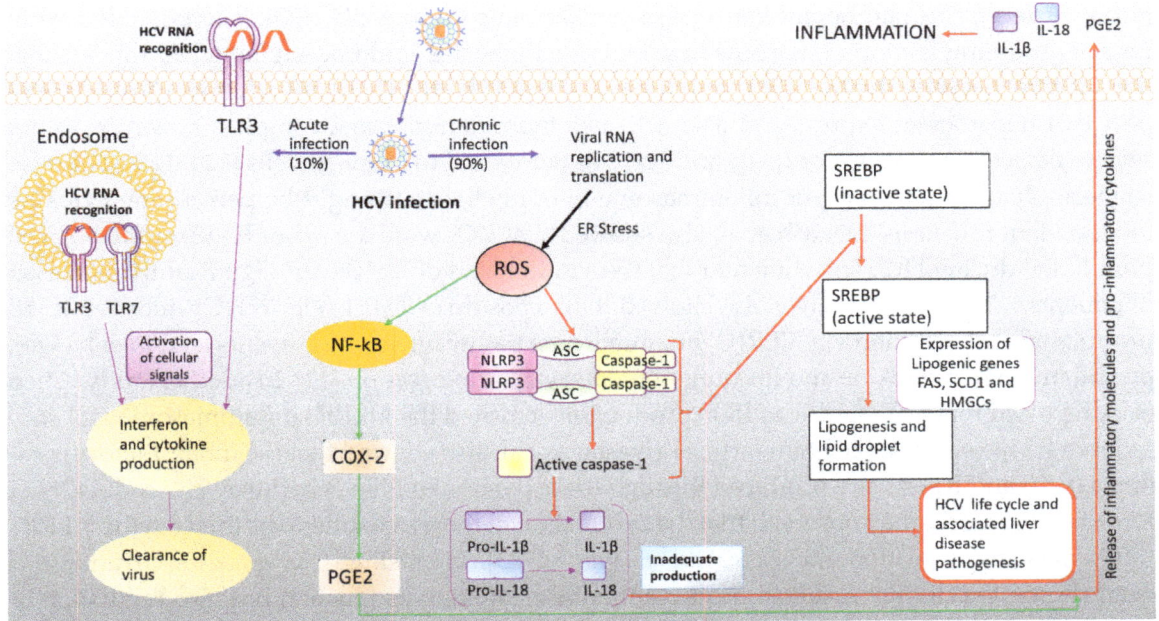

Figure 3. HCV-induced inflammasome regulates liver disease pathogenesis.

and NS5B [112] and also by decreasing the expression of TLR3 adaptor TRIF [113]. TLR7 activation leads to formation of a complex with MyD88, TRAF6, IRAK4 and IRAK1, which further activates IRF7 and induces interferon signaling.

During HCV infection HCV PAMPs are not only recognized by TLRs but also by RIG-I. It has been observed that HCV dsRNA is recognized by RIG-I during initial hours of HCV viral infection [114]. dsRNA binding to RIG-I initiates an interaction between 14-3-3ε and E3-ubiquitin ligase TRIM25 [115, 116]. This interaction leads to another interaction of RIG-I with MAVS, which contributes to IRF3 and NF-κB signalosome activation and production of IFNs [117, 118]. It was identified by Baril et al. that HCV prevents further signal transduction of RIG-I through proteolytic cleavage of MAVS by HCV NS3/NS4A protease [119]. MAVS cleavage results in disruption of RIG-I mediated IFN production during HCV infection [120].

HCV has also been shown to activate NLRP3 inflammasome in infected liver cells. A study has shown that HCV increases NLRP3 expression in liver [121]. In another study Burdette et al. for the first time showed induction and assembly of NLRP3 inflammasome in human hepatoma cells infected with HCV (JFH-1) (**Figure 3**) [15]. The study demonstrated that NLRP3, upon sensing the HCV, recruits an adaptor protein ASC for the assembly of the inflammasome complex. The study also highlighted that the activation of IL-1β in HCV infected cells was achieved by proteolytic processing of pro-caspase-1 into mature caspase-1 [15] and siRNA mediated cleavage of NALP3, ASC and caspase-1 abrogated the IL-1β secretion suggesting that HCV infected hepatoma cells (epithelial) activates NLRP3 inflammasome [15]. In another study by Boaru et al., it was shown that NLRP3 inflammasome was prominently assembled in liver sinusoidal endothelial cells and KCs, moderately in cultured HSCs and periportal myofibroblasts and almost absent in primary hepatocytes [122]. Studies have also shown that NLRP3 inflammasome was not activated in human hepatoma cells or primary hepatocytes [43, 123]. The possible reason for not observing the inflammasome in primary hepatocytes could be explained by the fact that the authors relied on the detection of mature IL-1β and IL-18. There are other studies that support that hepatocytes express and also activates the inflammasome complex, however do not secrete detectable amounts of IL-1β and IL-18 as compared to immune cells [124, 125]. This also suggests that the activation of inflammasome in epithelial cells might be performing cytokine independent functions. Negash et al. also showed that KCs were the major IL-1β-producing cell population during HCV infection and that the serum levels of IL-1β were significantly increased in patients with CHC [43]. They also showed that exposure of THP1 cells to HCV-induced IL-1β production and secretion via NLRP3 inflammasome pathway. All these events lead to enhanced proinflammatory cytokine and immune-regulatory gene expression [43]. In another study, Chen et al. reported that HCV-induced ROS production activated the NLRP3 inflammasome and subsequent IL-1β secretion [40]. Similarly, Shrivastava et al. also showed that the inflammatory cytokines IL-1β and IL-18 were produced through the activation of NF-κB pathway and induction of ROS. In THP-1 cells they observed that the production of these cytokines was through the NLRP3 inflammasome activation and caspase-1 cleavage [123]. Interestingly, caspase-1 activation has been shown to not only result in pro-inflammatory cytokine production but also regulation of many other cellular pathways. A study by Li et al. identified 40 genes regulated by caspase-1 in various tissues [126]. Previously, Grucel et al. showed caspase-1 induced activation of sterol regulatory element binding proteins (SREBP) in response to bacterial pore forming toxins. Thus, the contradicting results observed for the NLRP3 inflammasome activation in human hepatocytes cells and immune cells could be due to the possibility that activation of the NLRP3 inflammasome leads to regulation of other cellular genes or pathways other than production of pro-inflammatory cytokines. Therefore, the recent study from our lab has shown that HCV exploits the NLRP3 inflammasome to activate the SREBPs and host lipid metabolism for liver disease pathogenesis (**Figure 3**) [39]. In addition, IFN has been shown to inhibit NLRP3 inflammasome by blocking the caspase-1 dependent IL-1β maturation [127]. Thus therapeutically targeting NLRP3 inflammasome complex or IL-1β could provide better interventions in managing liver inflammation in CHC patients.

4. Therapeutic approaches to manage HCV-induced inflammation

HCV has been linked to several other diseases including the lymphoproliferative diseases [128], cardiovascular diseases [129], and atherosclerosis [130], and neuropsychiatric symptoms [131]. Since inflammation plays a key role in disease progression in chronic hepatitis C patients, a therapeutic method to anti-inflammatory approach would result in better management of the disease. Chen et al. have shown the beneficial effect of the aqueous extract of an edible seaweed *Gracilaria tenuistipitata* in inhibition of HCV replication by suppressing the Cox-2 protein and thus reducing inflammatory response [132]. Sorafenib is a chemotherapeutic agent that has been shown to inhibit the Raf/ERK pro-inflammatory and pro-fibrotic signaling pathways [133]. Similarly animal model have been used to show the effect of TNFα inhibitors on reduction of IL-6 and TGF-β [134], however the efficacy of such anti-inflammatory drugs will need extensive research owing to the risk of interference with the IFN therapy prescribed for HCV

Drugs	Disease	Role	Refs
Pre-existing treatments			
Sorafenib	Hepatocellular carcinoma	Inhibits Raf/ERK	[130]
Corticosteroids	Liver disorders	Anti-inflammatory	[138]
Cyclosporine	Autoimmune hepatitis	Calcineurin inhibitor, reduces cytokines, inhibits TGF-β and IL-4	[139]
Azathioprine	Autoimmune hepatitis	Anti-inflammatory	[140]
Budesonide	Autoimmune hepatitis	Anti-inflammatory synthetic corticosteroid	[141]
Tacrolimus	Autoimmune hepatitis	Calcineurin inhibitor	[142]
Emerging or possible treatments for liver inflammation			
Cenicriviroc	Non-alcoholic steatohepatitis (NASH) and liver fibrosis	Inhibits chemokine receptors CCR2/CCR5	[143]
Fresolimumab	Systemic sclerosis	Neutralizes TGF-β	[144]
Pioglitazone	Hepatic steatosis due to HIV/HCV infections	Acts as a PPARγ agonist, helps in reduction of ROS	[145]
Glycyrrhizin	Chronic hepatitis C and F2/F3 liver fibrosis	Anti-oxidant	[145]
Resveratrol	Non-alcoholic steatohepatitis (NASH)	Anti-oxidant	[146]
Humira	Certain arthritis such as rheumatoid and psoriatic	TNF-α blockers	[147]
Celecoxib	Pain and inflammation	Cox-2 inhibitor	[148]
Canakinumab	Acute and chronic non-infectious inflammatory diseases	IL-1β inhibitor	[135]
Pentoxifylline	Liver fibrosis, Non-alcoholic steatohepatitis (NASH), Primary biliary cirrhosis (PBC), Alcoholic liver disease	TNFα suppressing phosphodiesterase inhibitor	[136, 137]
Ursodeoxycholic acid	Primary biliary cirrhosis (PBC), Autoimmune hepatitis	Decreases TGF-β signaling and oxidative stress, TNF-α, IL-1α, IL-1β, and IL-6, IL-10 NF-κB	[149, 150]

Table 2. Pre-existing and emerging or possible treatments used against hepatic inflammation observed in various liver diseases.

mediated hepatitis. Microbial translocation in HCV infected resident KCs could also serve as a good platform to minimize the LPS-induced inflammasome response [135]. Dammacco et al. in their study showed that triple therapy with pegylated IFN-α, ribavirin, and rituximab (RTX) to patients with HCV-related cryoglobulinemia gave significantly better results than those who only got pegylated IFN-α and ribavirin [136]. Since IL-1β is directly involved in inflammatory response, and hence Canakinumab, a human monoclonal antibody that selectively inhibits IL-1β was shown to inhibit many inflammatory biomarkers [137].

Pentoxifylline (PTX) is a methylxanthine derivative with a variety of anti-inflammatory and antifibrotic effects, has been shown to be effective in liver diseases like the alcoholic liver disease [151], fibrosis/cirrhosis [152]. The drug also decreases the levels of TNF-α, IL-1, IL-6 and TGF-β which holds significant therapeutic potential [153]. There are few preexisting and possible emerging therapies against hepatic inflammation and liver disease available which are listed in **Table 2**.

5. Conclusions

Inflammation is a crucial part of human immune response that kicks into high gear during any tissue injury or invasion of harmful bacteria and viruses. When a cell dies, it stimulates a number of processes including the rapid recruitment of innate immune components from blood to generate an inflammatory response. This is a double-edged sword that in one hand protects and heals the injured tissues while on the other hand cause significant damage and disease progression. Both bacterial and viral infections have been well recognized as potent source of inflammation. Various studies have shown that these pathogens induce inflammation and in some cases the inflammation is continuous for several years ultimately contributing to cancer. With some oncogenic viruses, the unceasing inflammation significantly contributes to tumor formation. Growing evidences support the crucial role of HBV- and HCV-induced inflammatory responses in liver for both the reversal of disease as well as pathogenesis of hepatic and extrahepatic diseases. The persistent HCV infection leads to chronic inflammation which has been shown to be the primary cause of liver fibrosis and cancer. More importantly the epithelial cells mediate the progression from fibrotic to carcinogenic stage. It has been shown that during the chronic HCV infection, the hepatocytes show a transition from pSmad3C pathway, characteristics of mature epithelial cells, to JNK/pSmad3L pathway which favors the liver fibrosis and also increase the risk of cancer. Several studies have shown the roles of inflammatory mediator such as the IL-6, Cox-2, NF-κB and more recently the activation of inflammasomes, as major contributors in HCV pathogenesis. The HCV-induced inflammation still needs more studies to better elucidate the treatment options and to date, the novel therapeutic targets for inflammation, seems to be a good option for better management of disease, especially in non-responders to the standard antiviral treatment.

Acknowledgements

This work was supported by National Institutes of Health (NIH) grant DK106244 to Gulam Waris.

Author details

Binod Kumar, Akshaya Ramachandran and Gulam Waris*

*Address all correspondence to: gulam.waris@rosalindfranklin.edu

Department of Microbiology and Immunology, H.M. Bligh Cancer Research Laboratories, Chicago Medical School, Rosalind Franklin University of Medicine and Science, North Chicago, IL, USA

References

[1] Nathan C. Points of control in inflammation. Nature. 2002;**420**(6917):846-852

[2] Medzhitov R, Janeway Jr CA. Decoding the patterns of self and nonself by the innate immune system. Science. 2002;**296**(5566):298-300

[3] Janeway Jr CA, Medzhitov R. Innate immune recognition. Annual Review of Immunology. 2002;**20**:197-216

[4] Wilkins C, Gale Jr M. Recognition of viruses by cytoplasmic sensors. Current Opinion in Immunology. 2010;**22**(1):41-47

[5] Kawai T, Akira S. TLR signaling. Seminars in Immunology. 2007;**19**(1):24-32

[6] Kato H, Sato S, Yoneyama M, Yamamoto M, Uematsu S, Matsui K, et al. Cell type-specific involvement of RIG-I in antiviral response. Immunity. 2005;**23**(1):19-28

[7] Ting JP, Lovering RC, Alnemri ES, Bertin J, Boss JM, Davis BK, et al. The NLR gene family: A standard nomenclature. Immunity. 2008;**28**(3):285-287

[8] Roberts TL, Idris A, Dunn JA, Kelly GM, Burnton CM, Hodgson S, et al. HIN-200 proteins regulate caspase activation in response to foreign cytoplasmic DNA. Science. 2009;**323**(5917):1057-1060

[9] Pothlichet J, Meunier I, Davis BK, Ting JP, Skamene E, von Messling V, et al. Type I IFN triggers RIG-I/TLR3/NLRP3-dependent inflammasome activation in influenza A virus infected cells. PLoS Pathogens. 2013;**9**(4):e1003256

[10] Garlanda C, Dinarello CA, Mantovani A. The interleukin-1 family: Back to the future. Immunity. 2013;**39**(6):1003-1018

[11] Martinon F, Tschopp J. Inflammatory caspases and inflammasomes: Master switches of inflammation. Cell Death and Differentiation. 2007;**14**(1):10-22

[12] Martinon F, Burns K, Tschopp J. The inflammasome: A molecular platform triggering activation of inflammatory caspases and processing of proIL-beta. Molecular Cell. 2002;**10**(2):417-426

[13] Brodsky IE, Monack D. NLR-mediated control of inflammasome assembly in the host response against bacterial pathogens. Seminars in Immunology. 2009;21(4):199-207

[14] Rathinam VA, Jiang Z, Waggoner SN, Sharma S, Cole LE, Waggoner L, et al. The AIM2 inflammasome is essential for host defense against cytosolic bacteria and DNA viruses. Nature Immunology. 2010;11(5):395-402

[15] Burdette D, Haskett A, Presser L, McRae S, Iqbal J, Waris G. Hepatitis C virus activates interleukin-1beta via caspase-1-inflammasome complex. The Journal of General Virology. 2012;93(Pt 2):235-246

[16] Hornung V, Ablasser A, Charrel-Dennis M, Bauernfeind F, Horvath G, Caffrey DR, et al. AIM2 recognizes cytosolic dsDNA and forms a caspase-1-activating inflammasome with ASC. Nature. 2009;458(7237):514-518

[17] Reinholz M, Kawakami Y, Salzer S, Kreuter A, Dombrowski Y, Koglin S, et al. HPV16 activates the AIM2 inflammasome in keratinocytes. Archives of Dermatological Research. 2013;305(8):723-732

[18] Kuriakose T, Kanneganti TD. Regulation and functions of NLRP3 inflammasome during influenza virus infection. Molecular Immunology. 2017;86:56-64

[19] Poeck H, Bscheider M, Gross O, Finger K, Roth S, Rebsamen M, et al. Recognition of RNA virus by RIG-I results in activation of CARD9 and inflammasome signaling for interleukin 1 beta production. Nature Immunology. 2010;11(1):63-69

[20] Sun P, Fernandez S, Marovich MA, Palmer DR, Celluzzi CM, Boonnak K, et al. Functional characterization of ex vivo blood myeloid and plasmacytoid dendritic cells after infection with dengue virus. Virology. 2009;383(2):207-215

[21] Tsai YT, Chang SY, Lee CN, Kao CL. Human TLR3 recognizes dengue virus and modulates viral replication in vitro. Cellular Microbiology. 2009;11(4):604-615

[22] da Conceicao TM, Rust NM, Berbel AC, Martins NB, do Nascimento Santos CA, Da Poian AT, et al. Essential role of RIG-I in the activation of endothelial cells by dengue virus. Virology. 2013;435(2):281-292

[23] Nasirudeen AM, Wong HH, Thien P, Xu S, Lam KP, Liu DX. RIG-I, MDA5 and TLR3 synergistically play an important role in restriction of dengue virus infection. PLoS Neglected Tropical Diseases. 2011;5(1):e926

[24] Zhang L, Wang A. Virus-induced ER stress and the unfolded protein response. Frontiers in Plant Science. 2012;3:293

[25] Carroll TP, Greene CM, O'Connor CA, Nolan AM, O'Neill SJ, McElvaney NG. Evidence for unfolded protein response activation in monocytes from individuals with alpha-1 antitrypsin deficiency. Journal of Immunology. 2010;184(8):4538-4546

[26] Eizirik DL, Miani M, Cardozo AK. Signalling danger: Endoplasmic reticulum stress and the unfolded protein response in pancreatic islet inflammation. Diabetologia. 2013;56(2):234-241

[27] Smith JA. A new paradigm: Innate immune sensing of viruses via the unfolded protein response. Frontiers in Microbiology. 2014;**5**:222

[28] Schreck R, Rieber P, Baeuerle PA. Reactive oxygen intermediates as apparently widely used messengers in the activation of the NF-kappa B transcription factor and HIV-1. The EMBO Journal. 1991;**10**(8):2247-2258

[29] Wang G, Zhang J, Li W, Xin G, Su Y, Gao Y, et al. Apoptosis and proinflammatory cytokine responses of primary mouse microglia and astrocytes induced by human H1N1 and avian H5N1 influenza viruses. Cellular & Molecular Immunology. 2008;**5**(2):113-120

[30] Wang G, Li R, Jiang Z, Gu L, Chen Y, Dai J, et al. Influenza virus induces inflammatory response in mouse primary cortical neurons with limited viral replication. BioMed Research International. 2016;**2016**:8076989

[31] Eliopoulos AG, Stack M, Dawson CW, Kaye KM, Hodgkin L, Sihota S, et al. Epstein-Barr virus-encoded LMP1 and CD40 mediate IL-6 production in epithelial cells via an NF-kappaB pathway involving TNF receptor-associated factors. Oncogene. 1997;**14**(24):2899-2916

[32] Mosialos G, Birkenbach M, Yalamanchili R, VanArsdale T, Ware C, Kieff E. The Epstein-Barr virus transforming protein LMP1 engages signaling proteins for the tumor necrosis factor receptor family. Cell. 1995;**80**(3):389-399

[33] Maggio E, van den Berg A, Diepstra A, Kluiver J, Visser L, Poppema S. Chemokines, cytokines and their receptors in Hodgkin's lymphoma cell lines and tissues. Annals of Oncology. 2002;**13**(Suppl 1):52-56

[34] Punj V, Matta H, Schamus S, Yang T, Chang Y, Chaudhary PM. Induction of CCL20 production by Kaposi sarcoma-associated herpesvirus: Role of viral FLICE inhibitory protein K13-induced NF-kappaB activation. Blood. 2009;**113**(22):5660-5668

[35] Ensoli B, Sturzl M. Kaposi's sarcoma: A result of the interplay among inflammatory cytokines, angiogenic factors and viral agents. Cytokine & Growth Factor Reviews. 1998;**9**(1):63-83

[36] Falasca K, Ucciferri C, Dalessandro M, Zingariello P, Mancino P, Petrarca C, et al. Cytokine patterns correlate with liver damage in patients with chronic hepatitis B and C. Annals of Clinical and Laboratory Science. 2006;**36**(2):144-150

[37] Shukla R, Yue J, Siouda M, Gheit T, Hantz O, Merle P, et al. Proinflammatory cytokine TNF-alpha increases the stability of hepatitis B virus X protein through NF-kappaB signaling. Carcinogenesis. 2011;**32**(7):978-985

[38] Allen IC, Scull MA, Moore CB, Holl EK, McElvania-TeKippe E, Taxman DJ, et al. The NLRP3 inflammasome mediates in vivo innate immunity to influenza A virus through recognition of viral RNA. Immunity. 2009;**30**(4):556-565

[39] McRae S, Iqbal J, Sarkar-Dutta M, Lane S, Nagaraj A, Ali N, et al. The hepatitis C virus-induced NLRP3 inflammasome activates the sterol regulatory element-binding protein

(SREBP) and regulates lipid metabolism. The Journal of Biological Chemistry. 2016; **291**(7):3254-3267

[40] Chen W, Xu Y, Li H, Tao W, Xiang Y, Huang B, et al. HCV genomic RNA activates the NLRP3 inflammasome in human myeloid cells. PLoS One. 2014;**9**(1):e84953

[41] Rajan JV, Rodriguez D, Miao EA, Aderem A. The NLRP3 inflammasome detects encephalomyocarditis virus and vesicular stomatitis virus infection. Journal of Virology. 2011; **85**(9):4167-4172

[42] Lawrence TM, Hudacek AW, de Zoete MR, Flavell RA, Schnell MJ. Rabies virus is recognized by the NLRP3 inflammasome and activates interleukin-1beta release in murine dendritic cells. Journal of Virology 2013;**87**(10):5848-5857

[43] Negash AA, Ramos HJ, Crochet N, Lau DT, Doehle B, Papic N, et al. IL-1beta production through the NLRP3 inflammasome by hepatic macrophages links hepatitis C virus infection with liver inflammation and disease. PLoS Pathogens. 2013;**9**(4):e1003330

[44] Wu DL, Xu GH, Lu SM, Ma BL, Miao NZ, Liu XB, et al. Correlation of AIM2 expression in peripheral blood mononuclear cells from humans with acute and chronic hepatitis B. Human Immunology. 2013;**74**(5):514-521

[45] Saito T, Owen DM, Jiang F, Marcotrigiano J, Gale Jr M. Innate immunity induced by composition-dependent RIG-I recognition of hepatitis C virus RNA. Nature. 2008; **454**(7203):523-527

[46] Loo YM, Fornek J, Crochet N, Bajwa G, Perwitasari O, Martinez-Sobrido L, et al. Distinct RIG-I and MDA5 signaling by RNA viruses in innate immunity. Journal of Virology. 2008;**82**(1):335-345

[47] Ansari MA, Singh VV, Dutta S, Veettil MV, Dutta D, Chikoti L, et al. Constitutive interferon-inducible protein 16-inflammasome activation during Epstein-Barr virus latency I, II, and III in B and epithelial cells. Journal of Virology. 2013;**87**(15):8606-8623

[48] Ansari MA, Dutta S, Veettil MV, Dutta D, Iqbal J, Kumar B, et al. Herpesvirus genome recognition induced acetylation of nuclear IFI16 Is essential for its cytoplasmic translocation, inflammasome and IFN-beta responses. PLoS Pathogens. 2015;**11**(7):e1005019

[49] Johnson KE, Chikoti L, Chandran B. Herpes simplex virus 1 infection induces activation and subsequent inhibition of the IFI16 and NLRP3 inflammasomes. Journal of Virology. 2013;**87**(9):5005-5018

[50] Kufer TA, Fritz JH, Philpott DJ. NACHT-LRR proteins (NLRs) in bacterial infection and immunity. Trends in Microbiology. 2005;**13**(8):381-388

[51] He Y, Hara H, Nunez G. Mechanism and regulation of NLRP3 inflammasome activation. Trends in Biochemical Sciences. 2016;**41**(12):1012-1021

[52] Hornung V, Bauernfeind F, Halle A, Samstad EO, Kono H, Rock KL, et al. Silica crystals and aluminum salts activate the NALP3 inflammasome through phagosomal destabilization. Nature Immunology. 2008;**9**(8):847-856

[53] Cruz CM, Rinna A, Forman HJ, Ventura AL, Persechini PM, Ojcius DM. ATP activates a reactive oxygen species-dependent oxidative stress response and secretion of proinflammatory cytokines in macrophages. The Journal of Biological Chemistry. 2007;**282**(5):2871-2879

[54] Ichinohe T, Pang IK, Iwasaki A. Influenza virus activates inflammasomes via its intracellular M2 ion channel. Nature Immunology. 2010;**11**(5):404-410

[55] Kaushik DK, Gupta M, Kumawat KL, Basu A. NLRP3 inflammasome: Key mediator of neuroinflammation in murine Japanese encephalitis. PLoS One. 2012;**7**(2):e32270

[56] Ermler ME, Traylor Z, Patel K, Schattgen SA, Vanaja SK, Fitzgerald KA, et al. Rift Valley fever virus infection induces activation of the NLRP3 inflammasome. Virology. 2014;**449**:174-180

[57] Muruve DA, Petrilli V, Zaiss AK, White LR, Clark SA, Ross PJ, et al. The inflammasome recognizes cytosolic microbial and host DNA and triggers an innate immune response. Nature. 2008;**452**(7183):103-107

[58] Nour AM, Reichelt M, Ku CC, Ho MY, Heineman TC, Arvin AM. Varicella-zoster virus infection triggers formation of an interleukin-1beta (IL-1beta)-processing inflammasome complex. The Journal of Biological Chemistry. 2011;**286**(20):17921-17933

[59] Askari A, Nosratabadi R, Khaleghinia M, Zainodini N, Kennedy D, Shabani Z, et al. Evaluation of NLRC4, NLRP1, and NLRP3, as components of inflammasomes, in chronic hepatitis B virus-infected patients. Viral Immunology. 2016;**29**(9):496-501

[60] Yu X, Lan P, Hou X, Han Q, Lu N, Li T, et al. HBV inhibits LPS-induced NLRP3 inflammasome activation and IL-1beta production via suppressing the NF-kappaB pathway and ROS production. Journal of Hepatology. 2017;**66**(4):693-702

[61] Kolakofsky D, Kowalinski E, Cusack S. A structure-based model of RIG-I activation. RNA. 2012;**18**(12):2118-2127

[62] Yoneyama M, Kikuchi M, Natsukawa T, Shinobu N, Imaizumi T, Miyagishi M, et al. The RNA helicase RIG-I has an essential function in double-stranded RNA-induced innate antiviral responses. Nature Immunology. 2004;**5**(7):730-737

[63] Fernandes-Alnemri T, Yu JW, Juliana C, Solorzano L, Kang S, Wu J, et al. The AIM2 inflammasome is critical for innate immunity to *Francisella tularensis*. Nature Immunology. 2010;**11**(5):385-393

[64] Pan X, Xu H, Zheng C, Li M, Zou X, Cao H, et al. Human hepatocytes express absent in melanoma 2 and respond to hepatitis B virus with interleukin-18 expression. Virus Genes. 2016;**52**(4):445-452

[65] Choubey D. Interferon-inducible Ifi200-family genes as modifiers of lupus susceptibility. Immunology Letters. 2012;**147**(1-2):10-17

[66] Uchida K, Akita Y, Matsuo K, Fujiwara S, Nakagawa A, Kazaoka Y, et al. Identification of specific autoantigens in Sjogren's syndrome by SEREX. Immunology. 2005;**116**(1):53-63

[67] Mondini M, Vidali M, Airo P, De Andrea M, Riboldi P, Meroni PL, et al. Role of the interferon-inducible gene IFI16 in the etiopathogenesis of systemic autoimmune disorders. Annals of the New York Academy of Sciences. 2007;**1110**:47-56

[68] Kerur N, Veettil MV, Sharma-Walia N, Bottero V, Sadagopan S, Otageri P, et al. IFI16 acts as a nuclear pathogen sensor to induce the inflammasome in response to Kaposi Sarcoma-associated herpesvirus infection. Cell Host & Microbe. 2011;**9**(5):363-375

[69] Dutta D, Dutta S, Veettil MV, Roy A, Ansari MA, Iqbal J, et al. BRCA1 regulates IFI16 mediated nuclear innate sensing of herpes viral DNA and subsequent induction of the innate inflammasome and interferon-beta responses. PLoS Pathogens. 2015;**11**(6):e1005030

[70] Wang J, Alexander J, Wiebe M, Jones C. Bovine herpesvirus 1 productive infection stimulates inflammasome formation and caspase 1 activity. Virus Research. 2014;**185**:72-76

[71] Chevaliez S, Pawlotsky JM. HCV genome and life cycle. In: Tan SL, editor. Hepatitis C Viruses: Genomes and Molecular Biology. Norfolk (UK): Horizon Bioscience; 2006

[72] MacCallum PR, Jack SC, Egan PA, McDermott BT, Elliott RM, Chan SW. Cap-dependent and hepatitis C virus internal ribosome entry site-mediated translation are modulated by phosphorylation of eIF2alpha under oxidative stress. The Journal of General Virology. 2006;**87**(Pt 11):3251-3262

[73] Jaafar ZA, Oguro A, Nakamura Y, Kieft JS. Translation initiation by the hepatitis C virus IRES requires eIF1A and ribosomal complex remodeling. eLife. 2016;**5**:e21198

[74] Bradrick SS, Walters RW, Gromeier M. The hepatitis C virus 3'-untranslated region or a poly(A) tract promote efficient translation subsequent to the initiation phase. Nucleic Acids Research. 2006;**34**(4):1293-1303

[75] Appel N, Schaller T, Penin F, Bartenschlager R. From structure to function: New insights into hepatitis C virus RNA replication. The Journal of Biological Chemistry. 2006;**281**(15):9833-9836

[76] Pradere JP, Kluwe J, De Minicis S, Jiao JJ, Gwak GY, Dapito DH, et al. Hepatic macrophages but not dendritic cells contribute to liver fibrosis by promoting the survival of activated hepatic stellate cells in mice. Hepatology. 2013;**58**(4):1461-1473

[77] Tanaka H, Fujita N, Sugimoto R, Urawa N, Horiike S, Kobayashi Y, et al. Hepatic oxidative DNA damage is associated with increased risk for hepatocellular carcinoma in chronic hepatitis C. British Journal of Cancer. 2008;**98**(3):580-586

[78] Di Bisceglie AM. Natural history of hepatitis C: Its impact on clinical management. Hepatology. 2000;**31**(4):1014-1018

[79] Nunez O, Fernandez-Martinez A, Majano PL, Apolinario A, Gomez-Gonzalo M, Benedicto I, et al. Increased intrahepatic cyclooxygenase 2, matrix metalloproteinase 2, and matrix metalloproteinase 9 expression is associated with progressive liver disease in chronic hepatitis C virus infection: Role of viral core and NS5A proteins. Gut. 2004;**53**(11):1665-1672

[80] Huang YS, Hwang SJ, Chan CY, Wu JC, Chao Y, Chang FY, et al. Serum levels of cytokines in hepatitis C-related liver disease: A longitudinal study. Zhonghua Yi Xue Za Zhi (Taipei). 1999;**62**(6):327-333

[81] Matsuzaki K. Modulation of TGF-beta signaling during progression of chronic liver diseases. Frontiers in Bioscience (Landmark Ed). 2009;(14):2923-2934

[82] Okumoto K, Hattori E, Tamura K, Kiso S, Watanabe H, Saito K, et al. Possible contribution of circulating transforming growth factor-beta 1 to immunity and prognosis in unresectable hepatocellular carcinoma. Liver International. 2004;**24**(1):21-28

[83] Teicher BA. Malignant cells, directors of the malignant process: Role of transforming growth factor-beta. Cancer Metastasis Reviews. 2001;**20**(1-2):133-143

[84] Gong G, Waris G, Tanveer R, Siddiqui A. Human hepatitis C virus NS5A protein alters intracellular calcium levels, induces oxidative stress, and activates STAT-3 and NF-kappa B. Proceedings of the National Academy of Sciences of the United States of America. 2001;**98**(17):9599-9604

[85] Qadri I, Iwahashi M, Capasso JM, Hopken MW, Flores S, Schaack J, et al. Induced oxidative stress and activated expression of manganese superoxide dismutase during hepatitis C virus replication: Role of JNK, p38 MAPK and AP-1. Biochemical Journal. 2004;**378**(Pt 3):919-928

[86] Moriya K, Fujie H, Shintani Y, Yotsuyanagi H, Tsutsumi T, Ishibashi K, et al. The core protein of hepatitis C virus induces hepatocellular carcinoma in transgenic mice. Nature Medicine. 1998;**4**(9):1065-1067

[87] Okuda M, Li K, Beard MR, Showalter LA, Scholle F, Lemon SM, et al. Mitochondrial injury, oxidative stress, and antioxidant gene expression are induced by hepatitis C virus core protein. Gastroenterology. 2002;**122**(2):366-375

[88] Gotoh M, Sakamoto M, Kanetaka K, Chuuma M, Hirohashi S. Overexpression of osteopontin in hepatocellular carcinoma. Pathology International. 2002;**52**(1):19-24

[89] Patouraux S, Bonnafous S, Voican CS, Anty R, Saint-Paul MC, Rosenthal-Allieri MA, et al. The osteopontin level in liver, adipose tissue and serum is correlated with fibrosis in patients with alcoholic liver disease. PLoS One. 2012;**7**(4):e35612

[90] Iqbal J, McRae S, Banaudha K, Mai T, Waris G. Mechanism of hepatitis C virus (HCV)-induced osteopontin and its role in epithelial to mesenchymal transition of hepatocytes. The Journal of Biological Chemistry. 2013;**288**(52):36994-37009

[91] Iqbal J, McRae S, Mai T, Banaudha K, Sarkar-Dutta M, Waris G. Role of hepatitis C virus induced osteopontin in epithelial to mesenchymal transition, migration and invasion of hepatocytes. PLoS One. 2014;**9**(1):e87464

[92] Basu A, Meyer K, Lai KK, Saito K, Di Bisceglie AM, Grosso LE, et al. Microarray analyses and molecular profiling of Stat3 signaling pathway induced by hepatitis C virus core protein in human hepatocytes. Virology. 2006;**349**(2):347-358

[93] Nishitsuji H, Funami K, Shimizu Y, Ujino S, Sugiyama K, Seya T, et al. Hepatitis C virus infection induces inflammatory cytokines and chemokines mediated by the cross talk between hepatocytes and stellate cells. Journal of Virology. 2013;**87**(14):8169-8178

[94] Hosomura N, Kono H, Tsuchiya M, Ishii K, Ogiku M, Matsuda M, et al. HCV-related proteins activate Kupffer cells isolated from human liver tissues. Digestive Diseases and Sciences. 2011;**56**(4):1057-1064

[95] Polyak SJ, Khabar KS, Rezeiq M, Gretch DR. Elevated levels of interleukin-8 in serum are associated with hepatitis C virus infection and resistance to interferon therapy. Journal of Virology. 2001;**75**(13):6209-6211

[96] Li K, Foy E, Ferreon JC, Nakamura M, Ferreon AC, Ikeda M, et al. Immune evasion by hepatitis C virus NS3/4A protease-mediated cleavage of the Toll-like receptor 3 adaptor protein TRIF. Proceedings of the National Academy of Sciences of the United States of America. 2005;**102**(8):2992-2997

[97] Spanakis NE, Garinis GA, Alexopoulos EC, Patrinos GP, Menounos PG, Sklavounou A, et al. Cytokine serum levels in patients with chronic HCV infection. Journal of Clinical Laboratory Analysis. 2002;**16**(1):40-46

[98] Ramadori G, Saile B. Inflammation, damage repair, immune cells, and liver fibrosis: Specific or nonspecific, this is the question. Gastroenterology. 2004;**127**(3):997-1000

[99] Antonelli A, Ferri C, Ferrari SM, Ghiri E, Goglia F, Pampana A, et al. Serum levels of proinflammatory cytokines interleukin-1beta, interleukin-6, and tumor necrosis factor alpha in mixed cryoglobulinemia. Arthritis and Rheumatism. 2009;**60**(12):3841-3847

[100] Basha HI, Subramanian V, Seetharam A, Nath DS, Ramachandran S, Anderson CD, et al. Characterization of HCV-specific CD4+Th17 immunity in recurrent hepatitis C-induced liver allograft fibrosis. American Journal of Transplantation. 2011;**11**(4):775-785

[101] Kasprzak A, Zabel M, Biczysko W, Wysocki J, Adamek A, Spachacz R, et al. Expression of cytokines (TNF-alpha, IL-1alpha, and IL-2) in chronic hepatitis C: Comparative hybridocytochemical and immunocytochemical study in children and adult patients. The Journal of Histochemistry and Cytochemistry. 2004;**52**(1):29-38

[102] Moschen AR, Fritz T, Clouston AD, Rebhan I, Bauhofer O, Barrie HD, et al. Interleukin-32: A new proinflammatory cytokine involved in hepatitis C virus-related liver inflammation and fibrosis. Hepatology. 2011;**53**(6):1819-1829

[103] Knolle PA, Gerken G. Local control of the immune response in the liver. Immunological Reviews. 2000;**174**:21-34

[104] Waris G, Siddiqui A. Hepatitis C virus stimulates the expression of cyclooxygenase-2 via oxidative stress: Role of prostaglandin E2 in RNA replication. Journal of Virology. 2005;**79**(15):9725-9734

[105] Choi J, Lee KJ, Zheng Y, Yamaga AK, Lai MM, Ou JH. Reactive oxygen species suppress hepatitis C virus RNA replication in human hepatoma cells. Hepatology. 2004;**39**(1):81-89

[106] Bowman T, Garcia R, Turkson J, Jove R. STATs in oncogenesis. Oncogene. 2000;**19**(21): 2474-2488

[107] Waris G, Turkson J, Hassanein T, Siddiqui A. Hepatitis C virus (HCV) constitutively activates STAT-3 via oxidative stress: Role of STAT-3 in HCV replication. Journal of Virology. 2005;**79**(3):1569-1580

[108] Poli G. Pathogenesis of liver fibrosis: Role of oxidative stress. Molecular Aspects of Medicine. 2000;**21**(3):49-98

[109] Vidali M, Tripodi MF, Ivaldi A, Zampino R, Occhino G, Restivo L, et al. Interplay between oxidative stress and hepatic steatosis in the progression of chronic hepatitis C. Journal of Hepatology. 2008;**48**(3):399-406

[110] Presser LD, McRae S, Waris G. Activation of TGF-beta1 promoter by hepatitis C virus-induced AP-1 and Sp1: Role of TGF-beta1 in hepatic stellate cell activation and invasion. PLoS One. 2013;**8**(2):e56367

[111] Szabo G, Chang S, Dolganiuc A. Altered innate immunity in chronic hepatitis C infection: Cause or effect? Hepatology. 2007;**46**(4):1279-1290

[112] Wang Y, Li J, Wang X, Ye L, Zhou Y, Thomas RM, et al. Hepatitis C virus impairs TLR3 signaling and inhibits IFN-lambda 1 expression in human hepatoma cell line. Innate Immunity. 2014;**20**(1):3-11

[113] Wang N, Liang Y, Devaraj S, Wang J, Lemon SM, Li K. Toll-like receptor 3 mediates establishment of an antiviral state against hepatitis C virus in hepatoma cells. Journal of Virology. 2009;**83**(19):9824-9834

[114] Loo YM, Owen DM, Li K, Erickson AK, Johnson CL, Fish PM, et al. Viral and therapeutic control of IFN-beta promoter stimulator 1 during hepatitis C virus infection. Proceedings of the National Academy of Sciences of the United States of America. 2006; **103**(15):6001-6006

[115] Saito T, Hirai R, Loo YM, Owen D, Johnson CL, Sinha SC, et al. Regulation of innate antiviral defenses through a shared repressor domain in RIG-I and LGP2. Proceedings of the National Academy of Sciences of the United States of America. 2007;**104**(2):582-587

[116] Liu HM, Loo YM, Horner SM, Zornetzer GA, Katze MG, Gale Jr M. The mitochondrial targeting chaperone 14-3-3epsilon regulates a RIG-I translocon that mediates membrane association and innate antiviral immunity. Cell Host & Microbe. 2012;**11**(5):528-537

[117] Loo YM, Gale Jr M. Immune signaling by RIG-I-like receptors. Immunity. 2011;**34**(5): 680-692

[118] Gack MU, Shin YC, Joo CH, Urano T, Liang C, Sun L, et al. TRIM25 RING-finger E3 ubiquitin ligase is essential for RIG-I-mediated antiviral activity. Nature. 2007; **446**(7138):916-920

[119] Baril M, Racine ME, Penin F, Lamarre D. MAVS dimer is a crucial signaling component of innate immunity and the target of hepatitis C virus NS3/4A protease. Journal of Virology. 2009;**83**(3):1299-1311

[120] Horner SM, Liu HM, Park HS, Briley J, Gale Jr M. Mitochondrial-associated endoplasmic reticulum membranes (MAM) form innate immune synapses and are targeted by hepatitis C virus. Proceedings of the National Academy of Sciences of the United States of America. 2011;**108**(35):14590-14595

[121] Csak T, Ganz M, Pespisa J, Kodys K, Dolganiuc A, Szabo G. Fatty acid and endotoxin activate inflammasomes in mouse hepatocytes that release danger signals to stimulate immune cells. Hepatology. 2011;**54**(1):133-144

[122] Boaru SG, Borkham-Kamphorst E, Tihaa L, Haas U, Weiskirchen R. Expression analysis of inflammasomes in experimental models of inflammatory and fibrotic liver disease. Journal of Inflammation (Lond). 2012;**9**(1):49

[123] Shrivastava S, Mukherjee A, Ray R, Ray RB. Hepatitis C virus induces interleukin-1beta (IL-1beta)/IL-18 in circulatory and resident liver macrophages. Journal of Virology. 2013;**87**(22):12284-12290

[124] Sun Q, Gao W, Loughran P, Shapiro R, Fan J, Billiar TR, et al. Caspase 1 activation is protective against hepatocyte cell death by up-regulating beclin 1 protein and mitochondrial autophagy in the setting of redox stress. The Journal of Biological Chemistry. 2013;**288**(22):15947-15958

[125] Taxman DJ, Holley-Guthrie EA, Huang MT, Moore CB, Bergstralh DT, Allen IC, et al. The NLR adaptor ASC/PYCARD regulates DUSP10, mitogen-activated protein kinase (MAPK), and chemokine induction independent of the inflammasome. The Journal of Biological Chemistry. 2011;**286**(22):19605-19616

[126] Li YF, Nanayakkara G, Sun Y, Li X, Wang L, Cueto R, et al. Analyses of caspase-1-regulated transcriptomes in various tissues lead to identification of novel IL-1beta-, IL-18- and sirtuin-1-independent pathways. Journal of Hematology & Oncology. 2017;**10**(1):40

[127] Guarda G, Braun M, Staehli F, Tardivel A, Mattmann C, Forster I, et al. Type I interferon inhibits interleukin-1 production and inflammasome activation. Immunity. 2011;**34**(2):213-223

[128] Marcucci F, Mele A. Hepatitis viruses and non-Hodgkin lymphoma: Epidemiology, mechanisms of tumorigenesis, and therapeutic opportunities. Blood. 2011;**117**(6):1792-1798

[129] Ishizaka N, Ishizaka Y, Takahashi E, Tooda E, Hashimoto H, Nagai R, et al. Association between hepatitis C virus seropositivity, carotid-artery plaque, and intima-media thickening. Lancet. 2002;**359**(9301):133-135

[130] Adinolfi LE, Restivo L, Zampino R, Guerrera B, Lonardo A, Ruggiero L, et al. Chronic HCV infection is a risk of atherosclerosis. Role of HCV and HCV-related steatosis. Atherosclerosis. 2012;**221**(2):496-502

[131] Tillmann HL. Hepatitis C virus infection and the brain. Metabolic Brain Disease. 2004;**19**(3-4):351-356

[132] Chen KJ, Tseng CK, Chang FR, Yang JI, Yeh CC, Chen WC, et al. Aqueous extract of the edible Gracilaria tenuistipitata inhibits hepatitis C viral replication via cyclooxygenase-2 suppression and reduces virus-induced inflammation. PLoS One. 2013;**8**(2):e57704

[133] Wang Y, Gao J, Zhang D, Zhang J, Ma J, Jiang H. New insights into the antifibrotic effects of sorafenib on hepatic stellate cells and liver fibrosis. Journal of Hepatology. 2010;**53**(1):132-144

[134] Cohen-Naftaly M, Friedman SL. Current status of novel antifibrotic therapies in patients with chronic liver disease. Therapeutic Advances in Gastroenterology. 2011;**4**(6):391-417

[135] Sandler NG, Koh C, Roque A, Eccleston JL, Siegel RB, Demino M, et al. Host response to translocated microbial products predicts outcomes of patients with HBV or HCV infection. Gastroenterology. 2011;**141**(4):1220-1230. (e1-e3)

[136] Dammacco F, Tucci FA, Lauletta G, Gatti P, De Re V, Conteduca V, et al. Pegylated interferon-alpha, ribavirin, and rituximab combined therapy of hepatitis C virus-related mixed cryoglobulinemia: A long-term study. Blood. 2010;**116**(3):343-353

[137] Dinarello CA. A clinical perspective of IL-1beta as the gatekeeper of inflammation. European Journal of Immunology. 2011;**41**(5):1203-1217

[138] Uribe M, Go VL. Corticosteroid pharmacokinetics in liver disease. Clinical Pharmacokinetics. 1979;**4**(3):233-240

[139] Malekzadeh R, Nasseri-Moghaddam S, Kaviani MJ, Taheri H, Kamalian N, Sotoudeh M. Cyclosporin A is a promising alternative to corticosteroids in autoimmune hepatitis. Digestive Diseases and Sciences. 2001;**46**(6):1321-1327

[140] Johnson PJ, McFarlane IG, Williams R. Azathioprine for long-term maintenance of remission in autoimmune hepatitis. The New England Journal of Medicine. 1995; **333**(15):958-963

[141] Manns MP, Woynarowski M, Kreisel W, Lurie Y, Rust C, Zuckerman E, et al. Budesonide induces remission more effectively than prednisone in a controlled trial of patients with autoimmune hepatitis. Gastroenterology. 2010;**139**(4):1198-1206

[142] Larsen FS, Vainer B, Eefsen M, Bjerring PN, Adel Hansen B. Low-dose tacrolimus ameliorates liver inflammation and fibrosis in steroid refractory autoimmune hepatitis. World Journal of Gastroenterology. 2007;**13**(23):3232-3236

[143] Tacke F. Cenicriviroc for the treatment of non-alcoholic steatohepatitis and liver fibrosis. Expert Opinion on Investigational Drugs. 2018;**27**(3):301-311

[144] Rice LM, Padilla CM, McLaughlin SR, Mathes A, Ziemek J, Goummih S, et al. Fresolimumab treatment decreases biomarkers and improves clinical symptoms in systemic sclerosis patients. The Journal of Clinical Investigation. 2015;**125**(7):2795-2807

[145] Bansal R, Nagorniewicz B, Prakash J. Clinical advancements in the targeted therapies against liver fibrosis. Mediators of Inflammation. 2016;**2016**:7629724

[146] Kessoku T, Imajo K, Honda Y, Kato T, Ogawa Y, Tomeno W, et al. Resveratrol ameliorates fibrosis and inflammation in a mouse model of nonalcoholic steatohepatitis. Scientific Reports. 2016;**6**:22251

[147] Burmester GR, Panaccione R, Gordon KB, McIlraith MJ, Lacerda AP. Adalimumab: Long-term safety in 23 458 patients from global clinical trials in rheumatoid arthritis,

juvenile idiopathic arthritis, ankylosing spondylitis, psoriatic arthritis, psoriasis and Crohn's disease. Annals of the Rheumatic Diseases. 2013;**72**(4):517-524

[148] Tindall E. Celecoxib for the treatment of pain and inflammation: The preclinical and clinical results. The Journal of the American Osteopathic Association. 1999;**99** (11_suppl):S13-SS7

[149] Ko WK, Lee SH, Kim SJ, Jo MJ, Kumar H, Han IB, et al. Anti-inflammatory effects of ursodeoxycholic acid by lipopolysaccharide-stimulated inflammatory responses in RAW 264.7 macrophages. PLoS One. 2017;**12**(6):e0180673

[150] Liang TJ, Yuan JH, Tan YR, Ren WH, Han GQ, Zhang J, et al. Effect of ursodeoxycholic acid on TGF beta1/Smad signaling pathway in rat hepatic stellate cells. Chinese Medical Journal. 2009;**122**(10):1209-1213

[151] Hernandez E, Correa A, Bucio L, Souza V, Kershenobich D, Gutierrez-Ruiz MC. Pentoxifylline diminished acetaldehyde-induced collagen production in hepatic stellate cells by decreasing interleukin-6 expression. Pharmacological Research. 2002; **46**(5):435-443

[152] Austin AS, Mahida YR, Clarke D, Ryder SD, Freeman JG. A pilot study to investigate the use of oxpentifylline (pentoxifylline) and thalidomide in portal hypertension secondary to alcoholic cirrhosis. Alimentary Pharmacology & Therapeutics. 2004;**19**(1):79-88

[153] Raetsch C, Jia JD, Boigk G, Bauer M, Hahn EG, Riecken EO, et al. Pentoxifylline downregulates profibrogenic cytokines and procollagen I expression in rat secondary biliary fibrosis. Gut. 2002;**50**(2):241-247

6

HCV and Work Ability Assessment

Milan Milošević, Jelena Jakab, Lucija Kuna and
Martina Smolić

Abstract

Modifications to work and work ability assessment are required to prevent occupational transmission of hepatitis C virus (HCV). This is usually required in the health care setting, where exposure-prone procedures (EPPs) should not be carried out by infectious carriers of HCV. The risk of an individual surgeon acquiring HCV has been estimated at 0.001–0.032% per annum. Even in an area with a high prevalence of HCV among its population, the risk of acquiring HCV through occupational exposure is low. Rates of viral clearance with treatment of acute HCV infection are considerably higher than treatment of chronic HCV infection. Consequently, it is imperative that health care workers follow universal precautions and promptly report all exposures to blood or body fluid exposures according to their local policy. Health care workers who embark on, or transfer to, a career that requires EPP (exposure-prone procedures and dialysis work) should be assessed to ensure that they are free from infection with HCV. If the HCV antibodies are positive, the health care worker should be tested for HCV RNA PCR. If the HCV RNA PCR is negative on two separate occasions, the health care worker may be permitted to perform EPPs. If the HCV RNA PCR is positive, the health care worker should not be allowed to perform EPPs. Health care workers who already perform EPPs and who believe they may have been exposed to HCV infection should be advised to seek advice from their occupational health department for confidential advice on whether they should be tested.

Keywords: HCV, work ability assessment, fitness for work

1. Introduction

Work ability assessment or fitness to work refers to the process of ensuring that an employee can complete a task safely without presenting a risk to themselves, their colleagues, the company, or a third party. This term also refers to the impact of sickness and absence of employees in order to assess the possibility of having an employee return to work quickly and safely.

Work ability assessments are most often performed to determine medical fitness after an illness or injury, sometimes at the request of an employer after an offer of employment or as a condition of a job transfer.

Fitness to work assesses the capacity of an individual to perform physical and psychological work tasks according to the demands of the job. This demand may be directly associated with a task (e.g., carrying loads) or may be associated with a location that will impact the individual's health. Therefore, fitness to work addresses both the task and the location of the work to be done.

Reduced work productivity (WP) is a measure of the impact of illness and treatment burden in patients diagnosed with chronic diseases [1]. Patient's WP in the setting of a chronic condition presents a complex phenomenon that cannot be understood only by obtaining patient's clinical information. It is also important to collect patient-reported outcomes, especially ones that capture patients' energy and physical components. Hepatitis C (HCV) infection has a considerable negative impact on patient-reported outcomes (PRO) and patients' WP [2]. Numerous manifestations of HCV lead to an economic burden related to the complications and extrahepatic manifestation, thus decreasing WP [3]. For that reason, it is important to collect information that can help caregivers to develop a plan for maintaining patients' employment. Targeting important aspects of PROs has a substantial positive impact on patients' well-being as well as their WP, which results in notable economic benefits for the whole society [4].

2. Impact of HCV infection on work ability and productivity

Chronic HCV is a global health problem affecting 130–170 million people worldwide (80% of patients with acute HCV infections will develop chronic HCV). Every year, 3–4 million people are infected, and approximately 9 million patients have HCV infection in Europe, with greater prevalence in the southern and eastern European regions [5]. Around 2.7–4.1 million people have chronic HCV (HCV) in the United States. While frequently believed of as an asymptomatic disease, numerous studies have shown that those with chronic HCV experience increased work impairment revealed as decreased WP and increased absenteeism and presenteeism (attending work while being impaired) [6]. Risk factors identified included blood transfusion, injection drug use, employment in patient care or clinical laboratory work, exposure to a sex partner or household member who has had a history of hepatitis, exposure to multiple sex partners, and low socioeconomic level. These studies reported no association with military service or exposures resulting from medical, surgical, or dental procedures, tattooing, acupuncture, ear piercing, or foreign travel. If transmission from such exposures does occur, the frequency might be too low to detect [7].

Working in the health care, emergency medical (e.g., emergency medical technicians and paramedics), and public safety sectors (e.g., fire-service, law-enforcement, and correctional facility personnel) who have exposure to blood in the workplace are at high risk for being infected with bloodborne pathogens. Nevertheless, occurrence of HCV infection among health-care workers, including surgeons, is no greater than the general population, averaging 1–2%, and is 10 times lower than that for HBV infection [8]. In a single study that evaluated risk factors for infection, a history of unintentional needle-stick injury was the only occupational risk factor independently associated with HCV infection [9].

Among health care workers, the prevalence of HCV infection is about the same as that of the general population: 1.5%. Following percutaneous exposure of health care workers to infected blood, the risk of HCV seroconversion ranges from 0 to 10%, with an average of 1.8% [7].

HCV infection is a major cause of fatigue, muscle and joint pain, depression, and other psychological disorders, which decrease patient health-related quality of life (HRQL) and health utility [10]. Patients with chronic HCV infection demonstrated lower HRQL compared with the general population. Recently, investigators have turned their interest to the impact of HCV infection on absenteeism, work force participation, and overall work impairment.

Even if patients are employed, the complete participation productivity may be limited. Worker productivity is measured through two key concepts: presenteeism and absenteeism. Absenteeism is related to the percentage of work time missed, while presenteeism is related to the percentage of impairment experienced at work time missed because of one's health [6].

To date, numerous studies have demonstrated the impact of HCV on health care costs. Previous studies have evaluated health care costs associated with HCV to be $2470 per patient during the period from 1997 to 1999 [11, 12]. However, direct medical costs present only part of the societal burden of HCV infection. On the other hand, indirect costs related to work impairment have been ignored in the HCV literature for a long time. Previous models have omitted work impairment completely [13] or have evaluated productivity losses only in the premature mortality and disability as a consequence of projected late stage liver disease. Direct costs associated with HCV are fundamental. Also, indirect economic and humanistic costs are major and arise from the reduction of HRQL owing to both the disease and HCV treatments; this is related on the patient work, daily activities, and lifestyle [14].

Recent investigation has recognized a significant burden of HCV infection on work productivity, with infected patients missing 9% of working hours in the working week and reporting an average of 27% impairment while at work. Also, database study reported that HCV patients were 7.5% less productive based on work units per hour [15].

For better understanding of the societal impact of HCV, the association between the virus and work force participation and WP loss must be observed. It is also essential to investigate potential confusing variables that may contribute to a relationship between HCV and workplace activity. Nowadays, different studies have reviewed the impact comorbidities, and health behaviors may have on health outcomes among HCV patients, including psychiatric illness, fibrosis, fatigue, and depressive symptoms [16].

It would be educative and significant for some employers with a short-term focus to utilize a time series approach to document WP changes pre and post-HCV diagnosis. Although using a regression approach and a propensity scoring approach ensured a numerous series of results, other methodologies may be significant, especially when evaluating economic costs associated with HCV [16].

Patients with HCV infection have reduced WP, in terms of both presenteeism (impairment in WP while working) and absenteeism (productivity loss due to absence from work). The most important drivers of WP in HCV are impairment of physical aspects of PROs and clinical history of depression, anxiety, fatigue, and cirrhosis [4]. Some authors emphasize the impact of eradicating HCV virus on the WP of chronic HCV (CH-C) patients. Sensitivity analyses assessed the possibility that CH-C patients' labor costs were lower than the general populations and presented results by fibrosis stage. Before initiation of treatment, EU patients with CH-C genotype 1 (GT1) exhibited absenteeism and presenteeism impairments of 3.54 and 9.12%, respectively [17]. About 91.8% of EU patients in the ION trials achieved SVR and improved absenteeism and presenteeism impairments by 16.3 and 19.5%, respectively. Weighted average per-employed patient gains from treatment are projected to be higher in cirrhotic than in noncirrhotic patients. CH-C results in a significant economic burden to European society. Due to improvements in WP, sustained virologic response with treatment could provide substantial economic gains, partly offsetting the direct costs related to its widespread use [17].

HCV infection is generally considered an asymptomatic disease. However, studies have shown that HCV has a substantial negative impact on patients' quality of life and functioning. Su et al. [15] evaluated a total number of near 340,000 subjects. Workers with HCV had significantly more lost workdays per worker compared to the control cohort, including sick leave, short-term disability, and long-term disability. HCV-infected workers had 4.15 more days of absence per worker compared to the control cohort. Efficiency was measured by units of work processed per hour and workers with HCV processed 7.5% fewer units per hour than employees without HCV. All health care costs among HCV workers were significantly higher compared to the same costs among workers without HCV. This study provides evidence that there is a considerable secondary burden of disease and labels an association between HCV infection, efficiency, increased absenteeism, and higher health care benefit costs [15].

Gifford et al. [18] showed that at least 50% of the men had symptoms of HCV infection. Tiredness was the most common symptom, followed by nausea and pain in the liver. Men ignored symptoms of disease in higher percentage compared women. Thirty-five percent of men rated their health as 'fair' or 'poor' compared to 18% of men in the general population. Many were concerned about their ability to work and financial income, and more than half were worried about being unable to have a drink with their friends. Coughlan et al. presented a Dublin study documenting psychological well-being, mental health, and quality of life in 93 women diagnosed with medically acquired HCV infection. Overall, the women had significantly lower quality of life than the healthy female population. No significant difference was found between women who had a past or current HCV virus infection; they reported having low energy, poor health, and problems with work and other daily activities. Reduced quality of life can be related to the diagnostic process rather than HCV infection as such. While HCV have a significant physiological effect on the quality of life, it is imperative not to undervalue the social and psychological costs of being identified with a stigmatized chronic disease that has an unknown progression and outcome [19]. Gill et al. found that HCV compared to divorce, loss of source of income, or a move to another city diagnosis is a way more stressful. The authors suggested that pre-and post-test counseling and psychosocial support could help to decrease the stress related with HCV diagnosis [20]. HCV infection has a significant influence on the quality of life. Not only do symptoms such as fatigue lessen effective functioning but also living with a chronic stigmatized disease with an indeterminate future creates problems around expose, retrieving care, and satisfying confidence, employment, and relations.

3. The impact of the HCV antiviral therapy on work ability

A patient's ability to tolerate and adhere to HCV treatment has an impact to WP during the course of HCV treatment. This is important concern for patients considering treatment initiation because they will have to deal with the possibility of temporary reduced work participation during treatment [17].

Eradication of HCV may improve many different components of PRO, including HRQL and WP [21]. It is important that evaluation of new regimens for treatment of chronic hepatitis C (CHC) includes not only efficacy and safety reports but also data related to important PROs such as fatigue, HRQL, and WP [14]. The dual function of PRO is to represent patient experience with treatment and assess the indirect cost of treatment related to lower WP [22].

Treatment of HCV infection with the combination of peginterferon plus ribavirin (pegIFN/RBV) is a process with significant and sometimes dose-limiting adverse events. Those adverse effects further exacerbate the patient's already compromised productivity and consequently increase economic burden [17]. Brook et al. found that patients who received pegIFN/RBV took more sick leave, more long-term disability, and more workers' compensation than those without HCV treatment [3]. Perillo et al. designed a randomized control study and found that during treatment with peginterferon-alpha 2a, patients showed less impairment across all measures of work functioning and productivity when compared to patients who were treated with combination of interferon-alpha 2b plus ribavirin [23]. In a study conducted by McHutchison et al., randomly assigned patients who responded to therapy of IFN/RBV showed improvements across all measures of work functioning and productivity, in contrast with patients who received placebo. In addition, sustained responders work functioning and productivity decreased temporarily in approximately 46% of patients [14]. Patients who do not achieve an SVR are more likely to miss work or other commitments due to HCV infection or its treatment than those who achieve SVR. Aggrawal et al. confirmed that employed patients with genotype 1 chronic HCV infection receiving treatment have reduced work hours and reduced WP levels due to hepatitis or its treatment. This decline was observed early during the course of treatment, with return to baseline levels by week 72 post-treatment initiation, suggesting that WP losses can be considered a short-term outcome of HCV treatment [1].

To improve the tolerability and efficacy profile of anti-HCV treatment, a number of interferon-free regimens, such as sofosbuvir, have been developed. In a study by Younossi et al., subjects treated with the interferon-free regimen completely recovered by the end of 12 weeks of follow-up, their PRO scores returned to baseline values and showed further improvement. The impact on WP, especially presenteeism, was significantly more profound with the interferon-containing regimen than with the interferon-free regimen. Also, subjects who received the interferon-free regimen experienced substantially less fatigue compared with the subjects receiving interferon-containing regimens [22]. Another study by Younossi et al. showed that interferon and ribavirin-free regimen are associated with significant gains in most aspects of HRQL during treatment regardless of the stage of liver disease [24]. Expanding the access to a highly effective cure for all HCV-infected patients will improve the clinical outcomes but also patient-reported outcomes such as HRQL and work productivity, resulting in a superb comprehensive benefit to patients and society.

In conclusion, successful treatment and achieving SVR regardless of therapy have been associated with better economic outcomes [25]. For that reason, there is a strong evidence that this improvement can positively impact the indirect economic burden of HCV by improving WP.

4. Conclusions

In general, work-related activities should not pose a risk to patient with chronic liver disease [26]. The exception would be:

1. Patients with hepatic encephalopathy for whom certain task such as driving and operating heavy machinery may be risky due to impaired judgment and cognitive defects.

2. Working with hepatotoxic chemical such as carbon tetrachloride, vinyl chloride, and poly-chlorinated biphenyls (PCBs).

Patients with advanced liver disease have decreased exercise capacity from anemia, ascites, renal failure, or hepato-pulmonary syndrome, and work limitations are advised [26].

Modifications to work and work ability assessment are required to prevent occupational transmission of HCV. This is usually only required in the health care setting, where infectious carriers of HCV should not carry out exposure-prone procedures (EPP). Even in an area with a high prevalence of HCV among its population, the risk of acquiring HCV through occupational exposure is low—the risk of an individual surgeon acquiring the HCV has been estimated at 0.001–0.032% per annum [26, 27]. Rates of viral clearance with treatment of acute HCV infection are considerably higher than treatment of chronic HCV infection. Consequently, it is imperative that health care workers follow universal precaution and promptly report all exposures to blood or body fluid exposures according to their local policy.

Health care workers who embark on, or transfer to, a career that requires EPP (exposure-prone procedures and dialysis work) should be assessed to ensure that they are free from infection with HCV. Members of staff known to have been exposed to the blood of a HCV-positive patient through sharps injury should continue to work normally, but it is necessary to do the following procedure [26] that is also shown at **Figure** 1:

1. HCV RNA polymerase chain reaction test 6 weeks after exposure.

2. Twelve weeks after exposure, HCV RNA polymerase chain reaction test should be taken again, together with HCV antibody testing.

3. Six months after exposure, additional HCV antibody testing should be commenced (repeated negative testing designates infection absence).

Those who have positive test results should stop undertaking EPPs instantly and should be taken as soon as possible for specialist assessment by a gastroenterologist and/or infectologist. Health care workers who already perform EPPs and who believe they may have been exposed to HCV infection should be advised to seek advice from their occupational health department for confidential advice on whether they should be tested.

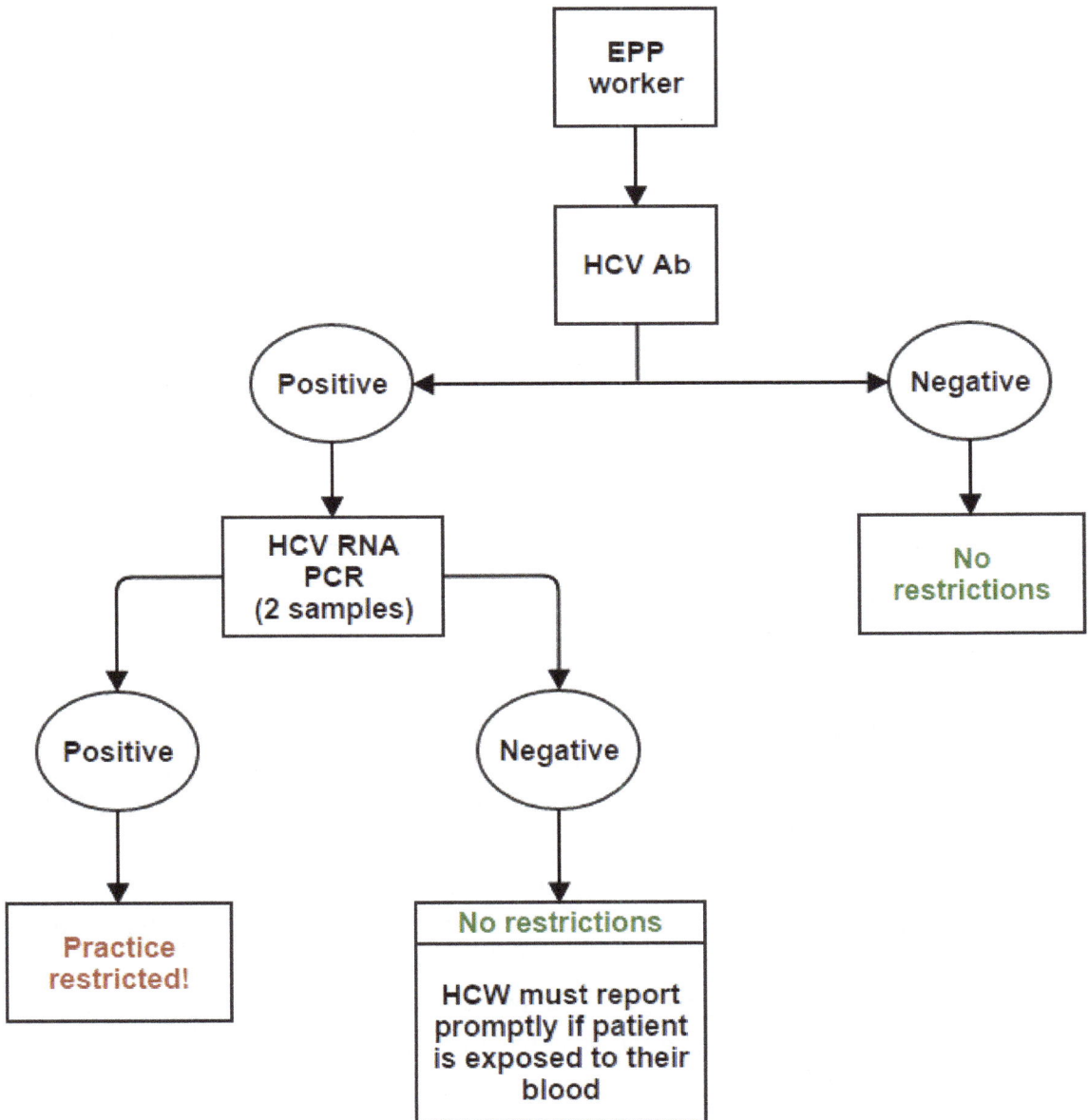

Figure 1. Investigation of HCV status in a worker performing exposure-prone procedures (Modified after Palmer et al. [26]).

Those health care workers who had HCV infection and have been treated with antiviral treatment may return to EPPs if they have tested negative to HCV RNA for at least 6 months after cessation of treatment. They should have one additional check for HCV RNA 6 months later. Present standard laboratory tests cannot demonstrate complete clearance of virus but can state that the virus is undetectable. In these situations, infectivity is likely to be so low that it is safe to return to EPPs and reactivation of infection is unlikely so no further testing is required. There is indication that infection remains within hepatocytes and can be reactivated following treatment with monoclonal antibodies (such as Rituximab) and other immunosuppressants (such as TNF-α inhibitors) including cancer chemotherapy. Recent data suggest that rituximab-based chemotherapy increases HCV expression in hepatic cells, can become a mark for a cell-mediated immune response after the treatment removal and the renewal of the immune control. Some studies have examined the incidence of HCV reactivation and related hepatic flare in patients with oncohematological diseases receiving R-CHOP (rituximab, cyclophosphamide, doxorubicin, vincristine, and prednisone). These studies suggest that the hepatic flares are often asymptomatic, but life-threatening liver failure occurs in closely 10% of cases [28].

Author details

Milan Milošević[1]*, Jelena Jakab[2], Lucija Kuna[2] and Martina Smolić[2]

*Address all correspondence to: milan.milosevic@snz.hr

1 University of Zagreb, School of Medicine, Andrija Stampar School of Public Health, WHO Collaborative Centre for Occupational Health, Zagreb, Croatia

2 Josip Juraj Strossmayer University of Osijek, Faculty of Medicine, Osijek, Croatia

References

[1] Aggarwal J, Vera-Llonch M, Donepudi M, Suthoff E, Younossi Z, Goss TF. Work productivity among treatment-naive patients with genotype 1 chronic hepatitis C infection receiving telaprevir combination treatment. Journal of Viral Hepatitis. 2015;**22**(1):8-17. DOI: 10.1111/jvh.12227

[2] Younossi Z, Henry L. Systematic review: Patient-reported outcomes in chronic hepatitis C – the impact of liver disease and new treatment regimens. Alimentary Pharmacology & Therapeutics. 2015;**41**(6):497-520. DOI: 10.1111/apt.13090

[3] Brook RA, Kleinman NL, Su J, Corey-Lisle PK, Iloeje UH. Absenteeism and productivity among employees being treated for hepatitis C. The American Journal of Managed Care. 2011;**17**(10):657-664

[4] Younossi ZM, Stepanova M, Henry L, Younossi I, Weinstein A, Nader F, Hunt S. Association of work productivity with clinical and patient-reported factors in patients

infected with hepatitis C virus. Journal of Viral Hepatitis. 2016;**23**(8):623-630. DOI: 10.1111/jvh.12528

[5] Vietri J, Prajapati G, El Khoury AC. The burden of hepatitis C in Europe from the patients' perspective: A survey in 5 countries. BMC Gastroenterology. 2013;**13**:16. DOI: 10.1186/1471-230X-13-16

[6] Manne V, Sassi K, Allen R, Saab S. Hepatitis C and work impairment: A review of current literature. Journal of Clinical Gastroenterology. 2014;**48**(7):595-599. DOI: 10.1097/MCG.0000000000000080

[7] Centers for Disease Control and Prevention. Recommendations for prevention and control of hepatitis C virus (HCV) infection and HCV-related chronic disease. MMWR – Recommendations and Reports. 1998;**47**(RR-19):1-39

[8] Cooper BW, Krusell A, Tilton RC, Goodwin R, Levitz RE. Seroprevalence of antibodies to hepatitis C virus in high-risk hospital personnel. Infection Control and Hospital Epidemiology. 1992;**13**(2):82-85

[9] Polish LB, Tong MJ, Co RL, Coleman PJ, Alter MJ. Risk factors for hepatitis C virus infection among health care personnel in a community hospital. American Journal of Infection Control. 1993;**21**(4):196-200

[10] Chong CA, Gulamhussein A, Heathcote EJ, Lilly L, Sherman M, Naglie G, Krahn M. Health-state utilities and quality of life in hepatitis C patients. The American Journal of Gastroenterology. 2003;**98**(3):630-638

[11] Leigh JP, Bowlus CL, Leistikow BN, Schenker M. Costs of hepatitis C. Archives of Internal Medicine. 2001;**161**(18):2231-2237

[12] Armstrong EP, Charland SL. Burden of illness of hepatitis C from a managed care organization perspective. Current Medical Research and Opinion. 2004;**20**(5):671-679. DOI: 10.1185/030079904125003485

[13] Touzet S, Kraemer L, Colin C, Pradat P, Lanoir D, Bailly F, Coppola RC, Sauleda S, Thursz MR, Tillmann H, Alberti A, Braconier JH, Esteban JI, Hadziyannis SJ, Manns MP, Saracco G, Thomas HC, Trépo C. Epidemiology of hepatitis C virus infection in seven European Union countries: A critical analysis of the literature. HENCORE group (Hepatitis C European Network for Co-operative Research). European Journal of Gastroenterology & Hepatology. 2000;**12**(6):667-678

[14] McHutchison JG, Ware JE, Bayliss MS, Pianko S, Albrecht JK, Cort S, Yang I, Neary MP, H I T Group. The effects of interferon alpha-2b in combination with ribavirin on health related quality of life and work productivity. Journal of Hepatology. 2001;**34**(1):140-147

[15] Su J, Brook RA, Kleinman NL, Corey-Lisle P. The impact of hepatitis C virus infection on work absence, productivity, and healthcare benefit costs. Hepatology. 2010;**52**(2):436-442. DOI: 10.1002/hep.23726

[16] DiBonaventura M, Wagner JS, Yuan Y, L'Italien G, Langley P, Ray Kim W. The impact of hepatitis C on labor force participation, absenteeism, presenteeism and non-work activities. Journal of Medical Economics. 2011;**14**(2):253-261. DOI: 10.3111/13696998.2011.566294

[17] Younossi Z, Brown A, Buti M, Fagiuoli S, Mauss S, Rosenberg W, Serfaty L, Srivastava A, Smith N, Stepanova M, Beckerman R. Impact of eradicating hepatitis C virus on the work productivity of chronic hepatitis C (CH-C) patients: An economic model from five European countries. Journal of Viral Hepatitis. 2016;**23**(3):217-226. DOI: 10.1111/jvh.12483

[18] Gifford SM, O'Brien ML, Smith A, Temple-Smith M, Stoove M, Mitchell D, Jolley D. Australian men's experiences of living with hepatitis C virus: Results from a cross-sectional survey. Journal of Gastroenterology and Hepatology. 2005;**20**(1):79-86. DOI: 10.1111/j.1440-1746.2004.03514.x

[19] Coughlan B, Sheehan J, Hickey A, Crowe J. Psychological well-being and quality of life in women with an iatrogenic hepatitis C virus infection. British Journal of Health Psychology. 2002;**7**(Pt 1):105-116. DOI: 10.1348/135910702169394

[20] Gill ML, Atiq M, Sattar S, Khokhar N. Psychological implications of hepatitis C virus diagnosis. Journal of Gastroenterology and Hepatology. 2005;**20**(11):1741-1744. DOI: 10.1111/j.1440-1746.2005.04061.x

[21] Kamal SM, Ahmed A, Mahmoud S, Nabegh L, El Gohary I, Obadan I, Hafez T, Ghoraba D, Aziz AA, Metaoei M. Enhanced efficacy of pegylated interferon alpha-2a over pegylated interferon and ribavirin in chronic hepatitis C genotype 4A randomized trial and quality of life analysis. Liver International. 2011;**31**(3):401-411. DOI: 10.1111/j.1478-3231.2010.02435.x

[22] Younossi ZM, Stepanova M, Henry L, Gane E, Jacobson IM, Lawitz E, Nelson D, Gerber L, Nader F, Hunt S. Effects of sofosbuvir-based treatment, with and without interferon, on outcome and productivity of patients with chronic hepatitis C. Clin Gastroenterol Hepatol. 2014;**12**(8):1349-1359.e13. DOI: 10.1016/j.cgh.2013.11.032

[23] Perrillo R, Rothstein KD, Rubin R, Alam I, Imperial J, Harb G, Hu S, Klaskala W. Comparison of quality of life, work productivity and medical resource utilization of peginterferon alpha 2a vs the combination of interferon alpha 2b plus ribavirin as initial treatment in patients with chronic hepatitis C. Journal of Viral Hepatitis. 2004;**11**(2):157-165

[24] Younossi ZM, Stepanova M, Afdhal N, Kowdley KV, Zeuzem S, Henry L, Hunt SL, Marcellin P. Improvement of health-related quality of life and work productivity in chronic hepatitis C patients with early and advanced fibrosis treated with ledipasvir and sofosbuvir. Journal of Hepatology. 2015;**63**(2):337-345. DOI: 10.1016/j.jhep.2015.03.014

[25] John-Baptiste AA, Tomlinson G, Hsu PC, Krajden M, Heathcote EJ, Laporte A, Yoshida EM, Anderson FH, Krahn MD. Sustained responders have better quality of life and productivity compared with treatment failures long after antiviral therapy for hepatitis C. The American Journal of Gastroenterology. 2009;**104**(10):2439-2448. DOI: 10.1038/ajg.2009.346

[26] Palmer KT, Brown I, Hobson J. Fitness for Work: The Medical Aspects. 5th ed. Oxford: Oxford University Press; 2013

[27] Yazdanpanah Y, De Carli G, Migueres B, Lot F, Campins M, Colombo C, Thomas T, Deuffic-Burban S, Prevot MH, Domart M, Tarantola A, Abiteboul D, Deny P, Pol S, Desenclos JC, Puro V, Bouvet E. Risk factors for hepatitis C virus transmission to health care workers after occupational exposure: A European case-control study. Clinical Infectious Diseases. 2005;**41**(10):1423-1430. DOI: 10.1086/497131

[28] Sagnelli E, Pisaturo M, Sagnelli C, Coppola N. Rituximab-based treatment, HCV replication, and hepatic flares. Clinical & Developmental Immunology. 2012;**2012**:945950. DOI: 10.1155/2012/945950

7

Micro-RNA in Hepatocellular Carcinoma - Related Hepatitis C Virus Patients in Correlation to Disease Progression

Moustafa Nouh Elemeery

Abstract

Hepatocellular carcinoma (HCC) is a multistep heterogeneous disease as it is related to the risk factors such as HBV and HCV infections, including uncontrolled hepatocyte proliferation, invasion of the neighboring tissue and metastasize to distant tissues. There are several factors affecting the course of HCC among the patients such as oncogenes and tumor suppressor genes. Recently, molecular mechanisms have cleared some of the underlying mechanisms of carcinogenesis, especially the microRNAs, the upstream regulators of a large number of critical genes. Mature miRNAs found to be mounted into RISC, which helps in recognizing the complementary binding sites in the 3' untranslated regions of target genes. That binding causes the degradation of/or inhibition of translation of mRNAs. miRNAs have been reported to be deregulated in human cancers demonstrating their double-edged role as a tumor suppressor and as an oncogene. miRNA deregulation is involved in modulating signal pathways of cellular transformation of a normal cell into a cancer cell. miRNAs have been reported to be associated with the processes of carcinogenesis including inflammation, cell-cycle, differentiation, apoptosis, and metastasis. miRNAs have been considered as potential biomarkers in HCC as their development has been attributed to the deregulation of many genes owing to abnormal expression of miRNAs. Herein, the current chapter will focus on studying the regulation of miRNAs in HCC-related HCV patients.

Keywords: miRNA, HCC, HCV, UTR, fibrosis progression

1. Introduction

MicroRNA (miRNA) has been proven as key regulator homeostasis for multiple biological systems, besides modulation of the disease pathology of many cancers. Experimental target miRNA biogenesis as key regulators using small molecules or other interferences sheds light on its crucial role in regulating posttranscriptional gene expression. Further studies reported the variability of their loci, the genetic organization, and their tissue specificity, besides controlling the translation of target protein and transcriptome in response to physiologic environmental cues, along with their vulnerability to become designated in diseases like cancer and fibrosis, including that related to infection viruses like HCV. Many pathways analysis of targeted genes performed using infection-associated miRNAs showed that the pathways related to signal transduction activation, DNA damage, and cell death were clearly observed in HBV-infected liver, while proteasome, lipid metabolism activation, immune response, and antigen presentation were predominantly in HCV-infected liver. These differences are associated with miRNAs' level in the infected liver and it was confirmed in cell line like Huh7.5 cells in which infectious HBV or HCV clones can be replicated, which proved that miRNAs act as key mediators of HCV and HBV infection and liver disease progression as well; therefore, miRNAs can act as liable therapeutic target molecules in the field of translational medicine.

2. Tissue-specific expression and variation level of miRNAs

MicroRNAs are a class of small, endogenous, conserved, non-coding RNAs with a length of 20–24 ribonucleotide RNA sequence that is biosynthesized through transcription of miRNA genes into primary transcripts (pri-miRNA), which are processed by the drosha, generating a precursor of a length of 70 nucleotides (pre-miRNA) with a hairpin-like structure. A remarkable mechanistic difference in canonical against noncanonical miRNAs is that canonical is drosha-dependent intronic miRNAs and so treated co-transcriptionally in the nucleus with protein-coding transcripts. Pre-miRNA is then processed by dicer in the cytoplasm generating mature miRNA duplexes. Mature miRNAs are then mounted into RISC (an miRNA-induced silencing complex) which helps in recognizing the complementary binding sites in the 3'UTR of target genes. Noncanonical intronic, ones called mirtrons, originate from small introns that are similar to pre-miRNAs and can detour the drosha-processing step [1, 2]. Noncanonical pathway affects common cellular response pathways like proliferation and apoptosis by targeting various mRNA transcripts [1]. miRNA binding causes the degradation of, or inhibition of, translation of mRNAs. miRNAs have been reported to be deregulated in human cancers demonstrating their double-edged role as a tumor suppressor and as an oncogene that offers miR clusters as complex and adaptive regulatory controllers for disease progression. Comparative research assessing the organizational structure for the mammalian genome has noticed enrichment in one of the following: copy number variation, chromosomal deletion or insertion, and single nucleotide polymorphisms (SNPs) that subsidize phenotypic diversity. This diversity is obvious in all aspects of human health and investigated diseases. No wonder there is a mounting gratitude to the variation in miRNAs and their target genes in phenotypic variability. Numerous solid malignancies that included hepatocellular carcinoma (HCC) proved to be correlated with miRNAs located at deleted, amplified, or translocated chromosomal regions [3]. Variation in gene expression or regulation affected by expression of the quantitative trait loci is caused due to genetic variants in either cis- or trans-acting SNPs [4]. A remarkable criterion of miRNA binding is their capability to distinguish binding site polymorphism (miRSNPs) in transcribed functional genes, as in the case of miR 214-5p that appears to be dysregulated in HCC [2] and miR-24 in the case of colorectal tumor by the targeting site of polymorphism in the dihydrofolate reductase gene [5]. This binding causes inhibition of translation for its transcripts and can phenocopy the phenotypic character of such a disease with genetic knockouts of the responsible gene [5].

Screening miRNA genetic variation and differential expression level across the human population in healthy and disease patients provides more insights on variable causes of disease progression and susceptibility in addition to physical functionalities [4]. Comparative genomic studies showed that the untranslated regions (UTRs) within the mRNA sequence act as a target sequence even for mRNA-UTR-displaying variants; during miRNA-mRNA adaptive coevolution, the co-expressed miRNA selects its cognate UTR mRNA, which depends on whether the dysregulation of protein output will be harmful, beneficial or inconsequential for the desired effect [6].

Evaluating reports on tissue-specific differential expression of miRNAs showed the cross-regulation feature of miRNAs and its correlation to stability of phenotype differentiation [7], as an example, regulation of neurite outgrowth, dendritic spine size, and neural differentiation that is regulated by overexpression of miR219, miR134, miR128, miR24, miR7, and others [7]. In the same strategy, miR499, miR486, miR208, miR206, miR133, and miR1 proved to control skeletal muscle growth, maintenance and differentiation [8], while miR133 proved to inhibit osteogenic cell-linage differentiation through controlling Runx2 that is required for bone development, differentiation, and formation. Not only the previously mentioned roles but miRNAs can also exert specialized functions as in case of hypothalamus; fine-tuning expression of oxytocin; and Fos controlled by hyper-expression of both miR24 and miR7 and hence they control lactation and parturition through controlling water in the body [9].

MicroRNA (miRNA) has been proven as key regulator homeostasis for multiple biological systems, besides modulation of the disease pathology of many cancers. Experimental target miRNA biogenesis key regulators using small molecules or other interferences sheds light on its crucial role in regulating posttranscriptional gene expression. Further studies reported the variability of their loci, the genetic organization, and their tissue specificity [10], besides controlling the translation of target protein and transcriptome in response to physiologic environmental cues, along with their vulnerability to become designated in diseases like cancer and fibrosis, including that related to infection viruses like HCV. Many pathways analysis of targeted genes performed using infection-associated miRNAs showed that the pathways related to signal transduction activation, DNA damage, and cell death are clearly observed in HBV-infected liver, while proteasome, lipid metabolism activation, immune response, and antigen presentation were predominantly in HCV-infected liver [2, 3]. These differences are associated with miRNAs' level in the infected liver and it was confirmed in cell line like Huh7.5 cells in which infectious HBV or HCV clones can be replicated, which proved that miRNAs act as key mediators of HCV and HBV infection and liver disease progression as well; therefore, miRNA can act as liable therapeutic target molecules in the field of translational medicine [11].

Since miRNA discovery as a liable promising class of small non-coding RNAs able to regulate protein translation and stability of mRNA, miRNAs have been implicated as key regulators in many diseases like cancer and autoimmune disease. So there is great effort to leverage knowledge of the miRNA regulatory system to these diseases, especially cancer [12].

3. MicroRNAs and disease susceptibility

Development in the pathobiology of miR Nas sheds light on its crucial character in transcriptome modulation which can reflect cancer state in addition to its application in attenuating possible risks that may be raised during cancer progression [13]. Currently, there is no doubt that down-regulating epithelial markers causes disruption in epithelial mesenchymal that is directly associated with differentiation of epithelial cells in lung cancer, a key developmental pathway in lung cancer progression and metastasis [14]. So expression of miRNA can be used as a progression marker for cancer disease depending on its differential expression during invasion, progression, and metastasis of cancer [3].

Reduction in dicer expression is often noticed in cancer stem cells like muscle stem cell tumors and rhabdomyosarcoma in periodic cases, shown to be correlated with the down-regulated level of myomiRNAs like miR 133 and miR 1 [15]. OncomiRNAs is a type of miRNA that can decrease tumor suppressor gene expression which leads to phenotype attenuation or promotion for oncogenic characters; miR92, miR21, and niR17 are members of that family that can modulate cell-cycle regulators like P21, PTEN, and E2F that can promote tumor proliferation [3, 12]. On the other hand, tumor-suppressor miRNAs, like let-7, target directly mRNA for silencing [3]; over-expressed Let7 has proved to modulate cell-cycle regulators that lead to tumor invasion and metastasis. So these miRNAs can be used as prognostic tools for cancer incidence or as a parameter for treatment susceptibility. In squamous cell carcinoma and adenocarcinoma, a comparative miRNA expression profiling revealed a significant difference that reached a specific signature to predict overall survival between male smoker patients in addition to the study performed by Liu et al. that clearly declared correlation between overall pathobiology in cancer and tissue-context miRNA expression [15]. Our team recently proved a small panel of four miRNAs that can act as a liable prognostic marker for HCC progression besides its ability to discriminate different stages in hepatocellular carcinoma [2].

3.1. miRNAs and hepatic diseases

Studies for understanding miRNAs in liver diseases showed a significant progression in that field, making liver a promising first organ to achieve precision and targeted therapy. Depending on accumulated studies of miRNA in liver disease, the unique vasculature of the liver, and the efficiently rapid accumulation of exogenous small RNAs, the liver showed a good target for RNAi targeted therapy. Manipulation of miRNAs in liver diseases proved great evidences in that field; as an example miR122 clearly illustrates a good effective target for ameliorating hepatic steatosis besides many studies that showed miR122 to be a good target in HCV targeted therapy through its role in production of neutralizing antagomirs. MicroRNAs as a key target for viral hepatitis afford another liable possibility for targeting HBV and HCV infection that, by one way or another, causes HCC progression and death upon chronic infection; this targeting prevention will help to reduce HCC risk incidence by regulating many oncogenic miRNAs like miR222, miR221, and miR21 or via tumor suppression ones like miR199 and miR122 that nowadays are used as liable biomarkers in HCC, besides many promising studies that showed its role as prognostic and a marker for therapy response.

3.1.1. miRNA as a metabolic modulator in hepatic diseases

Non-alcoholic fatty liver diseases (NAFLD) are characterized by increased liver fat content and progression to liver inflammation, fibrosis, and ultimately cancer [16, 17]. Obesity, insulin resistance, and diabetes mellitus are risk factors for this disease and it is estimated that NAFLD will be the most common problem in internal medicine by 2020 [18]. Despite the high prevalence of NAFLD, the biology behind the disease progression is not clear and importantly there is no specific treatment for this condition, so osculating necessity for liable biomarkers and discovery of potential drug targets, as researched by Benhamouche-Trouillet et al., showed that miR-21 may be implicated at various steps during the NAFLD disease progression in a cell-specific manner through modulation of PPARα [19]. Specific conditional dicer1 deletion from embryonic liver leads to disruption in maturation of microRNA from its pre-microRNA form which leads to striking of metabolic phenotypes that include steatosis together with triglyceride and fatty acid accumulation in addition to dysregulation of blood glucose in fasting mice under study [12]. On the other hand, miR-355 has been recently considered as a liable biomarker for hepatic lipid accumulation in rat experiments as its elevated level strongly correlated with obesity in mice in association with liver steatosis [15]; for that reason, a high-throughput screen for miRNAs as a predictor for lipid droplet formation in the liver metabolic disorder in humans is a great demand for disease progression, overall survival rate, and even for prognosis of possible hepatic disorder (as shown in **Figure 1** and **Table 1**).

The conflicting concerns about whether profile expression of miRNA correlated with NASH or NAFLD have also been well investigated. Sanyal [20] research group reported in double subject groups, including NASH and metabolic syndrome group, in addition to the control group; control groups were matched in BMI. His investigators reported 23 up-regulated miRNAs and the same number of down-regulated miRNAs, with detailed interpretation referring to the role of some miRNA expression dysregulation, that is, miR-34a and miR-146b up-regulation besides miR-122 down-regulation in NASH subjects. Odd findings were reported in human subjects with NASH-like decreased expression of miR-122. However, the protective feature arise from silencing of miR-122 specially in high fat-fed mice bears only indirect physiological matter differentiate steady-state cross-sectional investigations in overweight or obese humans subjects with such a fatty liver disease. This result includes the complexity of dissecting effects and causes cross-talk in hepatic expression of miR-122 and metabolic liver disease.

The importance of miRNAs cross-talk analysis was further elucidated in many publications where hepatic steatosis variations was evolved through application of an adenovirus encoding a dominant negative c-Jun and then testing changes in miRNA expression that is associated with it [21]. They found many miRNAs (miR-122 and miR-370 was common among many publications) to be differentially expressed (DE) in liver tissues of mice that were treated by adenovirus and showed that the elevated presence of miR-370 correlated with the osculating expression of hepatic lipogenic target mRNAs (e.g., FAS, SREBP-1c, and DGAT2); these findings suggest that dietary modulation of some miRNA expression is a relevant consideration [21].

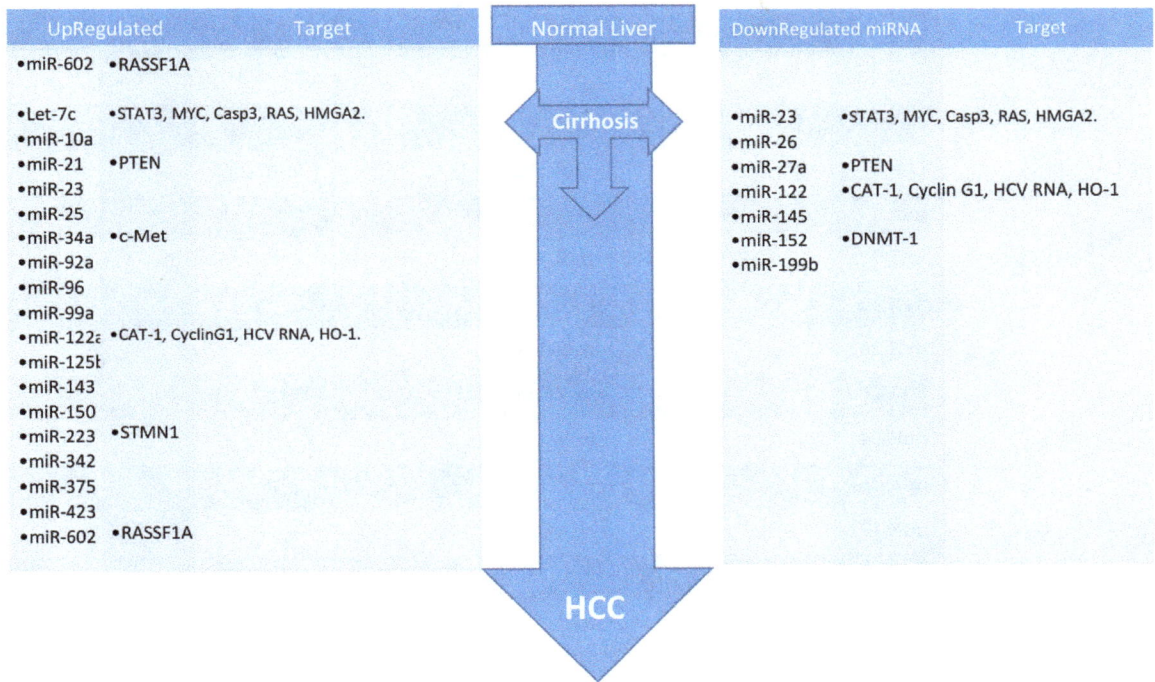

Figure 1. miRNA that either up-regulated or down-regulated with its target genes in different stages of HCC disease progression.

Liver diseases	Down-regulated miRNAs	Up-regulated miRNAs	Dysregulated miRNA
Steatohepatitis	miR-21	miR-17	miR-21
	miR-29a	miR-24	miR-33a/b
	miR-130a	miR-27	miR-122
	miR-185	miR-34a	miR-155
	miR-205	miR-103	
	miR-206	miR-107	
	miR-378	miR-122	
	miR-451		

Liver diseases	Down-regulated miRNAs	Up-regulated miRNAs	Dysregulated miRNA
HCV infection	Let-7	miR-21	miR-126
	miR-17	miR-122	miR-192
	miR-27a	miR-141	miR-198
	miR-29a,b,c	miR-146a	miR-345
	miR-130a	miR-192	
	miR-155	miR-215	
	miR-181a	miR-491	
	miR-194		
	miR-196		
	miR-199a		
	miR-221		
HCC	Let-7	miR-18a	miR-233
	miR-1	miR-21	
	miR-15a	miR-92a	
	miR-16	miR-130b	
	miR-26a	miR-141	
	miR-29	miR-155	
	miR-34a	miR-181	
	miR-101	miR-195	
	miR-122	miR-221	
	miR-124	miR-222	
	miR-125b	miR-224	
	miR-126	miR-494	
	miR-138	miR-1269	
	miR-141		
	miR-145		
	miR-146a		
	miR-148		
	miR-195		
	miR-199		
	miR-200		
	miR-223		
	miR-375		

Table 1. Liver diseases in association with the microRNA level in each stage.

3-hydroxy-3-methylglutaryl-CoA reductase (HMGCR), the enzyme that catalyzes mevalonic acid synthesis rate-limiting step in cholesterol and other isoprenoid production, showed both miR-21 and miR-34a as key player molecules in this step, through controlling dephosphorylation and activation of HMGCR [22]. One requirement for any effort to enhance miRNA levels as therapeutic tools is the well-established pro-oncogeneic characters for miRNAa in HCC and its related diseases, which will be discussed later here.

3.1.2. miRNA and HCV infection susceptibility

Hepatitis C virus is the sole member of hepacivirus C species that is known to be a blood-borne infectious viral disease causing the significant persistence of liver disease, with around 110–170 million infected patients globally, with nearly two-thirds of this number chronically infected and not less than one-third developing fibrosis and cirrhosis after 20 years of the onset of infection; most of them develop different stages of hepatocellular carcinoma [23]. Possible therapy for chronic hepatitis C (CHC) virus treatment has undergone a great transformation recently; discoveries in viral infections in humans have shown surprising findings that have broadened our understanding of miRNA function within human body.

In the setting of the HCV infection, the role of various miRNAs in modulating the viral infection response has been deeply studied, that clarifies causes of chronic hepatitis C progression in most infected patients and consequences of infection with its manipulation in the risk of developing cirrhosis and HCC [24]. The HCV virus is a positive-sense, single-stranded RNA virus of 9600 base [25]. It contains 5′ untranslated region (UTR) that contains four structurally conserved domains besides an internal ribosomal entry site (IRES) which allows viral RNA translation in a cap-independent manner with minimal dependence on canonical translation factors [26]. Translation of viral RNA leads to a polyprotein product that consists of six nonstructural and four structural viral proteins that undergo additional proteolysis by viral and host enzymes [27].

Subgenomic systems are easier to proceed after discovery of first sustainable cell-culture models for hepatitis viruses, in 1999 [28]. A noticed curious aspect in these early sustainable replicon systems was the successful sustainability of viral replication in Huh7 cell line but not HepG2, albeit both of these transformed cell lines have their origin in hepatocellular cancer in humans. The biologic declaration for this conflicted efficiency was first explained by Jopling et al. in 2005. When he verified that miR-122 has a detectable level in Huh7 but not HepG2 [29], in addition to that, he recently noticed that HCV contains a recognition site for the miR-122's seed sequence in the UTR area of viral genome. The miR-122-interacted viral elements have been mapped to two conserved points within 5′ UTR among stem-loop I and/or II, corresponding to the seed sequence of the miR-122 [30]. The finding was more astounding on the grounds that it appeared to be illogical to the customary thought of RNAi as an innate antiviral response like in invertebrates or plants [31]. Inhibition of RISC effector complex molecules like drosha, dicer1, DGCR8, and the RISC using small interfering RNA (siRNA) appears to inhibit HCV replication [32]. Although the mechanism underlying the miR-122 interaction with HCV is not precisely understood, miR-122 binding site position within the 5′ UTR proved to be critical, so translocation of this site to the 3′ UTR in a luciferase reporter mRNA causes up-regulation in reporter activity upon miR-122 diminished levels [30]. MiR-122 has been assumed to elevate both replication and translation of RNA, independently from viral replication [33]. Up-regulation of the translation step through miR122 dependent pathway is observed in reporter and full-length HCV genome constructs [34]. Also, Jangra et al. [35] deliberated the mutations of full-length HCV constructs that are capable of generating infectious virions in vitro. He found zero overlapped mutations within the miRNA or IRES binding site in distinct constructs. In those harboring mutations in IRES, infective viral production was down-regulated by more than 28-fold in comparison with constructs with the miR-122 binding site disruption that showed more than a 3000-fold reduction [35]. These observations are important in description of the role of miR-122 in HCV infection that requires searching beyond HCV replication, translation, and stability to investigate more pathways like liable RNA targets in HCV biology or posttranslational targets for it, as an example, heme oxygenase-1 (HO-1) which catalyzes the degradation of heme to biliverdin. Oxidative stress causes HO-1 elevation. Incubation of HCV-infected cell lines with biliverdin causes reduction in HCV amplicons via stimulation of interferon pathways [36]. Heterodimers of BACH1 and a member of the Maf protein family cause transcription repression of HO-1. It was observed that BACH1 3′ UTR contains miR-122 binding sites; its function was confirmed to be important by silencing miR-122 that leads to increased HO-1 mRNA levels double fold. Not only that but BATCH1 silencing using siRNA or other chemical means like heme or cobalt protoporphyrin also decreased HCV RNA level [37].

However, in these research-based findings, miR-122 proved to be essential in replication of HCV. Later cloned HCV from other genotypes proved to be replicated in some cell lines like HepG2 cells [38], liver cells (hepa1–6) [39], and cervical cancer-derived HeLa cell from humans [40]. In addition, the findings from cell culture are not yet completely correlated with outcomes from clinical infection, like miR-122 level in liver tissue of infected patients and viral load [41]. Moreover, HCV therapy non-responder (NR) patients showed lower pretreatment miR-122 levels in liver tissue biopsies rather than responders [41]. Another study showed inverse correlation between severity of hepatic fibrosis and hepatic miR-122 expression levels [42]. Even bearing in mind those conclusions, there is still convincing evidence that miR-122 targeted therapy may act as a liable strategy in HCV precision medicine. For example, Lanford et al. treated chronically infected chimpanzees with an LNA-modified oligonucleotide against miR-122 [43]. There was a significant drop by 2.6 orders of magnitude of HCV in the chimpanzee that received the optimal dose of this agent besides significant improvement in histologic examination of the liver specimens. Additionally, 5′ UTR sequencing indicated no signs for selection of adaptive mutations to the recognition site of miR-122. Similar findings were also reported in human clinical trials, phase II, that test the LNA-modified phosphorothioate antisense DNA oligonucleotide and the anti-miR-122 antagomir (Miravirsen) [44]. These findings were so encouraging to researchers, where the Miravirsen subcutaneous injection reduces serum HCV viral load in a dose-dependent manner, up to a 3-log reduction over 2–5 months [44]. Small molecules synthesis that targets miR-122 raises the possibility for new opportunities in HCV infection treatment [45].

However, miR-122 is the finest studied HCV-related miRNAs; it is not sole. There are others like MiR-199a that recognize HCV 5′ UTR and so suppress viral load [46]. Also, MiR196 down-regulates BACH1 [47], and MiR-196 is up-regulated in response to interferon signaling [48]. Besides, immune-regulatory miRNA-155 is induced by antiviral TLR3/4 signals [49]. Elevated MiR-155 levels in HCV-infected patients appeared to be inversely proportional to serum viral loads, signifying its relevant antiviral effect through suppression of Tim-3 (HAVCR2) that acts as an immune signaling modulator that is elevated in NK cells of HCV-infected patients where its up-regulation leads to inhibition of Tim-3 that causes an escalating production of interferon-γ (IFNγ) [50]. Not only that but MiR-155 also shows antiviral effects against other viruses like HIV infection through TLR3/TLR4 signaling pathway that prevents macrophage infection by HIV. Last but not least, miR-21, like many miRNAs, is induced by HCV infection but its induction aids HCV and escapes the immune response through directly suppressing interleukin-1 receptor-associated kinase 1 (IRAK1) and myeloid differentiation factor 88 (MyD88) [51] that is mandatory for mediating induced interferon response (type I) upon HCV infection. So, augmentation of miRNA expression levels and activity may prove a valuable aspect in HCV treatment and probably other viral infections.

4. MicroRNA inhibitors as a promising therapeutic approach

From the therapeutic point of view, silencing some miRNAs that encode potential vital or good protein-coding genes that is mandatory to preserve our health status. Inhibitors for these miRNAs have been considered for prospective therapeutic agents. Several approaches include direct delivery of miRNA-ASO or expressing it via mini-circle or viral vectors, which have been recognized for effective miRNA knockdown in vitro and in vivo too. Lately, miR-ASO-based therapy has been applied in humans and promising ongoing clinical trials considering liver sicknesses [52].

5. Conclusions

In conclusion, miRNA is a vital feature of assurance and monitoring throughout the tissue growth and disease states. In the near term, there will be much to be learned about adaptive or maladaptive states by an investigative way of differential expression of many miRNAs that is affected by the miRNA genetic architecture, mirtrons, and clusters in addition to SNP in miRNA or polymorphism in their target mRNA. There are diverse approaches of miRNA regulatory mechanism of action, for example negative, positive feedback and cross-regulatory through which various biological processes can be monitored, modulated or even resolved its signaling pathways, include fibrosis, viral infection and cancer. Possibly the micromanagement and homeostasis of these systems of regulatory miRNAs, when disturbed, can attain novel wannabe steady state of interacted interfaces that show an undesired effect in disease progression and severity especially in viral-related cancer cases like HCC. So, an enhanced sympathetic of these miRNA regulatory networks, in addition to improved therapeutic tools for controlling miRNA expression or their targets toward healthy regulatory states, will gain more interest over the coming years. Indeed, modern advanced miRNA precision-based medicine will undergo advanced phases of clinical trials that will afford more understandings into the biosafety and bioavailability in addition to the efficacy of miRNA as therapy and diagnostic tools.

Acknowledgements

I would like to express my deep thanks to Professor Ashraf Abdou Tabll, Head of Medical Biotechnology Department, National Research Centre, and Doaa Ahmed Ghareeb, Professor of Biochemistry, Faculty of Science, Beirut Arab University and Alexandria University, for their contribution in strengthening the field research.

Acronyms and abbreviations

CHC	chronic hepatitis C
E2F	elongation factor 2
HCC	hepatocellular carcinoma
HCV	hepatitis C virus
HO-1	heme oxygenase-1
HMG-CoA	3-hydroxy-3-methyl-glutaryl-CoA
IRES	internal ribosomal entry site
LNA	locked nucleic acid
miR	micro-ribonucleic acid
NAFLD	non-alcoholic fatty liver diseases
NASH	non-alcoholic steatohepatitis
PTEN	phosphatase and tensin homolog
RISC	RNA-induced silencing complex
UTR	untranslated region

Notes/Thanks/Other declarations

I would like to thank Mrs. Yasmin Ibrahim Hamed for her support while writing and editing this work.

Author details

Moustafa Nouh Elemeery[1,2,3]*

*Address all correspondence to: mn.badr@nrc.sci.eg

1 Center for Systemic Biotechnology, Korea Institute of Science and Technology, Gangneung, Gwang-do, Republic of Korea

2 Division of Biomedical Science and Technology, Korea University of Science and Technology, Daejeon, Republic of Korea

3 Microbial Biotechnology Department, Genetic Engineering and Biotechnology Research Division, National Research Centre, Dokki-Giza, Egypt

References

[1] Dai R, Ahmed SA. MicroRNA, a new paradigm for understanding immunoregulation, inflammation, and autoimmune diseases. Translational Research. 2011;**157**(4):163-179

[2] Elemeery MN et al. Validation of a serum microRNA panel as biomarkers for early diagnosis of hepatocellular carcinoma post-hepatitis C infection in Egyptian patients. World Journal of Gastroenterology. 2017;**23**(21):3864

[3] Nana-Sinkam SP, Croce CM. MicroRNAs as therapeutic targets in cancer. Translational Research. 2011;**157**(4):216-225

[4] Zhou T, Garcia JG, Zhang W. Integrating microRNAs into a system biology approach to acute lung injury. Translational Research. 2011;**157**(4):180-190

[5] Clop A et al. A mutation creating a potential illegitimate microRNA target site in the myostatin gene affects muscularity in sheep. Nature Genetics. 2006;**38**(7):813

[6] Bartel DP. MicroRNAs: Target recognition and regulatory functions. Cell. 2009;**136**(2):215-233

[7] Lian JB et al. MicroRNA control of bone formation and homeostasis. Nature Reviews Endocrinology. 2012;**8**(4):212

[8] Townley-Tilson WD, Callis TE, Wang D. MicroRNAs 1, 133, and 206: Critical factors of skeletal and cardiac muscle development, function, and disease. The International Journal of Biochemistry & Cell Biology. 2010;**42**(8):1252-1255

[42] Pineau P et al. miR-221 overexpression contributes to liver tumorigenesis. Proceedings of the National Academy of Sciences. 2010;**107**(1):264-269

[43] Fornari F et al. MiR-221 controls CDKN1C/p57 and CDKN1B/p27 expression in human hepatocellular carcinoma. Oncogene. 2008;**27**(43):5651

[44] Gramantieri L et al. MicroRNA-221 targets Bmf in hepatocellular carcinoma and correlates with tumor multifocality. Clinical Cancer Research. 2009;**15**(16):5073-5081

[45] Bae HJ et al. MicroRNA-221 governs tumor suppressor HDAC6 to potentiate malignant progression of liver cancer. Journal of Hepatology. 2015;**63**(2):408-419

[46] Morishita A, Masaki T. miRNA in hepatocellular carcinoma. Hepatology Research. 2015;**45**(2):128-141

[47] Jopling C. Liver-specific microRNA-122: Biogenesis and function. RNA Biology. 2012; **9**(2):137-142

[48] Wang B et al. Reciprocal regulation of microRNA-122 and c-Myc in hepatocellular cancer: Role of E2F1 and transcription factor dimerization partner 2. Hepatology. 2014; **59**(2):555-566

[49] Coulouarn C et al. Loss of miR-122 expression in liver cancer correlates with suppression of the hepatic phenotype and gain of metastatic properties. Oncogene. 2009;**28**(40):3526

[50] Zoni E et al. Epithelial plasticity in cancer: Unmasking a MicroRNA network for TGF-β-, Notch-, and Wnt-mediated EMT. Journal of Oncology. 2015;**2015**

[51] Liu S et al. MicroRNA-135a contributes to the development of portal vein tumor thrombus by promoting metastasis in hepatocellular carcinoma. Journal of Hepatology. 2012; **56**(2):389-396

[52] Kota SK, Balasubramanian S. Cancer therapy via modulation of micro RNA levels: A promising future. Drug Discovery Today. 2010;**15**(17-18):733-740

and were thus excluded from being considered as showing previous HBV infection; as a result, sixty patients were defined as having prior infection with HBV. The remaining 122 patients were not positive for any of HBsAg, HBcAb, or HBsAb. With the addition of the 5 vaccinated patients, a total of 127 patients were defined as showing no exposure to HBV. Clinical characteristics at baseline and outcomes such as SVR and incidence of HBV reactivation according to HBV infection status are shown in **Table 1**. No significant differences in clinical characteristics including age, sex, alanine aminotransferase, platelet count, HCV genotypes, and HCV viral load were evident between these three groups. SVR rate in HBV and HCV coinfected patients, HBV prior infection, and no exposure to HBV were 100, 95, and 97%, respectively. No significant differences in SVR were seen between groups. No cases representing definitive HBV reactivation were seen during and after DAA treatment. Clinical characteristics of the 12 patients with HBV and HCV coinfection are shown in **Table 2**. Concentrations of HBsAg were less than 100 IU/mL in most cases, and all titers of HBV-DNA were less than 5 log copies/mL. All patients were positive for hepatitis B e antibody (HBeAb). Four patients received entecavir (ETV) before DAA therapy.

4. Discussion

With the advent of novel agents for chemotherapy and immunotherapy, insufficient data have been accumulated regarding the incidence of HBV reactivation. The association between novel agents and HBV reactivation was noteworthy. At first glance, DAA therapy appears safe, since no HBV reactivation has been observed in several clinical trials. However, most clinical trials of DAA therapy for HCV infection have excluded patients with HBV coinfection, and this bias would obviously mask the incidence of HBV reactivation due to DAA therapy. Real-world experience has revealed HBV reactivation in patients with chronic hepatitis C treated using all-oral direct-acting antiviral regimens [13–16]. In the era of IFN-based therapy against HCV infection, HBV reactivation was not a noteworthy phenomenon for chronic hepatitis C. However, in the era of DAA therapy against HCV infection, HBV reactivation should be a concern in the treatment of patients with HCV infection. IFN rarely induces HBV reactivation, because IFN acts on both HBV and HCV, whereas DAAs act only on HCV. Viral interference between HCV and HBV is known to occur and HCV infection may suppress HBV replication. Rapid eradication of HCV by DAA would thus promote HBV replication and subsequent HBV reactivation. The small number of the total cohort and lack of incidence of HBV reactivation is of major concern for this study. Twelve patients infected with HBV and HCV were observed, and no cases showed definitive HBV reactivation during or after DAA treatment. Wang et al. reported that of 317 patients enrolled, 3 of the 10 patients with HBsAg showed HBV reactivation [18]. However, another study reported no evidence of HBV reactivation among patients treated with ledipasvir-sofosbuvir [19]. HBV reactivation thus remains controversial. Wang et al. speculated that DAAs, particularly NS3 polymerase inhibitors, carry a high risk of HBV reactivation because most reports of HBV reactivation related to DAA involved NS3 polymerase inhibitors [13, 14, 16, 18]. Ledipasvir is a NS5A replication complex inhibitor, and sofosbuvir is a NS5B polymerase inhibitor. The regimen with ledipasvir-sofosbuvir did not use NS3 polymerase inhibitors, which may be why their study found no cases of HBV reactivation. HBV reactivation induced by ledipasvir-sofosbuvir has been reported, in a patient infected with HIV who was receiving antiretroviral therapy including tenofovir [15]. However, that patient discontinued tenofovir because of osteoporosis 14 months before the onset of HBV reactivation. The effects of discontinuing tenofovir would thus have been relevant in that case. Further studies are needed to clarify whether HBV reactivation may occur irrespective of the class of DAA used. Another hypothesis that could explain the lack of HBV reactivation in this study was that the efficacy of prophylactic treatment with a nucleotide analog in preventing HBV reactivation among patients with HBV infection during and after chemotherapy and immunotherapy is well known. Four of twelve patients had received ETV before DAA therapy in our study and ETV would work as pre-emptive therapy in reducing the incidence of HBV reactivation. A second hypothesis for the absence of HBV reactivation in this study involves HBV status. All patients were negative for hepatitis B e antigen (HBeAg) and HBV-DNA titers were less than 5 log copies/mL. Several risk factors for HBV reactivation have been identified, including HBeAg positivity and high HBV DNA levels [20–22]. Thus, the majority of patients enrolled in our study were low-risk patients with HBeAg-negative status and low titers of HBV DNA.

We did not evaluate HBV genotypes in all patients because of low levels of both HBV DNA and HBsAg, but all our patients were Japanese, and we presumed the most prevalent types would be genotype B or C.

Two billion people have been exposed to HBV worldwide, and our study indicates that one-third of patients with HCV infection were defined as showing prior HBV infection. Most countries perform universal vaccination to prevent HBV infection, but only high-risk groups such as health care workers and household contacts of HBV carriers are selected for HBV vaccination in Japan [23]. Vaccinated patients were easily distinguished from those with resolved HBV infection in this study. Rituximab has become the standard of care for patients with malignant lymphoma, and HBV reactivation has also been reported in lymphoma patients with prior HBV infection [17]. A low level of HBV is well recognized as persisting in the liver and peripheral blood mononuclear cells in patients with resolved HBV infection and a functioning immune system. Immunosuppressive agents or chemotherapy may block the immune functions that suppress HBV replication, thus accelerating HBV replication. HBV reactivation thus occurred in patients with prior HBV infection. The incidence of HBV reactivation in patients with chronic hepatitis C treated by DAAs among patients with prior HBV infection is not yet fully understood, but we speculate that DAAs lead to HBV reactivation in patients with resolved HBV infection. However, we failed to identify any cases representing HBV reactivation among patients with resolved HBV infection in this study. We have previously report a case of acute hepatitis B in a patient with HCV infection after DAA therapy [16]. However, the presence of HBcAb or HBsAb was not determined before DAA therapy, so prior HBV infection status was unclear. This case is speculated to represent HBV reactivation in a patient with previously resolved HBV induced by DAA therapy, based on virologic analysis and clinical status. Amino acid substitutions in the S region as immune escape mutants and minority patterns for HBV genotype and serological subtype were virologic features of HBV reactivation [24, 25]. DAAs were suspected to induce HBV reactivation, and effective strategies to prevent HBV reactivation are needed. However, data on the incidence of HBV reactivation with DAA therapy are limited. Larger studies are needed to establish whether the risk of HBV reactivation is increased during and after DAA therapy.

Several factors have been identified, including age, liver fibrosis, HCV genotype, HCV RNA levels, race, amino acid substitutions in the core and NS5A regions, and interleukin 28B polymorphisms have been reported as predictors of response to IFN therapy [26–31]. This study investigated whether HBV coinfection affects response to DAA therapy. However, HBV infection was not associated with SVR from DAA therapy. DAA could eradicate over 95% of HCV, and identification of predictors for SVR is difficult. The limitation of the present study was the small sample size, and larger prospective cohorts are needed to confirm our results.

In conclusion, although relatively few cases have been reported in the literature, we suggest caution regarding HBV reactivation in HCV and HBV coinfected patients undergoing treatment with DAA.

Acknowledgements

This study received a research grant from AMED. Hidemi Goto received research grants from Abbvie, AstraZeneca, Astellas Pharma, Bristol-Myers Squibb, Chugai Pharmaceutical Co, Daiichi Sankyo, Dainippon Sumitomo Pharma, Mitsubishi Tanabe Pharma, MSD, Otsuka Pharmaceutical Co, and Takeda Pharmaceutical Co.

Author details

Kazuhiko Hayashi[1], Masatoshi Ishigami[1*], Yoji Ishizu[1], Teiji Kuzuya[1], Takashi Honda[1], Yoshihiko Tachi[2], Tetsuya Ishikawa[1], Yoshiaki Katano[3], Kentaro Yoshioka[4], Hidenori Toyoda[5], Takashi Kumada[5], Hidemi Goto[1] and Yoshiki Hirooka[1]

*Address all correspondence to: masaishi@med.nagoya-u.ac.jp

1 Department of Gastroenterology and Hepatology, Nagoya University Graduate School of Medicine, Nagoya, Japan

2 Department of Gastroenterology, Komaki City Hospital, Komaki, Japan

3 Department of Internal Medicine, Banbuntane Hotokukai Hospital, Fujita Health University, School of Medicine, Nagoya, Japan

4 Division of Liver and Biliary Diseases, Department of Internal Medicine, Fujita Health University, Toyoake, Japan

5 Department of Gastroenterology, Ogaki Municipal Hospital, Ogaki, Japan

References

[1] Seeff LB. Natural history of chronic hepatitis C. Hepatology. 2002;36:S35-S46. DOI: 10.1053/jhep.2002.36806

[2] Kumada H, Suzuki Y, Ikeda K, Toyota J, Karino Y, Chayama K, Kawakami Y, Ido A, Yamamoto K, Takaguchi K, Izumi N, Koike K, Takehara T, Kawada N, Sata M, Miyagoshi H, Eley T, McPhee F, Damokosh A, Ishikawa H, Hughes E. Daclatasvir plus asunaprevir for chronic HCV genotype 1b infection. Hepatology. 2014 Jun;59(6):2083-2091. DOI: 10.1002/hep.27113

[3] Mizokami M, Yokosuka O, Takehara T, Sakamoto N, Korenaga M, Mochizuki H, Nakane K, Enomoto H, Ikeda F, Yanase M, Toyoda H, Genda T, Umemura T, Yatsuhashi H, Ide T, Toda N, Nirei K, Ueno Y, Nishigaki Y, Betular J, Gao B, Ishizaki A, Omote M, Mo H, Garrison K, Pang PS, Knox SJ, Symonds WT, McHutchison JG, Izumi N, Omata M. Ledipasvir and sofosbuvir fixed-dose combination with and without ribavirin for 12 weeks in treatment-naive and previously treated Japanese patients with genotype 1 hepatitis C: An open-label, randomised, phase 3 trial. The Lancet Infectious Diseases. 2015 Jun;15(6):645-653. DOI: 10.1016/S1473-3099(15)70099-X

[4] Kumada H, Chayama K, Rodrigues L Jr, Suzuki F, Ikeda K, Toyoda H, Sato K, Karino Y, Matsuzaki Y, Kioka K, Setze C, Pilot-Matias T, Patwardhan M, Vilchez RA, Burroughs M, Redman R. Randomized phase 3 trial of ombitasvir/paritaprevir/ritonavir for hepatitis C virus genotype 1b-infected Japanese patients with or without cirrhosis. Hepatology. 2015 Oct;62(4):1037-1046. DOI: 10.1002/hep.27972

[5] Sulkowski M, Hezode C, Gerstoft J, Vierling JM, Mallolas J, Pol S, Kugelmas M, Murillo A, Weis N, Nahass R, Shibolet O, Serfaty L, Bourliere M, DeJesus E, Zuckerman E, Dutko F, Shaughnessy M, Hwang P, Howe AY, Wahl J, Robertson M, Barr E, Haber B. Efficacy and safety of 8 weeks versus 12 weeks of treatment with grazoprevir (MK-5172) and elbasvir (MK-8742) with or without ribavirin in patients with hepatitis C virus genotype 1 mono-infection and HIV/hepatitis C virus co-infection (C-WORTHY): A randomised, open-label phase 2 trial. Lancet. 2015 Mar 21;385(9973):1087-1097. DOI: 10.1016/S0140-6736(14)61793-1

[6] Forns X, Gordon SC, Zuckerman E, Lawitz E, Calleja JL, Hofer H, Gilbert C, Palcza J, Howe AY, DiNubile MJ, Robertson MN, Wahl J, Barr E, Buti M. Grazoprevir and elbasvir plus ribavirin for chronic HCV genotype-1 infection after failure of combination therapy containing a direct-acting antiviral agent. Journal of Hepatology. 2015 Sep;63(3):564-572. DOI: 10.1016/j.jhep.2015.04.009

[7] Roth D, Nelson DR, Bruchfeld A, Liapakis A, Silva M, Monsour H Jr, Martin P, Pol S, Londoño MC, Hassanein T, Zamor PJ, Zuckerman E, Wan S, Jackson B, Nguyen BY, Robertson M, Barr E, Wahl J, Greaves W. Grazoprevir plus elbasvir in treatment-naive and treatment-experienced patients with hepatitis C virus genotype 1 infection and stage 4-5 chronic kidney disease (the C-SURFER study): a combination phase 3 study. Lancet. 2015 Oct 17;386(10003):1537-1545. DOI: 10.1016/S0140-6736(15)00349-9

[8]   Leroy V, Dumortier J, Coilly A, Sebagh M, Fougerou-Leurent C, Radenne S, Botta D, Durand F, Silvain C, Lebray P, Houssel-Debry P, Kamar N, D'Alteroche L, Petrov-Sanchez V, Diallo A, Pageaux GP, Duclos-Vallee JC, Agence Nationale de Recherches sur le SIDA et les Hépatites Virales CO23 Compassionate Use of Protease Inhibitors in Viral C in Liver Transplantation Study Group. Efficacy of Sofosbuvir and Daclatasvir in patients with Fibrosing Cholestatic hepatitis C after liver transplantation. Clinical Gastroenterology and Hepatology. 2015 Nov;13(11):1993-2001. DOI: 10.1016/j.cgh.2015.05.030

[9]   Grebely J, Mauss S, Brown A, Bronowicki JP, Puoti M, Wyles D, Natha M, Zhu Y, Yang J, Kreter B, Brainard DM, Yun C, Carr V, Dore GJ. Efficacy and safety of Ledipasvir/ Sofosbuvir with and without ribavirin in patients with chronic HCV genotype 1 infection receiving opioid substitution therapy: Analysis of phase 3 ION trials. Clinical Infectious Diseases. 2016 Dec 1;63(11):1405-1411. DOI: 10.1093/cid/ciw580

[10] Akuta N, Sezaki H, Suzuki F, Fujiyama S, Kawamura Y, Hosaka T, Kobayashi M, Kobayashi M, Saitoh S, Suzuki Y, Arase Y, Ikeda K, Kumada H. Retreatment efficacy and predictors of ledipasvir plus sofosbuvir to HCV genotype 1 in Japan. Journal of Medical Virology. 2017 Feb;89(2):284-290. DOI: 10.1002/jmv.24617

[11] Wands JR, Chura CM, Roll FJ, Maddrey WC. Serial studies of hepatitis associated anti-gen and antibody in patients receiving antitumor chemotherapy for myeloproliferative and lymphoproliferative disorders. Gastroenterology. 1975;68:105-112

[12] Hoofnagle JH, Dusheiko GM, Schafer DF, Jones EA, Micetich KC, Young RC, Costa J. Reactivation of chronic hepatitis B virus infection by cancer chemotherapy. Annals of Internal Medicine. 1982;96:447-449

[13] Collins JM, Raphael KL, Terry C, Cartwright EJ, Pillai A, Anania FA, Farley MM. Hepatitis B virus reactivation during successful treatment of hepatitis C virus with sofosbuvir and simeprevir. Clinical Infectious Diseases. 2015;61:1304-1306. DOI: 10.1093/cid/civ474

[14] Takayama H, Sato T, Ikeda F, Fujiki S. Reactivation of hepatitis B virus during interferon-free therapy with daclatasvir and asunaprevir in patient with hepatitis B virus/hepatitis C virus co-infection. Hepatology Research. 2016 Mar;46(5):489-491. DOI: 10.1111/hepr.12578

[15] De Monte A, Courjon J, Anty R, Cua E, Naqvi A, Mondain V, Cottalorda J, Ollier L, Giordanengo V. Direct-acting antiviral treatment in adults infected with hepatitis C virus: Reactivation of hepatitis B virus coinfection as a further challenge. Journal of Clinical Virology. 2016;78:27-30. DOI: 10.1016/j.jcv.2016.02.026

[16] Hayashi K, Ishigami M, Ishizu Y, Kuzuya T, Honda T, Nishimura D, Goto H, Hirooka Y. A case of acute hepatitis B in a chronic hepatitis C patient after daclatasvir and asunaprevir combination therapy: Hepatitis B virus reactivation or acute self-limited hepatitis? Clinical Journal of Gastroenterology. 2016 Aug;9(4):252-256. DOI: 10.1007/s12328-016-0657-4

[17] Dervite I, Hober D, Morel P. Acute hepatitis B in a patient with antibodies to hepatitis B surface antigen who was receiving rituximab. The New England Journal of Medicine. 2001;344:68-69. DOI: 10.1056/NEJM200101043440120

[18] Wang C, Ji D, Chen J, Shao Q, Li B, Liu J, Wu V, Wong A, Wang Y, Zhang X, Lu L, Wong C, Tsang S, Zhang Z, Sun J, Hou J, Chen G, Lau G. Hepatitis due to reactivation of hepatitis B virus in endemic areas among patients with hepatitis C treated with direct-acting antiviral agents. Clinical Gastroenterology and Hepatology. 2017 Jan;15(1):132-136. DOI: 10.1016/j.cgh.2016.06.023

[19] Sulkowski MS, Chuang WL, Kao JH, Yang JC, Gao B, Brainard DM, Han KH, Gane E. No evidence of reactivation of hepatitis B virus among patients treated with Ledipasvir-Sofosbuvir for hepatitis C virus infection. Clinical Infectious Diseases. 2016 Nov 1;63(9):1202-1204. DOI: 10.1093/cid/ciw507

[20] Yeo W, Chan PK, Zhong S, Ho WM, Steinberg JL, Tam JS, Hui P, Leung NW, Zee B, Johnson PJ. Frequency of hepatitis B virus reactivation in cancer patients undergoing cytotoxic chemotherapy: A prospective study of 626 patients with identification of risk factors. Journal of Medical Virology. 2000;62:299-307

[21] Lau GK, Leung YH, Fong DY, Au WY, Kwong YL, Lie A, Hou JL, Wen YM, Nanj A, Liang R. High hepatitis B virus (HBV) DNA viral load as the most important risk factor for HBV reactivation in patients positive for HBV surface antigen undergoing autologous hematopoietic cell transplantation. Blood. 2002;99(7):2324-2330

[22] Zhong S, Yeo W, Schroder C, Chan PK, Wong WL, Ho WM, Mo F, Zee B, Johnson PJ. High hepatitis B virus (HBV) DNA viral load is an important risk factor for HBV reactivation in breast cancer patients undergoing cytotoxic chemotherapy. Journal of Viral Hepatitis. 2004;11:55-59

[23] Zanetti AR, Van Damme P, Shouval D. The global impact of vaccination against hepatitis B: A historical overview. Vaccine. 2008;26:6266-6273. DOI: 10.1016/j.vaccine.2008.09.056

[24] Salpini R, Colagrossi L, Bellocchi MC, Surdo M, Becker C, Alteri C, Aragri M, Ricciardi A, Armenia D, Pollicita M, Di Santo F, Carioti L, Louzoun Y, Mastroianni CM, Lichtner M, Paoloni M, Esposito M, D'Amore C, Marrone A, Marignani M, Sarrecchia C, Sarmati L, Andreoni M, Angelico M, Verheyen J, Perno CF, Svicher V. Hepatitis B surface antigen genetic elements critical for immune escape correlate with hepatitis B virus reactivation upon immunosuppression. Hepatology. 2015;61:823-833. DOI: 10.1002/hep.27604

[25] Hayashi K, Ishigami M, Ishizu Y, Kuzuya T, Honda T, Tachi Y, Ishikawa T, Katano Y, Yoshioka K, Toyoda H, Kumada T, Goto H, Hirooka Y. Clinical characteristics and molecular analysis of hepatitis B virus reactivation in hepatitis B surface antigen-negative patients during or after immunosuppressive or cytotoxic chemotherapy. Journal of Gastroenterology. 2016 Nov;51(11):1081-1089. DOI: 10.1007/s00535-016-1187-z

[26] Berg T, Sarrazin C, Herrmann E, Hinrichsen H, Gerlach T, Zachoval R, Wiedenmann B, Hopf U, Zeuzem S. Prediction of treatment outcome in patients with chronic hepatitis C: Significance of baseline parameters and viral dynamics during therapy. Hepatology. 2003;37:600-609. DOI: 10.1053/jhep.2003.50106

[27]   Conjeevaram HS, Kleiner DE, Everhart JE, Hoofnagle JH, Zacks S, Afdhal NH, Wahed AS, Virahep-C Study Group. Race, insulin resistance and hepatic steatosis in chronic hepatitis C. Hepatology. 2007 Jan;45(1):80-87. DOI: 10.1002/hep.21455

[28]   Tanaka Y, Nishida N, Sugiyama M, Kurosaki M, Matsuura K, Sakamoto N, Nakagawa M, Korenaga M, Hino K, Hige S, Ito Y, Mita E, Tanaka E, Mochida S, Murawaki Y, Honda M, Sakai A, Hiasa Y, Nishiguchi S, Koike A, Sakaida I, Imamura M, Ito K, Yano K, Masaki N, Sugauchi F, Izumi N, Tokunaga K, Mizokami M. Genome-wide association of IL28B with response to pegylated interferon-alpha and ribavirin therapy for chronic hepatitis C. Nature Genetics. 2009;41:1105-1109. DOI: 10.1038/ng.449

[29]   Akuta N, Suzuki F, Kawamura Y, Yatsuji H, Sezaki H, Suzuki Y, Hosaka T, Kobayashi M, Kobayashi M, Arase Y, Ikeda K, Kumada H. Predictive factors of early and sustained responses to peginterferon plus ribavirin combination therapy in Japanese patients infected with hepatitis C virus genotype 1b: Amino acid substitutions in the core region and low-density lipoprotein cholesterol levels. Journal of Hepatology. 2007;46:403-410. DOI: 10.1016/j.jhep.2006.09.019

[30]   Honda T, Katano Y, Shimizu J, Ishizu Y, Doizaki M, Hayashi K, Ishigami M, Itoh A, Hirooka Y, Nakano I, Urano F, Yoshioka K, Toyoda H, Kumada T, Goto H. Efficacy of peginterferon-alpha-2b plus ribavirin in patients aged 65 years and older with chronic hepatitis C. Liver International. 2010;30:527-537. DOI: 10.1111/j.1478-3231.2009.02064.x

[31]   Hayashi K, Katano Y, Honda T, Ishigami M, Itoh A, Hirooka Y, Ishikawa T, Nakano I, Yoshioka K, Toyoda H, Kumada T, Goto H. Association of interleukin 28B and mutations in the core and NS5A region of hepatitis C virus with response to peg-interferon and ribavirin therapy. Liver International. 2011 Oct;31(9):1359-1365. DOI: 10.1111/j.1478-3231.2011.02571.x

9

Approaches and Considerations for the Successful Treatment of HCV Infection

Robert Smolić, Jelena Jakab, Lucija Kuna,
Martina Smolić, Martina Kajić, Marinko Žulj and
Aleksandar Včev

Abstract

The complexity of the hepatitis C virus (HCV) infection is reflected in its therapy, and great efforts are needed from the patient and the physician to be successful in eliminating the infection. How HCV will progress depends a lot on patient characteristics and social factors, in addition to the timing of initiation, duration, and final results of the therapy. The first treatment approved for patients with chronic hepatitis C was interferon (IFN) which had a sustained viral response (SVR) rate in 20%. Due to side effects, the adherence to this treatment was limited and required a patient-tailored approach with various medical disciplines working together and intervening at the right time to minimize potential obstacles. The introduction of direct-acting antivirals (DAAs) has contributed to the advancement of HCV treatment. However, a major obstacle to wide use of DAAs is their high price which has largely limited access to treatment. Guidelines and recommendations on treatment of hepatitis C have been developed to assist physicians and other health care providers to determine priority. Despite that, the arrival of new oral therapies has been met with enthusiasm as shorter, simpler, safer treatment allows for the possibility of delivering antiviral therapy on a large scale.

Keywords: HCV treatment, patient-tailored approach, treatment development, treatment goals, treatment priority

1. Introduction

Nowadays, the complexity of HCV infection is reflected in its therapy, and great efforts are needed from the patient and the treating physician. As a chronic disease with potential progression to fibrosis and HCV-associated cirrhosis, therapy of HCV in patients with liver disease and post-liver transplant patients represents a challenge for physicians. Initiation, duration, and final results of the therapy depend on various factors such as viral factors, patient characteristics, and numerous social factors. The patient-tailored approach and close patient-physician cooperation as well as the role of various medical disciplines working together and intervening at the right time is important to decrease the potential barrier in the achieving an SVR.

2. HCV infection: complexity of infection

HCV is a single-stranded positive-sense RNA virus which belongs to the genus *Hepacivirus* of the Flaviviridae family. The most significant nonstructural (NS) proteins involved in virus replication include the NS3 helicase, NS3-NS4A serine protease, and the NS5B RNA-dependent RNA polymerase [1]. There are six known genotypes and a single known case of genotype 7 and more than 50 subtypes. Because the highest prevalence of genotype 1 is found in the most of middle-income countries, many DAAs have been primarily developed for use in those countries. Some DAAs are effective against multiple HCV genotypes. They are less effective for genotype 3 and cirrhosis [2].

The most significant clinical problems of chronic hepatitis C (CHC) involve the development of liver cirrhosis, hepatocellular carcinoma (HCC), or the need for liver transplantation [3, 4]. Progression of liver disease is more likely in patients with older age, male sex, longer duration of infection, advanced histologic stage and grade, genotype 1, increased hepatic iron, concomitant liver disorders, HIV infection, and obesity [5]. As many as 74% of people suffer from extrahepatic manifestations, and fatigue is the most common symptom. There are immune complex–mediated extrahepatic complications, glomerulonephritis, lymphoproliferative disorders such as B-cell lymphoma and extrahepatic complications unrelated to immune-complex injury (Sjögren's syndrome, lichen planus, porphyria cutanea tarda, type-II diabetes mellitus, and the metabolic syndrome) [2].

Recurrence of HCV following liver transplant occurs in more than 95% of patients and reinfection occurs within 72 h [2]. Not all patients can receive therapy instantly on the approval of new agents, so priority should be given to those patients with the most urgent necessity [6]. About 80% of patients treated with interferon-based treatment experience adverse effects. Hence, the close monitoring, timely preventive, therapeutic measures, and patient motivation are needed. Furthermore, adverse effects vary between drugs and range from poor general well-being to specific conditions affecting hematopoiesis, skin, behavior, thyroid, eyes, or lungs, and therefore, a multidisciplinary approach is necessary [7].

3. HCV treatment options goals and timeline development

CHC caused by infection with HCV is one of the major causes of liver disease. The goal of hepatitis C treatment is to achieve SVR defined as no detectable HCV in blood at least 12 weeks after finishing treatment. If a durable SVR can be achieved, the risks for liver-related morbidity and mortality are decreased [2].

In infected patients, IFN-mediated immune response is associated with the induction of IFN-stimulated genes (ISGs) in the liver [9] during the first 4–10 weeks of infection. This is followed by an HCV-specific T cell response [8]. However, the virus persists in 80% of infected patients. To boost the immune response, in 1989, interferon-alfa (IFN-α) was first developed, and in the decades that followed IFN-α, monotherapy was the standard therapy for hepatitis C. While developing the best regimen, various doses and durations of treatment were tested, but SVR rates remained modest (15–20%) [8].

The natural history of the HCV does not differ significantly among genotypes. However, HCV genotype 3 induces liver steatosis more often than the other genotypes. Patients with different genotypes can differ in their response to treatment with recombinant IFN-α and DAAs. Treatment efficacy has shown progressive improvement following the pegylation of IFN-α and its effect in combination with other antiviral drugs. However, viral escape mechanisms, IFN-α signaling in the liver, and substantial drug toxicity still restricted the efficacy of this treatment [9]. The restricted efficacy of IFN-α treatments stimulated considerable research efforts of academia and industry with the aim of understanding the mechanisms of nonresponse to IFN-α [10]. Recently, numerous studies showed association between genetic variants near the IFNL3 known as IL28B gene and the response to IFN-α treatments [11]. The molecular mechanisms that link genetic variation in the IFNL3 gene locus to the response to IFN-α remains to be investigated [12].

Combining IFN-α with ribavirin (RBV) became the new standard therapy in 1998. RBV had been used as a monotherapy for CHC in the 1990s, and it was discovered to transiently decrease serum alanine aminotransferase (ALT) levels during therapy [13, 14]. Subcutaneously injected interferon-α2b (INF-α2b) with daily oral RBV achieved an SVR in 38%. SVR was 54–56% after pegylated INF α (PEG-INF) was introduced. Until 2011, when the interferon-free era began, hepatitis C was treated with 6–12 months of weekly PEG-INF injections and twice-daily RBV tablets [2, 8]. Oral DAAs have simplified treatment procurement and delivery and improved HCV treatment outcomes. Numerous trials of interferon-free, oral DAA regimens have reported cure rate of more than 85% regardless of HCV genotype, many in only 12 weeks [5]. To date, it is assumed that high serum concentrations of IFN-α which are obtained after therapy with PEG-INF ensure a crucial advantage compared with nonpegylated forms of recombinant IFN-α [9].

In 2014, four classes of DAAs were described: NS3/4A protease inhibitors, non-nucleoside polymerase inhibitors, nucleoside/tide polymerase inhibitors, and NS5A inhibitors [5]. In general, DAA regimens are better tolerated and more effective than PEG-IFN and RBV. Boceprevir and telaprevir—two HCV protease inhibitors—were developed to be given in combination with RBV and PEG-IFN. This combination prevented emergence of HCV mutants with genetic resistance to the protease inhibitors. For the first time, an SVR could be achieved in more than 75% of individuals that were infected with the HCV genotype 1 [15, 16]. HCV non-nucleoside polymerase inhibitors (dasabuvir) are twice-daily drugs developed primarily for genotype1 [17, 18]. HCV nucleoside/tide polymerase inhibitors, such as sofosbuvir, are taken once daily and generally have a pangenotypic activity, potency, high resistance barrier, and low propensity for drug-drug interactions. HCV NS5A inhibitors

1989	1998	2001	2011	2013	2014			
IFNα	IFNα and ribavirin	peglFNα and ribavirin	peglFNα and ribavirin, telaprevir or boceprevir	Sofosbuvir. Used with peglFNα and RBV, or RBV alone;simeprevir or daclatasvir, with or without RBV	Simeprevir. Used with peglFNα and RBV, or sofosbuvir, with or without RBV	Daclatasvir. Used with peglFNα and RBV orsofosbuvir, with or without RBV	Sofosbuvir/ ledipasvir. Used with or without RBV	Ombitasvir/ paritaprevir/ ritonavir plus dasabuvir. Used with or without RBV

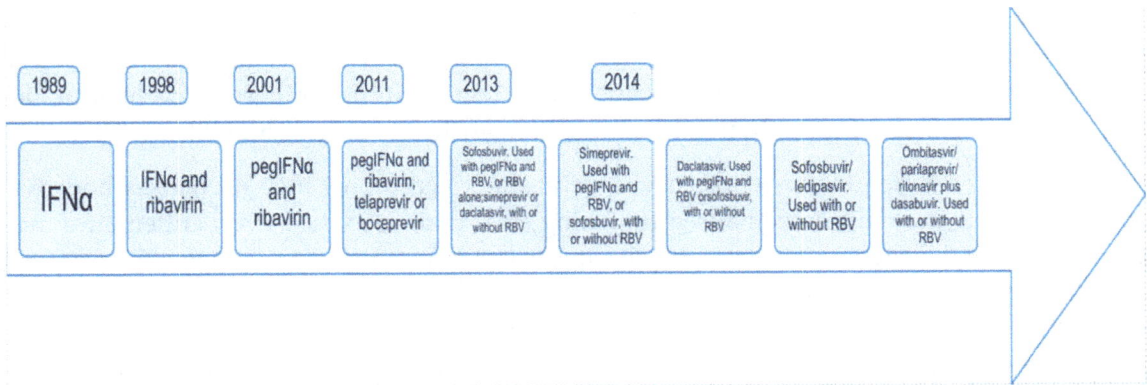

Figure 1. HCV Therapeutic Timeline.

(daclatasvir, ledipasvir, and ombitasvir) are novel drug class that are potent and have low barrier to resistance (**Figure 1**). So further research is needed to prevent or overcome drug resistance. On the other hand, daclatasvir and ledipasvir are pangenotypic and are well suited for combination with other DAAs [16].

4. Approach considerations in the IFN treatment era

Adherence to therapy is one of the most important factors for successful therapy [19]. It is important to reduce side effects and motivate patients to adhere to treatment in favor of optimizing treatment responses [20]. Due in part to the side effects, the adherence to interferon-based HCV treatment was limited, resulting in dosage reduction and sometimes discontinuation of therapy, which led to the frequent virus breakthrough [21]. Historically, the most predominant side effects have consisted of "flu"-like symptoms: fatigue, myalgia, fever, insomnia, and weakness [22]. Although up to two-thirds of patients complained of fatigue, it is important that the clinician distinguishes it from severe anemia, depression, or other metabolic disorders [23]. The "flu"-like symptoms were usually easily managed and did not lead to treatment discontinuation. On the other hand, cytopenias, particularly anemia, were the most troublesome side-effect, causing drug-dose reduction and early treatment discontinuation [24]. In addition, patients with HCV had other conditions that required treatment with medications that could cause hematologic toxicities. For that reason, a multifaceted approach was required, such as pretreatment screening, cardiac, and hematologic consultations when necessary, frequent laboratory monitoring, and dose reductions [25]. Erythropoietin and blood transfusions, as well as aggressive RBV dosage reductions, are effective for managing anemia [26].

Various types of dermatologic manifestations, such as dry skin and pruritus, have been reported during anti-HCV therapy. Dermatologic side effects seriously affect the skin barrier, quality of life, and sleep. A break in the skin can be the point of entry for a bacterial infection. Injection site reactions from interferon-based therapies may occur typically characterized by

local tenderness, erythema, and itching [27]. It is wise to eliminate any unnecessary medications before HCV therapy and to recommend good skin hygiene. For patients who develop
drug-related rash, use of topical antipruritics or systemic antihistamines can be helpful, but
sometimes dermatology consultation is required for further management [28].

Some of the most frequently reported gastrointestinal symptoms include nausea and dysgeusia. Patients may minimize nausea by taking RBV with food; however, antiemetics may
be needed [25]. Dysgeusia is treated by sipping water frequently. To maintain salivary flow
and oral hygiene, oral ointments and mouth washes are used [29]. Anal discomfort, with
or without diarrhea, may respond to barrier creams and hemorrhoidal ointments. Patients
presenting with a rectal bleed and abdominal pain should be worked-up for ischemic colitis,
which can be diagnosed by CT scan with contrast or colonoscopy [30].

Psychiatric effects of HCV therapy are relatively preventable through symptom monitoring,
frequent visits to assess clinical improvement, the use of selective serotonin reuptake inhibitors, and IFN dose reduction when needed. Patients who develop severe depression should
be taken off HCV therapy because suicide has been reported on combination therapy [31]. The
health care provider should observe symptoms that could be related to depression, such as
sleep disturbance, irritability, and decreased memory. Early consultation with a psychiatrist
is of great importance for defining a psychiatric diagnosis, selecting a treatment, and educat-
ing the patient about treatment expectations [32].

There are many ways a health care provider can help the patient manage side effects of the
treatment. A gentle modification of behavior or routine medical therapy is often the first step,
followed by dose reduction or adding additional medications. Patients are advised to rest
when required and to maintain a regular daily schedule. Also, encouraging physical activity
may help maintain emotional balance and promote energy levels [33]. Maintaining hydration
is important in boosting a sense of well-being. Providing a support network, such as availability of nurses and an after-hours telephone health link, improves adherence to treatment and
patient satisfaction. Additionally, the right timing and the adequate injection of the PEG-INF
injection can be helpful [29].

Patient quality of life (QOL) during HCV treatment affects medication adherence [34], which
is why it is necessary to think broadly about treatment management. In a study conducted by
Manos et al., serious financial consequences of the HCV treatment (job loss, decreased work
hours, difficulty paying for medications) were reported by 34.8% patients [35]. Over half of
the patients reported difficulty attending social functions. When asked to rank how helpful
different types of support might be for future patients undergoing treatment, the most highly
ranked options were more frequent provider contact by telephone and peer support availability. Overall, patients were more satisfied with a care provided by a nurse or clinical pharma-
cist rather than by physicians. Others have reported frustration with communication among
physicians and communication between the patient and the physician [36]. Furthermore, a
common desire among patients was access to multidisciplinary services [35]. Communication
quality is impacted by the time limitation of providers. To address such limitations, some
healthcare systems rely on nurse practitioners and physician assistants to care for patients
with hepatitis C [37]. The importance of nurses in patient QOL during HCV treatment and

their support has been rated highly [38]. Mental health providers are also helpful to maintain HCV treatment adherence, and a pilot study suggests effectiveness of the weekly telephone meetings with a mental health professional [39]. Other studies and guidelines suggest that interdisciplinary, integrated care models can help optimizing HCV treatment [40, 41].

In conclusion, the treatment of HCV should be undertaken by physicians with a broad clinical knowledge. Close clinical follow-up of patients is needed for early recognition and appropriate management of most of the side effects. Prescreening patients for potential clinical problems is crucial part of side effects anticipation which leads to involving specialists in a timely manner. The HCV provider is able to address side effects and monitor the efficacy of the regimen when patient visits twice monthly, at least in the beginning of therapy. Moreover, successful adherence to treatment can be enhanced by a strong support network, which includes specially trained hepatitis nurses and a multidisciplinary team consisting of pharmacists, counselors, and social workers.

5. Approach considerations in the IFN-free treatment era

The protease inhibitor boceprevir was approved in 2011, followed by the approval of telaprevir [42]. A third protease inhibitor, simeprevir, was approved in 2013 and is recommended as a part of combination therapy for chronic HCV infection. More recently, NS5B polymerase inhibitor sofosbuvir has emerged as an important component of currently recommended regimens [43]. In 2014, the FDA approved an all-oral regimen of simeprevir plus sofosbuvir for treatment-naïve or treatment-experienced patients [44]. DAAs are effective regardless of race, gender, or HIV status [45, 46]. They have few side effects, short durations of treatment, and high SVRs. Therefore, DAAs have the potential to lower mortality, improve QOL, and reduce long-term costs of complications in HCV infected individuals [47]. This is why every patient with chronic HCV infection should be considered for antiviral treatment with DAA agents, even if previous interferon-based therapy has failed [48].

There are certain settings where limited access to medications forces health practitioner to decide which patient should be treated first. In circumstances like this, practitioners rely on evidence-based medicine and guidelines. Treatment for CHC is based on guidelines from the Infectious Diseases Society of America (IDSA) and the American Associations for the Study of Liver Diseases (AASLD) [49]. Recommendations are evidence based and are constantly updated as new data from peer-reviewed evidence become available. The guidelines propose that treatment priority should be given to those with the most urgent need. The recommendations include the following:

1. The highest priority for treatment should be given to the patients with advanced fibrosis, compensated cirrhosis, and severe extrahepatic hepatitis, as well as liver transplant recipients.

2. Patients with high priority for treatment are the ones at high risk for liver-related complications and severe extrahepatic hepatitis C complications.

3. Certain subgroups of HCV patients, such as men who have high-risk sex with men, active injection drug users, incarcerated persons, and those on hemodialysis are patients whose risk of HCV transmission is high, and in whom, HCV treatment may result in a reduction in

transmission. In those patients, treatment decisions should balance the anticipated reduction in transmission versus the likelihood of reinfection.

Although antiviral therapy for CHC should be determined on a case-by-case basis, treatment is widely recommended for patients with elevated ALT levels who meet the following criteria [50]: older than 18 years, positive HCV antibody and serum HCV RNA, compensated liver disease, adequate hematologic and biochemical indices, willingness, and adherence to treatment, without contraindications.

In Europe, EASL Recommendations on Treatment of Hepatitis C assist physicians and other healthcare providers in the clinical decision-making process by providing information about the current optimal management of patients with acute and chronic HCV infections [51]. The recommendations have been based on evidence from existing publications and presentations at international meetings and the expert personal experiences. According to EASL, all treatment-naïve and treatment-experienced patients with compensated or decompensated chronic liver disease related to HCV, who have no contraindications to treatment, must be considered for therapy. The treatment must be available without delay in patients with significant fibrosis or cirrhosis, including decompensated cirrhosis; patients with clinically significant extrahepatic manifestations (e.g., symptomatic vasculitis, mixed cryoglobulinemia, nephropathy, and non-Hodgkin B-cell lymphoma); patients with HCV recurrence after liver transplantation; patients with concurrent comorbidities who are at risk of a rapid evolution of liver disease (non-liver solid organ or stem cell transplant recipients, diabetes); and individuals at risk of transmitting HCV (active injection drug users, men who have sex with men with high-risk sexual practices, women of childbearing age who wish to get pregnant, hemodialysis patients, incarcerated individuals) [51].

Prior to initiating DAA therapy, patients should undergo a thorough pre-treatment evaluation, which includes identifying the genotype of hepatitis C, evidence of cirrhosis, and previous treatment. Comorbid physical or psychological conditions should be optimized before commencing therapy because it will improve compliance. Evaluation for advanced fibrosis is recommended for all persons with HCV infection [49]. Another important consideration before starting therapy is the possibility of drug-drug interactions, as well as severe renal impairment [48].

Treatment of chronic HCV infection has two goals: to achieve SVR and to prevent progression of cirrhosis, hepatocellular carcinoma, and decompensated liver disease which can lead to the liver transplantation [49]. Patients who achieve an SVR experience numerous health benefits, including a decrease in liver inflammation levels, a reduction in the rate of progression of liver fibrosis [52], and reduced symptoms and mortality from severe extrahepatic manifestations [53]. Patients with normal liver function tests after SVR can be managed as if they had never been infected with HCV. Individuals who have failed to achieve SVR must be given an opportunity to pursue further therapeutic options [48].

6. Approach considerations in the near future

Currently, access to treatment for HCV is limited, with only a minority diagnosed patients, and even fewer assessed are initiated on treatment [54]. HCV therapy has the potential to ensure individual and health benefits, but high prices have stopped access to HCV therapy, even in high income countries and to people with advanced liver disease. If DAAs are to stop HCV-related mortality and decrease the global burden of HCV infection in the coming years, current HCV treatment rates of 1% to <5% must be increased [55]. Treating patients with fibrosis will decrease morbidity and mortality of HCV, but unless patients without advanced liver disease are treated too, the epidemic of HCV will continue [56].

7. Conclusion

Key desirable characteristics of the HCV therapy include high efficacy, tolerability, pan-genotypic activity, short duration, oral administration, affordability, and fixed-dose combination. The major reasons for limited treatment access are the cost, complexity, and limited effectiveness of treatment, as well as lack of access to reliable and affordable diagnostics. The improved safety profile and improved efficacy across genotypes of the new DAAs make the pre-treatment screening simple. In the future, HCV treatment could be initiated immediately after confirmation of infection and the presence of viremia, with only an initial assessment of the stage of liver disease. Future development of pan-genotypic regimens with minimal side effects that will be available at an affordable price holds the greatest potential for expanding access to treatment to all HCV patients.

Author details

Robert Smolić[1,2]*, Jelena Jakab[2], Lucija Kuna[2], Martina Smolić[2], Martina Kajić[3], Marinko Žulj[2] and Aleksandar Včev[1,2]

*Address all correspondence to: robert.smolic@mefos.hr

1 University Hospital Center Osijek, Osijek, Croatia

2 Faculty of Medicine, Josip Juraj Strossmayer University of Osijek, Osijek, Croatia

3 Pharmaceutical Company Pliva, Zagreb, Croatia

References

[1] Poustchi H, Esmaili S, Mohamadkhani A, Nikmahzar A, Pourshams A, Sepanlou SG, et al. The impact of illicit drug use on spontaneous hepatitis C clearance: Experience from a large cohort population study. PloS One. 2011;**6**(8):

[2] Longo DL, Kasper DL, Jameson JL, Fauci AS, Hauser SL, Loscalzo J. Harrison's Principles of Internal Medicine. USA: McGraw Hill Medical; 2012.

[3] Lee MH, Yang HI, SN L, Jen CL, You SL, Wang LY, et al. Chronic hepatitis C virus infection increases mortality from hepatic and extrahepatic diseases: A community-based long-term prospective study. The Journal of Infectious Diseases. 2012;**206**(4):469-477

[4] Maasoumy B, Wedemeyer H. Natural history of acute and chronic hepatitis C. Best Practice & Research. Clinical Gastroenterology. 2012;**26**(4):401-412

[5] Swan T. Overview of New Treatments for Hepatitis C Virus: Moving Towards a Public Health Agenda. Geneva: World Health Organization; 2017. Available from: http://www.who.int/selection_medicines/committees/expert/20/reviews/overview-new-treatments-HEP-C

[6] Garcia-Retortillo M, Forns X, Feliu A, Moitinho E, Costa J, Navasa M, et al. Hepatitis C virus kinetics during and immediately after liver transplantation. Hepatology. 2002;**35**(3):680-687

[7] Strazzula L, Pratt DS, Zardas J, Chung RT, Thiim M, Kroshinsky D. Widespread morbilliform eruption associated with telaprevir: Use of dermatologic consultation to increase tolerability. JAMA Dermatology. 2014;**150**(7):756-759

[8] Bigger CB, Brasky KM, Lanford RE. DNA microarray analysis of chimpanzee liver during acute resolving hepatitis C virus infection. Journal of Virology. 2001;**75**(15):7059-7066

[9] Heim MH. 25 years of interferon-based treatment of chronic hepatitis C: An epoch coming to an end. Nature Reviews Immunology. 2013;535-542

[10] Heim MH. Innate immunity and HCV. Journal of Hepatology. 2013;**58**(3):564-574

[11] Rauch A. Genetic variation in IL28B is associated with chronic hepatitis C and treatment failure: A genome-wide association study. Gastroenterology. 2010;1338-1345

[12] Prokunina-Olsson L. A variant upstream of IFNL3 (IL28B) creating a new interferon gene IFNL4 is associated with impaired clearance of hepatitis C virus. Nature Genetics. 2013;**45**(2):164-171

[13] Reichard O, Andersson J, Schvarcz R, Weiland O. Ribavirin treatment for chronic hepatitis C. Lancet. 1991;**337**(8749):1058-1061

[14] Di Bisceglie AM, Shindo M, Fong TL, Fried MW, Swain MG, Bergasa NV, et al. A pilot study of ribavirin therapy for chronic hepatitis C. Hepatology. 1992;**16**(3):649-654

[15] Poordad F, McCone J, Bacon BR, Bruno S, Manns MP, Sulkowski MS, et al. Boceprevir for untreated chronic HCV genotype 1 infection. The New England Journal of Medicine. 2011;**364**(13):1195-1206

[16] Jacobson IM, McHutchison JG, Dusheiko G, Di Bisceglie AM, Reddy KR, Bzowej NH, et al. Telaprevir for previously untreated chronic hepatitis C virus infection. The New England Journal of Medicine. 2011;**364**(25):2405-2416

[17] Everson GTSK, Rodriguez-Torres M. Efficacy of an interferon- and ribavirin-free regimen of daclatasvir, asunaprevir, and BMS-791325 in treatment-naive patients with HCV genotype 1 infection. Gastroenterology. 2014;**146**(2):420-429

[18] Kowdley KVLE, Poordad F, et al. Phase 2b trial of interferon-free therapy for hepatitis C virus genotype 1. The New England Journal of Medicine. 2014;**370**(3):222-232

[19] McHutchison JG, Manns M, Patel K, Poynard T, Lindsay KL, Trepo C, et al. Adherence to combination therapy enhances sustained response in genotype-1-infected patients with chronic hepatitis C. Gastroenterology. 2002;**123**(4):1061-1069

[20] Manns MP, Wedemeyer H, Cornberg M. Treating viral hepatitis C: Efficacy, side effects, and complications. Gut. 2006;**55**(9):1350-1359

[21] Perales C, Quer J, Gregori J, Esteban JI, Domingo E. Resistance of hepatitis C virus to inhibitors: Complexity and clinical implications. Virus. 2015;**7**(11):5746-5766

[22] Tsai SM, Kao JT, Tsai YF. How hepatitis C patients manage the treatment process of pegylated interferon and ribavirin therapy: A qualitative study. BMC Health Services Research. 2016;**16**:247

[23] Group GBOHCW. Global burden of disease (GBD) for hepatitis C. Journal of Clinical Pharmacology. 2004;**44**(1):20-29

[24] Pontali E, Angeli E, Cattelan AM, Maida I, Nasta P, Verucchi G, et al. Cytopenias during treatment of HIV-HCV-coinfection with pegylated interferon and ribavirin: Safety analysis of the OPERA study. Antiviral Therapy. 2015;**20**(1):39-48

[25] Slim J, Afridi MS. Managing adverse effects of interferon-alfa and ribavirin in combination therapy for HCV. Infectious Disease Clinics of North America. 2012;**26**(4):917-929

[26] Hézode C. Management of anaemia and other treatment complications. Digestive and Liver Disease. 2013;**45**(Suppl 5):S337-S342

[27] Fortune BE, Francis S, Forman LM, Hepatitis C. Virus therapy-related skin manifestations. Gastroenterol Hepatol (N Y). 2010;**6**(5):326-328

[28] Veluru C, Atluri D, Chadalavada R, Burns E, Mullen KD. Skin rash during chronic hepatitis C therapy. Gastroenterol Hepatol (N Y). 2010;**6**(5):323-325

[29] Chopra A, Klein PL, Drinnan T, Lee SS. How to optimize HCV therapy in genotype 1 patients: Management of side-effects. Liver International. 2013;**33**(Suppl 1):30-34

[30] Baik SJ, Kim TH, Yoo K, Moon IH, Cho MS. Ischemic colitis during interferon-ribavirin therapy for chronic hepatitis C: A case report. World Journal of Gastroenterology. 2012;**18**(31):4233-4236

[31] Lucaciu LA, Dumitrascu DL. Depression and suicide ideation in chronic hepatitis C patients untreated and treated with interferon: Prevalence, prevention, and treatment. Annals of Gastroenterology. 2015;**28**(4):440-447

[32] Lotrich F. Management of psychiatric disease in hepatitis C treatment candidates. Current Hepatitis Reports. 2010;**9**(2):113-118

[33] Payen JL, Pillard F, Mascarell V, Rivière D, Couzigou P, Kharlov N. Is physical activity possible and beneficial for patients with hepatitis C receiving pegylated interferon and ribavirin therapy? Gastroentérologie Clinique et Biologique. 2009;33(1 Pt 1):8-14

[34] Rodis JL, Kibbe P. Evaluation of medication adherence and quality of life in patients with hepatitis C virus receiving combination therapy. Gastroenterology Nursing. 2010;33(5):368-373

[35] Manos MM, Ho CK, Murphy RC, Shvachko VA. Physical, social, and psychological consequences of treatment for hepatitis C : A community-based evaluation of patient-reported outcomes. Patient. 2013;6(1):23-34

[36] Zickmund S, Hillis SL, Barnett MJ, Ippolito L, LaBrecque DR. Hepatitis C virus-infected patients report communication problems with physicians. Hepatology. 2004;39(4):999-1007

[37] Gujral H, Viscomi C, Collantes R. The role of physician extenders in managing patients with chronic hepatitis C. Cleveland Clinic Journal of Medicine. 2004;71(Suppl 3):S33-S37

[38] Grogan A, Timmins F. Patients' perceptions of information and support received from the nurse specialist during HCV treatment. Journal of Clinical Nursing. 2010;19(19-20):2869-2878

[39] Silberbogen AK, Ulloa E, Mori DL, Brown K. A telehealth intervention for veterans on antiviral treatment for the hepatitis C virus. Psychological Services. 2012;9(2):163-173

[40] Evon DM, Simpson K, Kixmiller S, Galanko J, Dougherty K, Golin C, et al. A randomized controlled trial of an integrated care intervention to increase eligibility for chronic hepatitis C treatment. The American Journal of Gastroenterology. 2011;106(10):1777-1786

[41] Yee HS, Chang MF, Pocha C, Lim J, Ross D, Morgan TR, et al. Update on the management and treatment of hepatitis C virus infection: Recommendations from the Department of Veterans Affairs Hepatitis C Resource Center Program and the National Hepatitis C Program Office. The American Journal of Gastroenterology. 2012;107(5):669-689 quiz 90

[42] Alexopoulou A, Karayiannis P. Interferon-based combination treatment for chronic hepatitis C in the era of direct acting antivirals. Annals of Gastroenterology. 2015;28(1):55-65

[43] Stedman C. Sofosbuvir, a NS5B polymerase inhibitor in the treatment of hepatitis C: A review of its clinical potential. Therapeutic Advances in Gastroenterology. 2014;7(3):131-140

[44] Lawitz E, Matusow G, DeJesus E, Yoshida EM, Felizarta F, Ghalib R, et al. Simeprevir plus sofosbuvir in patients with chronic hepatitis C virus genotype 1 infection and cirrhosis: A phase 3 study (OPTIMIST-2). Hepatology. 2016;64(2):360-369

[45] Afdhal N, Reddy KR, Nelson DR, Lawitz E, Gordon SC, Schiff E, et al. Ledipasvir and sofosbuvir for previously treated HCV genotype 1 infection. The New England Journal of Medicine. 2014;370(16):1483-1493

[46] Afdhal N, Zeuzem S, Kwo P, Chojkier M, Gitlin N, Puoti M, et al. Ledipasvir and sofosbuvir for untreated HCV genotype 1 infection. The New England Journal of Medicine. 2014;370(20):1889-1898

[47] Cousien A, Tran VC, Deuffic-Burban S, Jauffret-Roustide M, Dhersin JS, Yazdanpanah Y. Hepatitis C treatment as prevention of viral transmission and liver-related morbidity in persons who inject drugs. Hepatology. 2016;**63**(4):1090-1101

[48] Khoo A, Tse E. A practical overview of the treatment of chronic hepatitis C virus infection. Australian Family Physician. 2016;**45**(10):718-720

[49] Panel. AIHG. Recommendations for Testing, Managing, and Treating Hepatitis C. 2016. Available from: http://www.hcvguidelines.org/

[50] Ly KN, Xing J, Klevens RM, Jiles RB, Ward JW. Holmberg SD. The increasing burden of mortality from viral hepatitis in the United States between 1999 and 2007. Annals of Internal Medicine. 2012;**156**(4):271-278

[51] EASL recommendations on treatment of hepatitis C 2016. Journal of Hepatology. 2017; **66**(1):153-194

[52] Poynard T, McHutchison J, Manns M, Trepo C, Lindsay K, Goodman Z, et al. Impact of pegylated interferon alfa-2b and ribavirin on liver fibrosis in patients with chronic hepatitis C. Gastroenterology. 2002;**122**(5):1303-1313

[53] Sise ME, Bloom AK, Wisocky J, Lin MV, Gustafson JL, Lundquist AL, et al. Treatment of hepatitis C virus-associated mixed cryoglobulinemia with direct-acting antiviral agents. Hepatology. 2016;**63**(2):408-417

[54] Ford N, Swan T, Beyer P, Hirnschall G, Easterbrook P, Wiktor S. Simplification of anti-viral hepatitis C virus therapy to support expanded access in resource-limited settings. Journal of Hepatology. 2014;**61**(1 Suppl):S132-S138

[55] Dore GJ, Ward J, Thursz M. Hepatitis C disease burden and strategies to manage the burden (Guest Editors Mark Thursz, Gregory Dore and John Ward). Journal of Viral Hepatitis. 2014;**21**(Suppl 1):1-4

[56] Gane E, Kershenobich D, Seguin-Devaux C, et al. Strategies to manage hepatitis C virus (HCV) infection disease burden. Journal of Viral Hepatitis. 2015;46-73

10

Hepatitis C Virus (HCV) Treatment in Croatia: Recent Advances and Ongoing Obstacles

Marko Duvnjak, Nina Blažević and
Lucija Virović Jukić

Abstract

The prevalence of hepatitis C virus (HCV) antibodies in Croatia is low in the general population (reported <1%), similar to the prevalence rates of many European countries, but is higher in the populations at risk, especially among intravenous drug users. With the development of new classes of direct-acting antiviral agents and interferon-free regimens, the landscape of HCV treatment has completely changed. Management of HCV infection in Croatia is in accordance with the European Association for the Study of the Liver (EASL) recommendations published in 2015, recently updated Croatian Guidelines (published in April 2016) and the recommendations of Croatian Health Insurance Fund (HZZO) which covers the costs of treatment. HZZO approved simeprevir at the beginning of 2015. By the end of the 2015 sofosbuvir, combination of sofosbuvir + ledipasvir and the combination of ombitasvir, paritaprevir and ritonavir ± dasabuvir became available. Although the drawback of these new highly effective treatments is their price, prioritization of patients on a national level offers equal opportunities to patients in need for treatment. Due to improvements in therapy and prevention, clinical care for patients with HCV in Croatia advanced significantly during the last two years.

Keywords: hepatitis C virus, Croatia, epidemiology, treatment, direct-acting antivirals (DAAs)

1. Introduction

The prevalence of hepatitis C virus (HCV) antibodies in Croatia is low in the general population (reported <1%). HCV seroprevalence in the Croatian adult general population is similar to the prevalence rates of many European countries (for example Spain, France, Belgium,

Poland, and Bulgaria) [1–5]. In comparison with other European countries, there have also been changes in the HCV epidemiology in Croatia over the past few decades. According to the published data, the estimated number of HCV-infected patients in Croatia is around 39,000, although the experts' opinion is that the real numbers are significantly smaller [6, 7]. There was no significant difference in the HCV seropositivity between males and females in the Croatian population, with the highest prevalence in the 30–39 age group (1.7%) [8]. Routine HCV screening of blood products was introduced in Croatia in 1992.

The prevalence of HCV infection in some population groups in Croatia is shown in **Table 1** [9–21]. Patients requiring multiple transfusions have a high prevalence of HCV infection, but with the implementation of mandatory anti-HCV and HCV RNA screening of blood/blood donations, the risk of transfusion-associated hepatitis C has virtually been eliminated. [22]. HCV seroprevalence in the Croatian pregnant women is comparable to data reported in Switzerland and Spain [23, 24]. In this population, injecting drug users (IDU), history of blood products transfusion before 1992 and hospitalization with surgical procedures were identified as most common risk factors [25]. Since blood donors represent a strictly controlled group, it is expected that the HCV prevalence is lower than in the general population [26]. There are no published data on the HCV prevalence in the Croatian healthcare workers who have sustained contaminated needle stick injuries (occupationally exposed groups) [27].

Population group	Prevalence of HCV infection in Croatia
General population	<1%
Injecting drug users (IDUs)	40%
Prison populations	8–44%
Human immunodeficiency virus-infected patients	15%
Persons with high-risk sexual behavior	4.6%
Alcohol abusers	2.4%
Pregnant women	0.5–1.5%
Pregnant IDUs	40–50%
Hemodialysis patients	2.3–3.2%
Children and adolescents	0.3%
First-time blood donors	0.1%
Healthcare workers (occupationally exposed groups)	No published data

Table 1. Prevalence of HCV infection in Croatia in different population groups.

Prevalence of HCV genotypes in Croatia varies by different population groups and regions. The prevalence of genotypes in Croatian population is shown in **Table 2**. In the general population, genotype 1 is the most widely distributed, while genotype 3 is predominant among IDUs. The most commonly detected subtype is 1b and it is predominant in hemodialysis patients. In prison population, genotype 1 and 3 are equally distributed and similar genotype distribution is found in groups with high-risk sexual behavior [28–31]. Similar pattern of genotype distribution is found in other European countries, where genotypes 1 and 3 also account for the majority of HCV infections with the most frequent subtype 1b [32]. The prevalence of genotype 4 is rising in Europe (in countries such as France, Germany, Greece, Italy, Poland, Portugal, Spain, Sweden, and Switzerland) due to immigration in these areas [33].

HCV genotype	Prevalence
Genotype 1	60.4–79.8%
Genotype 1, subtype 1b	41.6%
Genotype 3	12.9–47.9%
Genotype 3 (IDUs)	60.5–83.9%

Table 2. Prevalence of HCV genotypes in Croatia.

2. Indications for treatment in Europe and Croatia

Following new trends in the management of viral hepatitis, an expert panel held the first Croatian Consensus Conferences on Viral Hepatitis in 2005, and later in 2009 and 2013. With the development of new classes of direct-acting antiviral agents (DAAs) and interferon-free regimens, the landscape of HCV treatment has significantly changed. The European Association for the Study of the Liver (EASL) published its recommendations in 2015, with the latest update in September 2016, and the World Health Organization in May 2016 adopted the first-ever Global Health Sector Strategy on viral hepatitis with the longer-term aim to reduce new viral hepatitis infection by 90% by 2030. Management of HCV infection in Croatia is in accordance with the EASL Guidelines published in 2015, Croatian Guidelines (published by the Croatian Referral Centre for the Diagnostics and Treatment of Viral Hepatitis at University Hospital for Infectious diseases 'Dr. Fran Mihaljević' and updated in April 2016), and the recommendations of the Croatian Health Insurance Fund (HZZO) which covers the costs of treatment for all patients in accordance with the recommended guidelines. These recommendations are based on currently licensed drugs and updated regularly, following approval of new drug regimens.

There are some differences comparing EASL and Croatian Guidelines, which are listed as following. According to EASL Guidelines from 2015 and Croatian Guidelines, treatment should be prioritized (considered without delay) in patients with significant fibrosis or cirrhosis (METAVIR Score F3 or F4), including decompensated (Child-Pugh B or C) cirrhosis, in patients with clinically significant extra-hepatic manifestations, in patients with HCV recurrence after liver transplantation, and in HBV/HIV-coinfected patients (not in latest EASL Guidelines in 2016). Compared with EASL Guidelines, in Croatia, treatment is also prioritized in patients before or after solid organ transplantation and justified for individuals at risk of transmitting HCV (IDU, men who have sex with men with high-risk sexual practices, women of child bearing age who wish to get pregnant, hemodialysis patients, and incarcerated patients); in EASL Guidelines, they are in prioritized category. In Croatia, treatment is justified in patients with moderate cirrhosis (METAVIR F2) and in patients with long disease duration (>20 years), regardless of fibrosis (not in EASL recommendations; indication of moderate cirrhosis was in previous EASL recommendations from 2015.). Treatment can be deferred in Croatian patients (not in EASL Guidelines) with no or mild disease (METAVIR Score F0 and F1) and in patients with none of the clinically significant extra-hepatic manifestations. The latest EASL recommendations from 2016 (not in Croatian Guidelines) say that treatment should be considered without delay in patients with significant fibrosis or cirrhosis (METAVIR score F2, F3, or F4), including decompensated (Child-Pugh B or C) cirrhosis, in patients with clinically significant extra-hepatic manifestations (e.g., symptomatic vasculitis associated with HCV-related mixed cryoglobulinemia, HCV immune complex-related nephropathy, and non-Hodgkin B cell lymphoma), in patients with HCV recurrence after liver transplantation, and in individuals at risk of transmitting HCV (active injection drug users, men who have sex with men with high-risk sexual practices, women of child-bearing age who wish to get pregnant, hemodialysis patients, and incarcerated individuals). In all recommendations, treatment is not recommended in patients with limited life expectancy due to non-liver-related comorbidities [34–38].

3. Therapeutic protocol

The goal of therapy is to cure HCV infection to prevent hepatic cirrhosis, decompensation of cirrhosis, hepatocellular carcinoma, severe extrahepatic manifestations, and death. The endpoint of therapy is undetectable HCV RNA in blood by a sensitive assay 12 weeks (SVR12—sustained virologic response) and/or 24 weeks (SVR24) after the end of treatment [37].

For decision-making related to therapies/drug selection, various factors are important: age, duration of infection, stage of fibrosis/cirrhosis, response to previous antiviral therapy, extra-hepatic manifestations, comorbidities (HBV/HIV coinfection, autoimmune disease), concomitant therapy, genotype (1, 2, 3, 4), subgenotype (1a, 1b), HCV RNA viral load, presence of mutations that confer resistance to certain antiviral drugs and IL-28B genotype (CC, CT, TT) if interferon-based therapies are being considered.

With the introduction of the first two protease inhibitors (PI) in 2011, the new era of HCV therapy began. Boceprevir and telaprevir as the first-generation of oral direct-acting antiviral agents (DAAs) became available in Croatia in 2013, for the treatment of genotype 1 HCV patients who failed PegIFN and ribavirin therapy.

Croatia is a member of the European Union and all drugs registered by European Medicines Agency are also approved for use in Croatia. Available drugs for the treatment of HCV in Croatia (with costs covered directly by Croatian Health Insurance Fund—HZZO) in 2016 are: PegIFN, ribavirin, simeprevir, sofosbuvir, combination of ombitasvir + ritonavir-boosted paritaprevir ± dasabuvir, and sofosbuvir + ledipasvir. In the European Union, there are some drugs that are not yet available in Croatia: velpatasvir, daclatasvir, grazoprevir, and elbatasvir.

Croatian Guidelines for the treatment are based on EASL and AASLD recommendations, but are somewhat more restrictive. For the treatment of naive patients with genotype 1 in 2016, it was still recommended to use the combination therapy with PegIFN and ribavirin (24–48 weeks) for patients with mild fibrosis and favorable predictors of response. For those patients with unfavorable predictors, if they achieve rapid virologic response (RVR), standard PegIFN and ribavirin combination is also recommended, otherwise a protease inhibitor (PI)—simeprevir or sofosbuvir should be added. In those with advanced fibrosis (F3), simeprevir or sofosbuvir should be added to PegIFN + ribavirin. Patients with significant (F4) fibrosis, who have contraindications to IFN therapy, presence of extrahepatic manifestations, HIV-coinfection or in transplanted patients, IFN-free regimens should be used for 12 weeks (ombitasvir, ritonavir-boosted paritaprevir, dasabuvir ± ribavirin; sofosbuvir and ledipasvir ± ribavirin; sofosbuvir and simeprevir ± ribavirin). For patients with decompensated cirrhosis, the combination of sofosbuvir and ledipasvir with or without ribavirin should be used, which is the same as recommended by the EASL and AASLD Guidelines. The main difference to EASL Guidelines is that, according to EASL, naive patients with or without compensated cirrhosis are treated with fixed-dose combination of sofosbuvir and ledipasvir without ribavirin.

For the treatment of experienced patients with genotype 1, triple combination of PegIFN, ribavirin, and a PI (simeprevir or sofosbuvir) is recommended in those with previous relapse or partial response (F1-F3 fibrosis). For nonresponders to PegIFN-ribavirin treatment (regardless of fibrosis) and for patients with F4 fibrosis (regardless of type of response), as well as for patients with TT IL-28B genotype, contraindications to IFN therapy, presence of extrahepatic manifestations, HIV-coinfection and transplanted patients, IFN-free regimens are offered (previously mentioned for treatment of naive patients). For patients with decompensated cirrhosis, the only treatment option currently available is the combination of sofosbuvir and ledipasvir with ribavirin for 12 weeks or without ribavirin for 24 weeks. This is also the only available option for patients previously treated with the triple combination of PegIFN + ribavirin + first-generation PIs (boceprevir or telaprevir) (in Croatia, there are only a few patients that have not responded to treatment with new-generation DAAs, as they have recently become available). According to EASL, experienced, DAA-naive patients with genotype 1b with or without compensated cirrhosis should be treated with fixed-dose combination of sofosbuvir and ledipasvir without ribavirin, and with ribavirin in those patients with genotype 1a. In EASL Guidelines, for the treatment of naive and experienced patients with genotype 1, there are two more options (not available in Croatia): fixed-dose combination of sofosbuvir and velpatasvir without ribavirin, ritonavir-boosted paritaprevir, ombitasvir and dasabuvir with or without ribavirin, grazoprevir and elbasvir with or without ribavirin, and sofosbuvir and daclatasvir with or without ribavirin.

For the treatment of patients with genotype 4, the same recommendations as for genotype 1 apply, with the exception of fixed combination of ombitasvir, paritaprevir, and ritonavir, which is used without dasabuvir. In patients with cirrhosis, duration of treatment is 24 weeks.

In EASL Guidelines, for the treatment of these patients, there are few more options available: sofosbuvir and velpatasvir without ribavirin, grazoprevir and elbasvir with or without ribavirin, and sofosbuvir and daclatasvir with or without ribavirin.

For the treatment of naive patients with genotype 2, with F1-F3 fibrosis, the use of standard combination treatment with PegIFN and ribavirin for 24 weeks is still recommended. Naive patients with F4 fibrosis, nonresponders (regardless of fibrosis), patients with contraindications to IFN therapy, with presence of extrahepatic manifestations, HIV-coinfection and transplanted patients are treated with combination of sofosbuvir and ribavirin (12 weeks without cirrhosis and 16–20 weeks with cirrhosis). In EASL recommendations, for the treatment of these patients there are two options: sofosbuvir and velpatasvir without ribavirin and sofosbuvir and daclatasvir without ribavirin.

For the treatment of naive patients with genotype 3, with F1-F3 fibrosis, it is still recommended to use PegIFN and ribavirin for 24 weeks. Naive patients with F4 fibrosis and nonresponders to PegIFN + ribavirin therapy (regardless of fibrosis) are treated with combination of sofosbuvir, PegIFN, and ribavirin for 12 weeks. Patients with F1-F3 fibrosis and with contraindication to IFN therapy are treated with combination of sofosbuvir and ribavirin for 24 weeks. Those patients with F4 fibrosis and with contraindication to IFN therapy are treated with combination of sofosbuvir and daclatasvir for 12 weeks or combination of sofosbuvir, ledipasvir, and ribavirin for 24 weeks. In EASL Guidelines, for treatment of naive and experienced patients there are two options: sofosbuvir and velpatasvir with or without ribavirin and sofosbuvir and daclatasvir with or without ribavirin [37, 38].

4. Croatian Health Insurance Fund (HZZO)—reimbursement requirements

Croatian Health Insurance Fund (HZZO) is covering over 99% of the population. HCV treatments are funded from a separate budget for expensive medicines [39]. HZZO has listed conditions that patients have to fulfill in order for HCV treatment to be covered from the before-mentioned fund: age between 18 and 70 years, HCV RNA positive, with a specified genotype, histologic evidence of chronic inflammation (biopsy finding) or fibroscan result larger than 8 kPa, and abstinence of IDU and significant alcohol consumption for the past 12 months. In patients with normal alanine aminotransferase (ALT) level, treatment is indicated with fibrosis F ≥ 2 or fibroscan finding >8 kPa. Patients who are IDUs need to have evidence of abstinence from illegal substances for at least one year and documented psychiatrist's finding and results of toxicology testing every 3 months during medical treatment. Treatment reimbursement requirements in Croatia include: specialist recommendation for treatment, Hospital's drug committee approval, and request for treatment sent to Expert committee for the treatment of hepatitis C of HZZO for final approval of treatment modality and duration (respect priorities among patients). All other Croatian patients with chronic hepatitis C (not fulfilling the above-mentioned requirements) can also be treated based on the judgment of the treating physician, but with a more restricted reimbursement options.

5. Conclusion

Regarding improvements in therapy and prevention, clinical care for patients with HCV in Croatia has advanced significantly during the past two years. Comparing epidemiology, indications for the treatment, available drugs, and therapeutic protocols, it is clear that Croatia accompanies European trends in HCV treatment. In future, rapid changes in the treatment of chronic HCV infection with the innovation of new drugs will lead to more effective, shorter treatment courses and PegIFN-free modalities.

Author details

Marko Duvnjak[1,2]*, Nina Blažević[1] and Lucija Virović Jukić[1,2]

*Address all correspondence to: marko.duvnjak1@gmail.com

1 Division of Gastroenterology and Hepatology, Department of Internal Medicine, Sestre Milosrdnice University Hospital Center, Zagreb, Croatia

2 University of Zagreb School of Medicine, Zagreb, Croatia

References

[1] Muñoz-Gámez JA, Salmerón J. Prevalence of hepatitis B and C in Spain – further data are needed. Revista Española de Enfermedades Digestivas. 2013;105:245-248

[2] Meffre C, Le Strat Y, Delarocque-Astagneau E, et al. Prevalence of hepatitis B and hepatitis C virus infections in France in 2004: Social factors are important predictors after adjusting for known risk factors. Journal of Medical Virology. 2010;82:546-555

[3] Van Damme P, Thyssen A, Van Loock F. Epidemiology of hepatitis C in Belgium: Present and future. Acta Gastro-Enterologica Belgica. 2002;65:78-79

[4] Gańczak M, Szych Z. Rationale against preoperative screening for HIV in Polish hospitals: A prevalence study of anti-HIV in contrast to anti-hepatitis C virus and hepatitis B surface antigen. Infection Control and Hospital Epidemiology. 2009;30:1227-1229

[5] Atanasova MV, Haydouchka IA, Zlatev SP, et al. Prevalence of antibodies against hepatitis C virus and hepatitis B coinfection in healthy population in Bulgaria. A seroepidemiological study. Minerva Gastroenterologica e Dietologica. 2004;50:89-96

[6] Civljak R, Kljakovic-Gaspic M, Kaic B, Bradaric N. Viral hepatitis in Croatia. Journal of Viral Hepatitis. 2014;20:49-56

[7] Kaić B, Vilibić-Cavlek T, Filipović SK, et al. Epidemiology of viral hepatitis. Acta Medica Croatica. 2013;67:273-279

[8] Vilibić-Cavlek T, Kucinar J, Ljubin-Sternak S, et al. Prevalence of viral hepatitis in Croatian adult population undergoing routine check-up, 2010-2011. Central European Journal of Public Health. 2014;22:29-33

[9] Kolarić B, Stajduhar D, Gajnik D, et al. Seroprevalence of blood-borne infections and population sizes estimates in a population of injecting drug users in Croatia. Central European Journal of Public Health. 2010;18:104-109

[10] Medić A, Dzelalija B, Sonicki Z, Zekanović D. Characteristics of hepatitis C infection in injecting drug users in Zadar County, Croatia. Collegium Antropologicum. 2008;32:697-702

[11] Kolovrat A, Jurisić I, Marić Z, Cvitković A. Prevalence of hepatitis B, hepatitis C and HIV among injecting drug users treated outpatiently and in therapeutic community in Brod-Posavina County, Croatia. Acta Medica Croatica. 2010;64:287-296

[12] Cavlek TV, Marić J, Katicić L, Kolarić B. Hepatitis C virus antibody status, sociodemographic characteristics, and risk behaviour among injecting drug users in Croatia. Central European Journal of Public Health. 2011;19:26-29

[13] Trisler Z, Seme K, Poljak M, et al. Prevalence of hepatitis C and G virus infections among intravenous drug users in Slovenia and Croatia. Scandinavian Journal of Infectious Diseases. 1999;31:33-35

[14] Vilibic-Cavlek T, Gjenero-Margan I, Retkovac B, et al. Sociodemographic characteristics and risk behaviors for HIV, hepatitis B and hepatitis C virus infection among Croatian male prisoners. International Journal of Prisoner Health. 2011;7:28-31

[15] Burek V, Horvat J, Butorac K, Mikulić R. Viral hepatitis B, C and HIV infection in Croatian prisons. Epidemiology and Infection. 2010;138:1510-1620

[16] Seme K, Poljak M, Begovac J, et al. Low prevalence of hepatitis C virus infection among human immunodeficiency virus type 1-infected individuals from Slovenia and Croatia. ActaVirologica. 2002;46:91-94

[17] Cavlek TV, Margan IG, Lepej SZ, et al. Seroprevalence, risk factors, and hepatitis C virus genotypes in groups with high-risk sexual behavior in Croatia. Journal of Medical Virology. 2009;81:1348-1353

[18] Crnjaković-Palmović J, Jeren-Strujić B, Gudel-Gregurić J, et al. Hepatitis virus infection among hemodialysis patients. Acta Medica Croatica. 2005;59:113-116

[19] Istria County Institute of Public Health. Data on the Health Status of the Population and the Work of Health Care Services in the Istria County in 2013 [Internet]. 2013. Available from: http://www.zzjziz.hr/uploads/media/2013_uvod.pdf. [Accessed: December 30, 2016]

[20] Indolfi G, Bartolini E, Casavola D, Resti M. Chronic hepatitis C virus infection in children and adolescents: Epidemiology, natural history, and assessment of the safety and efficacy of combination therapy. Adolescent Health, Medicine and Therapeutics. 2010;1:115-128

[21] Gerner P, Wirth S, Wintermeyer P, et al. Prevalence of hepatitis C virus infection in children admitted to an urban hospital. The Journal of Infection. 2006;52:305-308

[22] Busch MP. Closing the windows on viral transmission by blood transfusion. In: Stramer SL, editor. Blood Safety in the New Millennium. Bethesda: American Association of Blood Banks; 2001. pp. 33-54

[23] Santiago B, Blázquez D, López G, et al. Serological profile of immigrant pregnant women against HIV, HBV, HCV, rubella, *Toxoplasma gondii, Treponema pallidum,* and *Trypanosoma cruzi.* Enfermedades Infecciosas Y Microbiologica Clinica. 2012;30:64-69

[24] Suárez González A, Viejo De La Guerra G, Oterro Guerra L, Solís Sánchez G. Antibody determination for the human immunodeficiency virus in pregnant women in the public health care area of Gijón, Spain. Medicina Clínica (Barcelona). 2001;116:517-519

[25] Aniszewska M, Kowalik-Mikołajewska B, Pokorska-Lis M, et al. Seroprevalence of anti-HCV in pregnant women. Risk factors of HCV infection. Przegląd Epidemiologiczny. 2009;63:293-298

[26] Transfusion Medicine Newsletter. (In Croatian). No. 53, 2013 [Internet]. 2013. Available from: http://www.hztm.hr/glasilo/53/index.html

[27] Vilibic-Cavlek T, Kucinar J, Kaic B, et al. Epidemiology of hepatitis C in Croatia in the European context. The World Journal of Gastroenterology. 2015;21(32):9476-9493

[28] Vince A, Iscić-Bes J, ZidovecLepej S, et al. Distribution of hepatitis C virus genotypes in Croatia – A 10 year retrospective study of four geographic regions. Collegium Antropologicum. 2006;30(Suppl 2):139-143

[29] Davila S. Comparison of hepatitis C virus genotypes distribution in prison population and injecting drug users in northwest Croatia [thesis in Croatian]. Zagreb: School of Medicine University of Zagreb; 2013

[30] Bingulac-Popović J, Babić I, Dražić V, Grahovac B. Distribution of hepatitis C virus genotypes in the Croatian population. Biochemia Medica. 2000;3-4:175-180

[31] Golubić D, Vurusić B, Kessler HH. Prevalence and significance of hepatitis C virus (HCV) genotypes in anti-HCV positive patients in northwest Croatia. Acta Medica Croatica. 1997;51:79-82

[32] MohdHanafiah K, Groeger J, Flaxman AD, Wiersma ST. Global epidemiology of hepatitis C virus infection: new estimates of age-specific antibody to HCV seroprevalence. Hepatology. 2013;57:1333-1342

[33] Quer J and Esteban Mur JI. Epidemiology and prevention. In: Thomas HC, Lok ASF, Locarnini A, Zuckerman A, editors. Viral Hepatitis. 4th ed. Chichester: John Wiley & Sons; 2014. pp. 256-265

[34] Vince A, Hrstić I, Begovac J, et al. Viral hepatitis – Croatian Consensus Statement 2013. Acta Medica Croatica. 2013;67: 273-279

[35] World Health Organization. Guidelines for Screening, Care and Treatment of Persons with Hepatitis C Infection [Internet]. 2016. Available from: http://www.who.int/hepatitis/publications/hepatitis-c-guidelines-2016/en/. [Accessed: December 30, 2016]

[36] World Health Organization. Global Health Sector Strategy on Viral Hepatitis 2016-2021 [Internet]. 2016. Available from: http://www.who.int/hepatitis/strategy2016-2021/ghss-hep/en/. [Accessed: December 30, 2016]

[37] European Association for the Study of the Liver. EASL recommendations on treatment of hepatitis C 2016. Journal of Hepatology. 2017;66:153-194

[38] Ministry of Health Referral Centre for Diagnosis and Treatment of Viral Hepatitis. Hepatitis C Treatment Recommendations [Internet]. 2016. Available from: www.bfm.hr/page/hepatitis-c [Accessed: December 30, 2016]

[39] De Bruijn W, Ibanez C, Frisk P, et al. Introduction and utilization of high priced HCV medicines across Europe: Implications for the future. Frontiers in Pharmacology. 2016;7:197

11

Metabolic Factors and their Influence on the Clinical Course and Response to HCV Treatment

Livia M Villar, Cristiane A Villela-Nogueira, Allan P da Silva and Letícia P Scalioni

Abstract

Nowadays, direct-acting antivirals (DAA) have been used for hepatitis C virus (HCV) treatment leading to cure in 90–95% of non-cirrhotic patients depending on genotype, treatment experience, and regimen used. It was observed rates of antiviral response above 90% in compensated cirrhotic patients that should be treated for long time and/or ribavirin may be required. Metabolic syndrome, obesity, and insulin resistance are increasing worldwide and further contribute to hepatic steatosis and have long been recognized as a cause of lipid deposition in the liver. These factors affect the rate of antiviral response to interferon-based therapy, but it seems not impact DAA treatment. The effect of HCV eradication on hepatic steatosis and progression to fibrosis, cirrhosis, and hepatocellular carcinoma warrants further study in the era of direct-acting antivirals. Other factors that could be related to increase liver damage are vitamin D and associated polymorphisms. Patients with low concentration of total vitamin D [25(OH)D] presented high degree of fibrosis and high values of total cholesterol and triglycerides. In this chapter, we review the challenges and metabolic pathology associated with HCV infection and, discuss the influence of some metabolic factors which can cause liver damage.

Keywords: hepatitis C, metabolic syndrome, insulin resistance, vitamin D, genetic polymorphism

1. Introduction

Hepatitis C virus (HCV) infection is a serious health problem with an estimated 71 million of people having chronic HCV worldwide [1]. During chronic hepatitis C (CHC), it is observed many extrahepatic manifestations that could lead to rapid progression of the

disease, increasing the risk of developing hepatocellular carcinoma (HCC) and advanced fibrosis [2, 3]. The effect of HCV eradication on hepatic steatosis and progression to fibrosis, cirrhosis, and hepatocellular carcinoma warrants further study in the era of direct-acting antivirals. Now, with HCV eradication possible in virtually everyone, the sequelae of steatosis, fibrosis and its drivers will garner more attention. People infected by HCV genotype other than three presenting high BMI and visceral obesity have high risk of hepatic steatosis. It is believed that insulin resistance (IR) is the primary pathologic mechanism that leads to abnormal lipid accumulation within hepatocytes. But it is not defined if IR is due to host factors, presence of HCV infection, or a combination. These data become extremely relevant due to the high prevalence of obesity and metabolic syndromes observed worldwide [3].

Nowadays antiviral treatment for HCV demonstrated to be very effective (>90%), but it is important to recognize and identify irreversible and associated metabolic damage, thereby reducing the morbidity and mortality associated with HCV [3]. IR has been associated to CHC [4, 5], which is characterized by hyperinsulinemia in patients with normal fasting blood glucose and with an increased risk of developing diabetes mellitus type II (DM2), heart disease, and nonalcoholic fatty liver disease [6–8].

One of the consequences of persistent IR may be the development of DM2. DM2 is a metabolic disease characterized by hyperglycemia that can occur due to defects in insulin secretion and/or action involving specific pathogenic processes, such as the destruction of insulin-producing pancreatic beta cells or resistance to insulin action. It is the most common metabolic disease and the one with the highest prevalence among individuals with hepatitis C compared to those infected with the hepatitis B virus (HBV), for example [9, 10]. DM2 comprises approximately 90% of cases and may have a genetic and environmental component. Type 1 diabetes, comprising about 10% of the cases, results in the destruction of beta cells, which may lead to absolute insulin deficiency, thus requiring the exogenous administration of it to avoid ketoacidosis and coma.

HCV core protein is involved in the development of IR, however little is known about the clinical impact of HCV core region on IR [11, 12]. Patients infected with HCV genotype 1b who had 70Q core mutation had higher rates of IR compared to those without the mutation, indicating that this substitution is associated with the development of IR [11]. Mutation at core 70Q have been associated to higher incidence of HCC and mutations in 70 and/or 91 core HCV are important predictors of IR in patients without cirrhosis or DM [13, 14]. However, this finding was not seen in Brazilian population [12].

Other factor that could be related to increase liver damage is vitamin D and associated polymorphisms. Vitamin D, whose active form is 1,25-dihydroxy vitamin D3, is essential for calcium and bone homeostasis, and its deficiency has been associated to several diseases, such as cancer, cardiovascular and autoimmune diseases, IR, and infectious disease [15–19].

Vitamin D is an important immunomodulator and plays an important role in metabolic and inflammatory diseases in the liver, including HCV infection. Vitamin D deficiency is common in healthy worldwide populations [20]. Despite this, patients with liver diseases such as CHC are at substantially higher risk for hypovitaminosis D [15, 21, 22]. The polymorphism of the vitamin D receptor (VDR) gene was associated with rapid progression to fibrosis [bAt haplotype (CCA)] among HCV patients [23]. This information together demonstrates the potential of VDR-vitamin D axis association in viral hepatitis and highlights the importance of vitamin D as an immunomodulator, indicating an association between vitamin D deficiency and the absence of sustained virological response (SVR) in patients with hepatitis C [24, 25].

Studies have found a relationship between vitamin D concentration and decreased response to antiviral treatment in hepatitis C patients with genotype 1, 2 and 3 in double therapy with peg-interferon (PEG-IFN) and ribavirin [15, 24]. Bitetto et al. [26] observed that the vitamin D concentration and polymorphism in rs12979860 of IL28B gene were independent predictors of response to treatment. Patients who did not present the CC (IL28B) and vitamin D deficient genotype presented a greater risk of not responding to antiviral treatment. In addition, vitamin D concentration supplementation improves response to antiviral treatment in double therapy with PEG-IFN and ribavirin for recurrent hepatitis C [27]. Scalioni et al. [28] demonstrated that patients with lower concentration of 25(OH)D presented high degree of fibrosis and higher values of total cholesterol and triglycerides.

Currently, studies have been conducted correlating vitamin D and SVR levels in patients under direct-acting antivirals (DAAs) treatment. Backsteadt et al. [29] evaluated the association of vitamin D levels with cirrhosis in an HCV-infected cohort. In addition, they assessed pre-treatment vitamin D levels up to week 12. A higher prevalence of vitamin D deficiency was observed in cohorts of HCV-cirrhotic patients, but changes in vitamin D levels did not influence SVR rates [29]. Belle et al. [30] evaluated the impact of vitamin D levels in treatment-naive genotype 1 patients and submitted to conventional double therapy (PEG-IFN + ribavirin) in a French cohort. No impact was observed between vitamin D levels and response to antiviral therapy [30]. Studies have also evaluated genetic polymorphisms related to vitamin D cascade in Thai population and have observed that polymorphism in the DHCR7 gene may be a predictive marker of response to dual therapy (PEG-IFN + ribavirin) in a patient with HCV genotype 1 [31].

Egypt has the highest prevalence rate of HCV infection in the world, where hepatitis C is considered a major health problem. The standard treatment of HCV is combination therapy of PEG-IFN and ribavirin where SVR is only achieved in 30% of the patients. Due mainly to the adverse effects and cost of treatment, discontinuation of treatment is an important approach. In this way, Abdelsalam et al. [32] evaluated the association between vitamin D concentration and VDR polymorphisms with SVR acquisition, where the concentration of vitamin D, FokI and TaqI was considered as predictors for the antiviral response with the combination of pegylated interferon and ribavirin.

2. HCV disease progression in patients with metabolic alterations

Recently, epidemiological, clinical, and experimental studies have related HCV to liver steatosis and several metabolic derangements [33–35]. There is also evidence that HCV infection can induce IR through different mechanisms [34]. Insulin metabolism is affected by HCV directly and indirectly leading to the production of several proinflammatory cytokines. The process of replication, assembly, and release of HCV from hepatocytes depend on close interactions with lipid droplets and host lipoproteins. The role of HCV in lipid metabolism of hepatocytes can lead to hepatic steatosis, especially in HCV patients infected by genotype 3 [36].

In genotype-1 patients, liver steatosis is directly related to metabolic factors including IR [37]. The impact of IR on the progression of liver disease has been debated and many evidence suggest that patients who have IR have a worse prognosis concerning multiple disease outcomes including progression of hepatic fibrosis and development of hepatocellular carcinoma [37]. Before the era of DAA for HCV infection treatment, IR also had an impact on treatment response, which has now been overcome by the high efficacy of these drugs. However, even with DAA treatment, IR is improved after the achievement of SVR [33].

There are several studies that analyze the association of HCV infection with IR and a meta-analysis of 34 studies found a positive correlation between HCV infection and increased risk of DM2 in comparison to the general population in both retrospective and prospective studies [38].

Regarding the studies that evaluated response to HCV treatment with interferon-containing regimens, it was observed that attaining SVR was associated with the improvement of IR defined by a lower homeostatic model assessment (HOMA)-IR after treatment [39, 40]. In addition, among patients submitted to treatment, those with a lower HOMA-IR had a higher chance of SVR [41].

Many studies found an association between higher HOMA-IR and fibrosis as well as the association of hepatocellular carcinoma with IR. Petit et al. [42] studied 123 HCV infected patients to investigate the host and viral specific factors associated with diabetes mellitus and IR in chronic hepatitis C patients. In diabetic patients, a score F4 was one of the factors related to the presence of diabetes mellitus and in patients without diabetes the HOMA-IR of METAVIR F 0 and F1 patients was significantly different compared to F2 and F3/F4 patients. They concluded that IR in non-diabetic HCV-infected patients was related to grading of liver fibrosis and occurred already at an early stage during HCV infection [42].

Hickman et al. [43] hypothesized that host metabolic factors might be associated with increased body mass index (BMI) and might play a role in liver disease progression. Thus, they studied 160 HCV patients at the time of liver biopsy and collected their serum for the assessment of the levels of insulin, c-peptide and leptin. They found that insulin was independently associated to fibrosis (P = 0.046) but not inflammation (P = 0.83). In addition, serum leptin levels were not associated to stage of fibrosis. So, in HCV patients infected by any genotype, increasing circulating insulin levels may be a factor responsible for the association between BMI and fibrosis [43].

Cua et al. [44] confirmed the impact of IR on fibrosis where they found that increased steatosis was related to high viral load ($p = 0.001$) but was not related to fibrosis ($p = 0.1$) in HCV genotype 3 patients. In HCV genotype I, body mass index ($p = 0.04$) and HOMA-IR (p = 0.01) contributed directly to steatosis. HOMA-IR was independently associated to fibrosis for HCV genotype 1 (OR, 3.22; p = 0.02) and genotype 3 (OR, 3.17; $p = 0.04$). [44].

Petta et al. [45] aimed to assess whether increasing degrees of IR, up to overt diabetes, were associated to steatosis and higher stages of fibrosis in patients with CHC resulting from genotype 1 HCV. About 201 genotype −1 HCV-infected patients were evaluated by liver biopsy and anthropometric and metabolic measurements, including IR, by the HOMA-IR (nondiabetic patients were defined as insulin resistant if HOMA-IR was >2.7). They evaluated three different groups concerning IR profile: 96 patients were noninsulin resistant (group 1), 76 were insulin resistant without diabetes (group 2), and 29 were diabetic (group 3). At multivariate analysis, fibrosis of >/=3 was independently associated with high necroinflammatory activity, low platelets, low cholesterol, high ferritin, and a high prevalence of IR. Diabetic patients were twice as likely to have severe fibrosis (60%) than those with IR but no diabetes (30%) ($p = 0.006$). This study concluded that in genotype 1 HCV infected patients, IR and overt diabetes are major determinants of advanced fibrosis, regardless of the degree of steatosis, mainly in the presence of severe necroinflammation.

Mohammed et al. [46] also concluded in a study that evaluated HCV infected patients compared to control group of non-infected HCV patients that IR may increase the rate of fibrosis progression in non-diabetic patients with chronic HCV. They suggested that follow up of hyperinsulinemia by serial assessment of HOMA-IR in non-diabetic HCV infected patients may be a biochemical indicator for progression of liver fibrosis [46]. On the other hand, some studies found no association between insulin resistance and liver fibrosis, like the one from Carvalho et al. who concluded that patients with chronic hepatitis C have significant metabolic alterations (hyperadiponectinemia and high HOMA-IR values) that are independent of HCV viremia and liver fibrosis [47].

Another issue that deserves discussion is the association of HCC and IR. Although the exact delineated mechanism is not yet established, there are some evidences to emphasize the involvement of HCV induced chronic inflammation, oxidative stress, IR, endoplasmic reticulum stress, liver steatosis and liver fibrosis in the progression of HCV chronic disease to hepatocellular carcinoma [48]. Possibly, IR is only one step involved among a complex interplay among factors that lead to HCC development. The impact of IR on HCC development is possible related to the fact that HCV interferes with insulin signaling by degradation of insulin receptor substrate 1 (IRS-1) and IRS-2 by suppressor of cytokine signaling (SOCS) protein or PI3K/Akt/mTOR pathway. IRS-1 is inactivated by TGF-α and PI3K/Akt also [49]. Based on these facts, the early stage of chronic HCV infection with increasing steatosis and IR creates an environment to develop hepatocarcinogenesis.

To investigate the role of IR and serum adiponectin level in hepatocellular carcinoma associated with chronic hepatitis C. Hung et al. analyzed three groups of patients and found that diabetes mellitus was more prevalent among HCV patients (35.6%, n = 59) compared to those infected by hepatitis B virus (HBV; 12.7%, n = 63), and non-HBV, non-HCV patients (7.1%, n = 28). Among HCV patients, age, serum insulin, HOMA-IR, DM and male gender were independently associated with HCC. This result was similar even when diabetic individuals were excluded from the analysis [50].

Noteworthy, most studies that evaluated the association of IR and HCV fibrosis are transversal studies. Longitudinal studies evaluating truly fibrosis progression and HCC development in patients with and without insulin resistance are needed to better understand this link. However, in the new DAA era one must reevaluate the impact of IR in fibrosis progression since the elimination of the virus per se will probably improve liver histology as well.

3. HCV treatment in patients with metabolic syndrome and vitamin D deficiency

HCV infection may contribute to hepatic steatosis and to metabolic syndrome, forming a positive feedback that may further increase steatosis and culminate in steatohepatitis and fibrosis. As HCV infection is considered a curable disease, fibrosis can regress in some patients after therapy response [51, 52]. However, based on data from IFN era, infected patients have comorbidities, as metabolic syndrome, that may prevent fibrosis regression, leading eventually to a continued liver damage, even after viral eradication.

Vitamin D is an important physiological regulator that contributes to various biological, immunological, and metabolic functions in liver diseases. Previous in vitro results indicated that 25-OH vitamin D appeared to be significant associated with treatment response, particularly in the aspect of the rapid virological response (RVR) [53], which is an important predictive factor for SVR achievement [54, 55]. Patients with RVR have an approximately 90% of chance of treatment success after receiving PegIFN/RBV combined therapy, regardless of the viral genotypes [56–58]. The achievement of this early goal provides greater flexibility for tailoring the treatment duration on an individual basis and enhances the cost-effectiveness of treatment [55]. However, the impact of 25-OH vitamin D deficiency on RVR and the precise mechanisms underlying the inhibition of HCV replication were not thoroughly elucidated.

Some cross-sectional studies have shown associations between a higher 25-OH vitamin D level and response to therapy with PEG-IFN and ribavirin [15, 59, 60], while low levels are associated with poor response and its supplementation improves SVR rates. On the other hand, studies conducted in French HCV patients did not observed an impact of vitamin D levels in response to double therapy [30]. No causality can be established by cross-sectional studies and discordant results have been observed [61]. Associations may occur because healthier people are more exposure to sunlight and perform more physical exercises, which lead to a higher 25-OH vitamin D level. Also, chronic inflammation can shorten the half-life of 25-OH vitamin D and hepatic production of vitamin D-binding protein is reduced in patients with advanced liver disease and this may accelerate vitamin D turnover. Indeed, some studies pointed that its level before antiviral therapy has no impact on the efficacy of antiviral therapy, regardless the genotype [62]. On the other hand, an Italian study found high frequency of vitamin D deficiency among decompensated cirrhosis showing that vitamin D may play a role in the development of infections in patients affected by liver cirrhosis [63].

Potential relationship of vitamin D gene pathway has been suggested in the pathophysiology of HCV infection. Studies conducted in Asian and Latin America population did not find an association of VDR gene polymorphism to SVR in double therapy [28, 64]. On the other, studies conducted among European patients infected by genotypes 1, 2 and 3 found that VDR gene polymorphisms are independently related to the response to Peg-IFN + RBV therapy in CHC. These differences could be related to genetic differences among these studies [65, 66].

Few studies have evaluated the impact of vitamin D metabolism in therapy with direct-acting antivirals (DAAs). Recently, Cusato et al. [67] evaluated the impact of polymorphisms in genes (CYP27B1, CYP24A1, VDBP and VDR) related to vitamin D pathway on sofosbuvir and GS-331007 plasma levels in HCV mono-infected patients at 1 month of treatment. They found that genetic polymorphisms involved in vitamin D pathway influenced drug concentration. In future, it might be useful to understand if these polymorphisms can affect other DAAs concentrations; and to understand their role in the prediction of clinical variables, such as the probability to develop hepatocarcinoma or to influence the viral load decay.

High rates of early tumor recurrence were recently reported after therapy with DAAs in 103 HCV-infected patients with prior HCC [68]. Despite therapy with DAAs, the occurrence of liver cancer could not be reduced in cirrhotic patients with SVR [69]. Recently, a study conducted in Italy found an association of HCC risk factors to age, ribavirin administration, IL28B rs12979860 CC and previous treatments; VDR FokI CC, sex and insulin resistance were protective factors [67]. However, three distinct prospective cohorts showed no increased risk of HCC recurrence in 267 patients after DAA treatments [70]. Whether DAA treatments increase HCC occurrence or recurrence rates will remain a subject for debate until have emerged with a proper control arm to assess this important question [71].

With the efficacious DAAs regimens, comorbidities appear not to impair SVR. Long-term studies in very large patient cohorts treated with DAAs will elucidate the degree to which steatosis, steatohepatitis, and/or fibrosis reverse with SVR. The persistence of these comorbidities may prevent complete return to health in HCV-cured patients.

4. Conclusion

In conclusion, several metabolic alterations, such as, insulin resistance and DM2 have been observed among CHC patients. During double therapy with PEG-IFN and ribavirin, IR and vitamin D levels were important to define high successful rates of virological response. Nowadays, with the advent of DAAs, the rate of SVR have been increased, however high rates of early tumor recurrence were recently reported after therapy with DAAs. In addition, the role of vitamin D levels and genetic polymorphisms involved in vitamin D metabolism could be important predictors for viral response and evolution of clinical cases. Further studies should be necessary to confirm the impact of these factors during new antiviral regimens.

Acknowledgements

The authors would like to thank the financial support of Fundação de Amparo a Pesquisa do Estado do Rio de Janeiro (FAPERJ), Brazilian National Counsel of Technological and Scientific Development (CNPq), and Oswaldo Cruz Foundation (FIOCRUZ).

Author details

Livia M Villar[1]*, Cristiane A Villela-Nogueira[2], Allan P da Silva[1] and Letícia P Scalioni[1]

*Address all correspondence to: liviafiocruz@gmail.com

1 Viral Hepatitis Laboratory, Oswaldo Cruz Institute, FIOCRUZ, Rio de Janeiro, Brazil

2 University Hospital Clementino Fraga Filho, School of Medicine, Federal University of Rio de Janeiro, Rio de Janeiro, RJ, Brazil

References

[1] World Health Organization (WHO). [Internet]. 2017. Available from: http://www.who.int/mediacentre/factsheets/fs164/en/. [Accessed: March 22, 2018]

[2] CDC. Hepatitis C Information for Health Professionals. Atlanta, GA, USA: Department of Health and Human Services, CDC; 2008. Available online: http://www.cdc.gov/hepatitis/HCV/index.htm (Accessed on)

[3] Wong RJ, Gish RG. Metabolic manifestations and complications associated with chronic hepatitis C virus infection. Journal of Gastroenterology and Hepatology. 2016;**12**:293-299

[4] Cannon CP. Mixed dyslipidemia, metabolic syndrome, diabetes mellitus, and cardiovascular disease: Clinical implications. The American Journal of Cardiology. 2008;**102**:5-9. DOI: 10.1016/j.amjcard.2008.09.067

[5] Lavanchy D. The global burden of hepatitis C. Liver International. 2009;**29**:74-81. DOI: 10.1111/j.1478-3231.2008.01934.x

[6] Alter MJ, Mast EE, Moyer LA, Margolis HS. Hepatitis C. Infectious Disease Clinics of North America. 1998;**12**:13-26

[7] Parvaiz F, Manzoor S, Tariq H, Javed F, Fatima K, Qadri I. Hepatitis C virus infection: Molecular pathways to insulin resistance. Virology Journal. 2011;**8**:474. DOI: 10.1186/1743-422X-8-474

[8] Hung CH, Lee CM, Lu SN. Hepatitis C virus associated insulin resistance: Pathogenic mechanisms and clinical implications. Expert Review of Anti-Infective Therapy. 2011;**9**:525-533. DOI: 10.1586/eri.11.33

[9] Fraser GM, Harman I, Meller N, Niv Y, Porath A. Diabetes mellitus is associated with chronic hepatitis C but not chronic hepatitis B infection. Israel Journal of Medical Sciences. 1996;**32**:526-530

[10] Serfaty L, Capeau J. Hepatitis C, insulin resistance and diabetes: Clinical and pathogenic data. Liver International. 2009 Mar;**29**(Suppl 2):13-25. DOI: 10.1111/j.1478-3231.2008.01952.x. Review. PubMed PMID: 19187069

[11] Akuta N, Suzuki F, Hirakawa M, Kawamura Y, Yatsuji H, Sezaki H, Suzuki Y, Hosaka T, Kobayashi M, Kobayashi M, et al. Amino acid substitutions in the hepatitis C virus core region of genotype 1b are the important predictor of severe insulin resistance in patients without cirrhosis and diabetes mellitus. Journal of Medical Virology. 2009;**81**:1032-1039. DOI: 10.1002/jmv.21473

[12] Scalioni LP, da Silva AP, Miguel JC, Espírito Santo MPD, Marques VA, Brandão-Mello CE, Villela-Nogueira CA, Lewis-Ximenez LL, Lampe E, Villar LM. Lack of association between hepatitis C virus core gene variation 70/91aa and insulin resistance. International Journal of Molecular Sciences. 2017 Jul 21;**18**(7). pii: E1444. DOI: 10.3390/ijms18071444

[13] Akuta N, Suzuki F, Hirakawa M, Kawamura Y, Sezaki H, Suzuki Y, Hosaka T, Kobayashi M, Kobayashi M, Saitoh S, et al. Amino acid substitutions in the hepatitis C virus core region are the important predictor of hepatocarcinogenesis. Hepatology. 2007;**46**:1357-1364. DOI: 10.1002/jmv.22094

[14] El-Shamy A, Shindo M, Shoji I, Deng L, Okuno T, Hotta H. Polymorphisms of the core, NS3, and NS5A proteins of hepatitis C virus genotype 1b associate with development of hepatocellular carcinoma. Hepatology. 2013;**58**:555-563. DOI: 10.1002/hep.26205

[15] Petta S, Cammà C, Scazzone C, Tripodo C, Di Marco V, Bono A, Cabibi D, et al. Low vitamin D serum level is related to severe fibrosis and low responsiveness to interferon-based therapy in genotype 1 chronic hepatitis C. 15. Hepatology. 2010;**51**:1158-1167

[16] Steinvil A, Leshem-Rubinow E, Berliner S, Justo D, Finn T, Ish-shalom M, Birati EI, et al. Vitamin D deficiency prevalence and cardiovascular risk in Israel. European Journal of Clinical Investigation. 2011;**41**:263-268

[17] Fleet JC, DeSmet M, Johnson R, Li Y. Vitamin D and cancer: A review of molecular mechanisms. The Biochemical Journal. 2012;**441**:61-76

[18] O'Brien MA, Jackson MW. Vitamin D and the immune system: Beyond rickets. Veterinary Journal. 2012;**194**:27-33

[19] Sung CC, Liao MT, Lu KC, Wu CC. Role of vitamin d in insulin resistance. Journal of Biomedicine & Biotechnology. 2012;**2012**:634195

[20] Rosen CJ. Vitamin D and falls--are intermittent, high doses better? Nature Reviews. Endocrinology. 2011 Nov 1;**7**(12):695-696. DOI: 10.1038/nrendo.2011.185

[21] Bitetto D, Fabris C, Falleti E, Toniutto P. Vitamin D deficiency and HCV chronic infection: What comes first? Journal of Hepatology. 2011 Oct;**55**(4):944-5; author reply 945. DOI: 10.1016/j.jhep.2011.01.044

[22] Melo-Villar L, Lampe E, de Almeida AJ, de P Scalioni L, Lewis-Ximenez LL, Miguel JC, Del Campo JA, Ranchal I, Villela-Nogueira CA, Romero-Gomez M. Hypovitaminosis D and its relation to demographic and laboratory data among hepatitis C patients. Annals of Hepatology. 2015 Jul-Aug;**14**(4):457-463

[23] Baur K, Mertens JC, Schmitt J, Iwata R, Stieger B, Frei P, Seifert B, Bischoff Ferrari HA, von Eckardstein A, Müllhaupt B, Geier A, Swiss Hepatitis C Cohort Study Group.

antivirals on the recurrence of hepatocellular carcinoma: Data from three ANRS cohorts. Journal of Hepatology. 2016 Oct;**65**(4):734-740. DOI: 10.1016/j.jhep.2016.05.045

[71] Llovet JM, Villanueva A. Liver cancer: Effect of HCV clearance with direct-acting antiviral agents on HCC. Nature Reviews. Gastroenterology & Hepatology. 2016 Oct;**13**(10):561-562. DOI: 10.1038/nrgastro.2016.140

12

The Molecular Basis of Anti-HCV Drug Resistance

Shaina M. Lynch and George Y. Wu

Abstract

Hepatitis C virus (HCV) is a significant medical problem and has become one of the leading causes of chronic liver disease. HCV replicates at a high rate, and due to inherently inaccurate nucleotide incorporation and lack of proofreading and post-replication repair, mutations are inevitable. In the era of direct acting antivirals (DAAs), treatment for HCV has become highly effective, but there are still about 5–10% of treated patients who do not achieve sustained virological response (SVR). There are many factors that affect SVR rates including the absorption and metabolism of DAAs, genetic make-up, the presence or absence of cirrhosis, and severity and resistance of HCV to DAAs. An important factor influencing treatment failure is HCV resistance. The majority of treatment failures while on DAAs are not due to on-treatment failures, but due to relapses. The exact mechanism for mutation-associated relapse is unclear, but possible theories include persistent intrahepatocytic viral replication and/or differences in the levels of host immune response.

Keywords: HCV, molecular, treatment, drug resistance, mutation

1. Introduction

Hepatitis C virus (HCV) is an important medical problem, affecting millions of people worldwide [1]. HCV is one of the leading causes of chronic liver disease with one third of those affected eventually developing liver cirrhosis or hepatocellular carcinoma [2]. Additionally, HCV infection is asymptomatic in the majority of cases, and persons often do not receive necessary medical care as they are unaware of their infection. [3] Worldwide, HCV-related complications are responsible for about 350,000 deaths annually [2, 4].

HCV is an enveloped, positive-strand RNA virus and encodes a single polyprotein. This single polyprotein is cotranslationally and post-translationally processed by host and viral proteases to create 10 viral proteins: N terminus, Core, E1, E2, p7, NS2, NS3, NS4A, NS4B,

NS5A, NS5B, C-terminus. Of these, NS3, NS4A, NS4B, NS5A, and NS5B are nonstructural proteins that are the major players in RNA viral replication (**Figure 1**). The life cycle and replication of HCV is similar to other positive-strand RNA viruses. First, the virus enters the hepatocyte by receptor-mediated endocytosis, and after fusion and uncoating of the virion, it is released into the cytoplasm. The viral genome is then used as mRNA for translation of the viral polyprotein. After cleavage and processing of the viral polyprotein, the nonstructural proteins involved in replication (NS3-NS5B) are incorporated into a membranous web to make replication complexes. Replication occurs by the synthesis of a negative-strand RNA from the positive-strand RNA, from which multiple copies of positive-strand RNA are synthesized. Infectious viral particles are then assembled by combining the structural proteins and positive-strand viral RNA. The infectious viral particles are then able to be transported out of the cell using the host VLDL-secretory pathway [1].

The high rate of HCV replication and low fidelity of the HCV polymerase results in heterogeneous virus populations [5]. Due to these factors, mutations are inevitable and the genomic composition is constantly changing. For RNA viruses, the mutation rate is about 10^{-3}–10^{-5} per nucleotide copied. The low fidelity of HCV RNA polymerases is due to the inherent inaccuracy in nucleotide incorporation and lack of proofreading and post-replication repair [6, 7].

With the advent of direct acting antivirals (DAAs), treatment for HCV has become highly effective. However, even with these new treatments, still about 5–10% of people with HCV fail treatment [1, 3]. Treatment success is measured based on sustained virological response (SVR), which is defined as an undetectable level of HCV RNA at 12 weeks or 24 weeks after the completion of treatment. For those who do not achieve SVR, there are many types of treatment failures that are described. Null responders are persons who fail to suppress HCV RNA by at least two logs by completion of treatment, whereas partial responders refer to those who achieve a decrease in HCV RNA levels by ≤2 logs, but never become undetectable. There are also treatment failures whose HCV RNA becomes undetectable, but then reappears in the serum. Of these, viral breakthrough refers to HCV RNA reemerging in the serum while still on treatment reappearance of HCV RNA in the serum occurs after treatment completion is referred to as virological relapse [8].

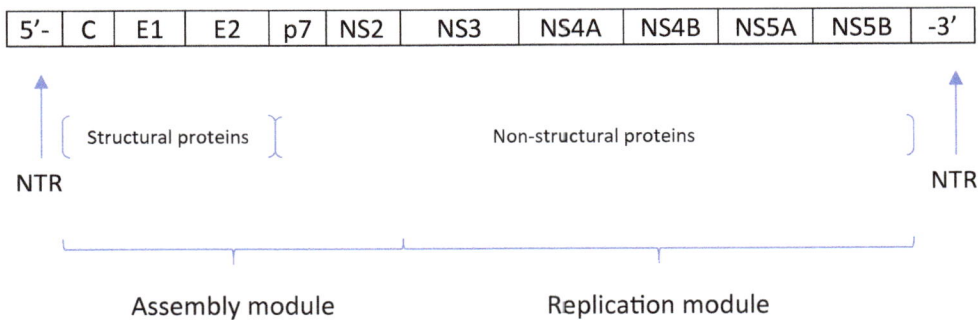

Figure 1. Hepatitis C viral genome configuration. The 5'- and 3'- designations indicate nontranslational regions (NTRs), and the 5'-region contains the internal ribosome entry site (IRES). The structural proteins (C, E1, E2) along with p7 and NS2 encompass the assembly module. The remainder of the nonstructural proteins makes up the replication complex.

The ability to achieve SVR depends on a combination of viral and host genetic factors. [5] Until recently, little evidence was available to explain host differences associated with chronic HCV infection. The discovery of a human polymorphism at the IL28B gene, a variation in a single nucleotide polymorphism (SNP) on chromosome 19 that is associated with the poor interferon response, has been crucial in distinguishing responders and nonresponders to interferon-based antiviral therapy [5, 9].

The DAAs currently target the proteins involved in HCV RNA replication, specifically NS3, NS5A, and NS5B (**Table 1**) [1]. Given high mutation rate, HCV is predisposed to the development of resistance to DAAs. Large numbers of genetically distinct HCV viral variants are generated daily in infected individuals. Collectively, these variants can create unique "quasispecies," possibly resulting in reduced susceptibility to DAAs if polymorphisms are created in drug-targeted genes [7].

Viral resistance is an important factor associated with HCV treatment failure. Resistant variants may be selected or enriched, and drug resistance may emerge during HCV antiviral treatment. While viral resistance is a consequence of treatment failure, it is not always the cause. Resistant variants occur naturally and often exist before antiviral drug treatment [10]. The prevalence of intrinsically resistant variants is partially related to replicative fitness. In viral quasispecies, a dominant variant is usually identified along with other less fit variants, which exist at lower frequencies. These small groups of resistance-associated substitutions (RASs) apparent before the initiation of treatment can become dominant in the presence of selective treatment with DAAs. This, in turn, may affect treatment outcomes, leading to virological breakthrough or more commonly, relapse after treatment cessation [7, 11].

Of note, there is a discrepancy in the term used to describe amino acid substitutions that reduce susceptibility of a virus to a drug or drug class, or the viral variants that carry the substitution resulting in reduced susceptibility. The term resistance-associated variants (RAVs) have been used previously to describe these mutants. Some investigators have stated that this term should be replaced by a different term, resistance-associated substitutions (RASs), to refer to the amino acid substitutions that confer resistance [11].

NS3	NS5A	NS5B
Boceprevir	Daclatasvir	Sofosbuvir
Telaprevir	Ledipasvir	Dasabuvir
Simeprevir	Ombitasvir	Beclabuvir
Asunaprevir	Elbasvir	
Paritaprevir	Velpatasvir	
Grazoprevir	Pibrentasvir	
Glecaprevir		

Table 1. Primary targets for DAAs for the treatment of HCV.

2. Identification of mutations

To identify barriers to resistance of experimental antiviral drugs, *in vitro* resistance selection studies are utilized. Many tests have been developed to identify HCV resistance including replicon systems in hepatoma cell lines, *in vitro* cell-free biochemical assays, and structural studies. However, these *in vitro* studies are not necessarily predictive of clinical resistance [7].

2.1. Replicon systems

Cell culture systems were developed to identify specific HCV mutations and how they affect drug resistance. The first cell culture replicon system was described in 1999 and is now available for the majority of HCV genotypes. This replicon system supports HCV replication in Huh7 hepatoma cells. Some replicons are unable to support the production of infectious virus particles, while more recent models are. The HCV pseudoparticle system, a cell culture replicon assay, was developed in 2003. This system works by creating a retrovirus coated with HCV envelope glycoproteins E1 and E2, which allows investigators to follow the steps of the specific HCV entry pathway. With this method, the entry of the virus can be monitored either visually or quantitatively by integrating reporter genes. In 2005, the first cell culture-infectious clone was introduced using the genotype 2a JFH1 isolate. With this method, the entire HCV viral life cycle is replicated in cell culture [1].

2.2. Cell-free biochemical assays

Cell-free assays are useful to examine the susceptibility of HCV to treatment with DAAs. This method can detect the effects of individual and complex substitutions on HCV enzyme activity under the influence of an investigational drug [7]. One such test is the NS3/4a enzyme assay, which uses a purified NS3 protease *in vitro*. In this assay, the NS3/4A fragment is cloned into an *Escherichia coli* expression plasmid for protein synthesis [7]. The protease activity is compared to various drug concentrations, and resistance is measured as inhibitory concentrations of either 50 and 90% (IC50 and IC90, respectively), drug concentrations that inhibit by 50 and 90%, respectively. [7]

Enzyme-based assays can be expensive and time consuming. These tests are based on coupled *in vitro* transcription/translation systems and have a turnaround time of about 10 hours. Several tools have been developed to study HCV replication, which evaluate viral enzyme efficacy and resistance to an RdRp inhibitor. The RdRp enzyme catalyzes the synthesis of both positive- and negative-strand RNAs. As for NS3/4A assays, the IC50 and IC90 can be calculated [7].

Studies have shown that some mutations reduce affinity for NS5A and decrease replication because NS5A regulates RdRp activity, although NS5A has no intrinsic enzyme activity [7].

2.3. Structural studies

Structural studies used to determine the structure of HCV proteins, and interactions with potential drugs include X-ray crystallography, nuclear magnetic resonance (NMR) spectroscopy, and computational methods [7].

X-ray crystallography was used to examine the conformational flexibility and interaction of the investigational drug with conserved or mutated viral structures. By using crystallography, insight can be obtained into the cross-resistance of drugs in relation to a specific viral protein as well as the genetic barrier to resistance can be measured [7].

The NMR spectroscopy method provides data on proteins in solution without requiring protein crystallization and, therefore, allows for structural and functional studies. For unstable disordered proteins such as NS5, this is a particularly useful method [7].

Computational methods involve creating a software-based structural modeling analysis that analyze the X-ray structures of mutated NS3 or NS5B proteins. Using wild-type structures obtained from the Protein Data Bank, three-dimensional analyses of drug-binding sites and the impact of varying amino acid substitutions can be determined [7].

It is the data from structural studies that led to the modeling and understanding of structure–function relationships that ultimately led to development of highly effective DAAs with few side effects. However, the factors involved in clinical resistance could only be identified by clinical studies.

3. Clinical resistance studies

Samples from treatment failure patients have been sequenced and compared to known mutations identified from cell culture phenotypic analysis. In this way, mutations and amino acid substitutions known to impact drug susceptibility have been correlated [5, 11]. The RdRp and NS5B proteins have high barriers, whereas NS5A inhibitors and NS34A protease inhibitors have low barriers to resistance [11]. Information on the prevalence of RASs at baseline has been heterogeneous. This is not only due to differences in methods but also because studies generally select which RASs to study and which can affect their clinical significance [11]. Furthermore, most studies have been performed on HCV genotype 1 with very little data on other genotypes.

3.1. NS3/NS4A

The HCV NS3/NS4A protease cleaves four sites along the encoded protein. Rapid development of resistance due to NS3/NS4A mutations is common in patients on treatment with protease inhibitor therapy. In patients with genotype 1 infection, the most frequent substitution noted was Q80K, which was found in 13.6% of cases [11]. The R155K mutation, which is seen in genotype 1a virus, causes resistance against nearly all protease inhibitors. In genotype 1b, various resistance mutations can arise based on the protease inhibitor class to which the patient has been exposed. In response to ketoamide protease inhibitors, A156, V36, T54, and V36 + A155 mutations have been observed. When macrocyclic inhibitors were used, however, mutations in R155K and D168A were seen. Given this information, even though NS3/NS4A inhibitors have been very effective in the treatment of HCV, it is evident that drug resistance challenges the success of these agents [5].

The majority of drug-resistant mutations in the NS3/NS4A protease occur at the active site, as alterations in these areas can modify drug binding while also having minimal impact on substrate binding and viral fitness. Danoprevir, simeprevir, and boceprevir, all project from the substrate envelope in areas known to have resistant mutations, leading to multi-drug-resistant variants. For instance, the large P2 moieties of danoprevir and simeprevir bind at the S2 subsite resulting in high interaction rates with the R155, D168, and A156 residues. It is not completely understood how these molecular alterations reduce inhibitor binding without affecting the binding of viral substrates [5] (**Figure 2**).

3.2. NS5A/NS5B

Substitutions in NS5B affecting efficacy of nucleoside analogs and non-nucleoside RdRp Palm-1 inhibitors are rare at baseline, while NS5A RASs are often detected in treatment naïve

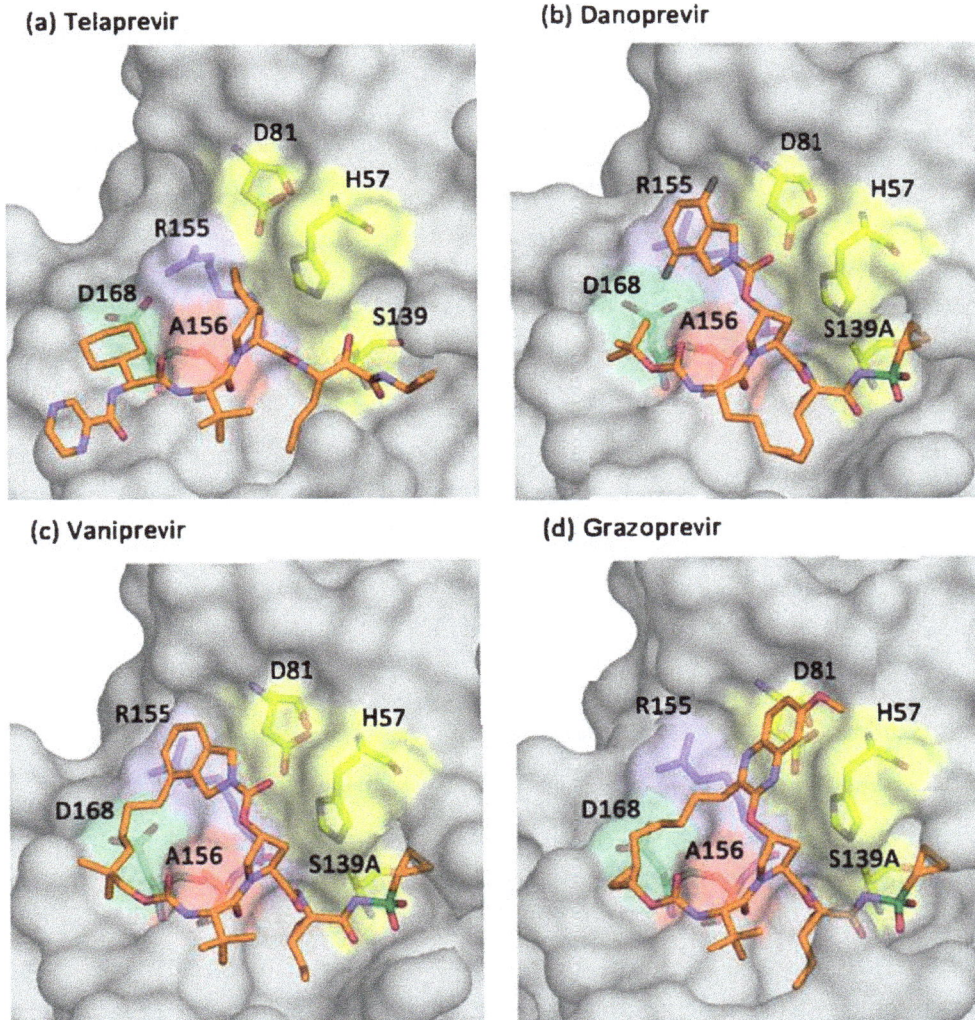

Figure 2. The binding conformations of telaprevir, danoprevir, vaniprevir, and grazoprevir. Surface representations of the wild-type protease in complex with (a) telaprevir, (b) danoprevir, (c) vaniprevir, and (d) grazoprevir. The catalytic triad consists of D81, H57, and S139A. The R155, A156, and D168 side chains are also labeled for each binding conformation. (Adapted from Romano et al. [5]).

patients. By using a 15% clinically relevant cutoff in patients with genotype 1a, one or more RASs were found in 13, 14, 7, and 16% of cases in North America, Europe, Asia-Pacific, and Oceania, respectively [11].

4. Clinical trial results

In patients treated with sofosbuvir/ledipasvir for genotype 1 infection, resistance has been examined in the ION 1–3 and ELECTRON studies. The presence of NS3-4A protease RASs at baseline did not affect the clinical response to treatment. NS5A RASs had no effect on the SVRs in naïve patients with or without cirrhosis and with or without ribavirin. They did, however, lead to a high level of resistance to ledipasvir. This resulted in a low SVR for treatment-experienced patients infected with genotype 1a. It was noted that all patients who relapsed had this RAS leading to reduced susceptibility to ledipasvir with an SVR of only 72%. Adding ribavirin improved SVR from 88 to 94% in cirrhotic patients treated for 12 weeks and from 85 to 100% for patients treated for 24 weeks. Ribavirin appears to reduce the effects of pre-existing NS5A RASs [11, 12].

A phase 2 study with combination of ombitasvir, paritaprevir, and ritonavir (ombitasvir/parita-previr/ritonavir) plus dasabuvir showed that patients with HCV genotype 1a infection with RASs at baseline had an SVR of 86% compared to 92% to those without RASs [13]. Researchers have reported SVR in HCV genotype 1-infected patients with and without cirrhosis who had baseline RASs. Treatment consisted of combinations of ombitasvir/paritaprevir/ritonavir plus dasabuvir with or without ribavirin for 12 or 24 weeks. Patients treated with HCV genotype 1b without riba-virin had 100% SVR. However, this was a small study with only four patients. The RAS region in these patients was NS3 protease- and paritaprevir-specific, which may explain the efficacy with-out ribavirin. The patients without baseline RASs treated with ombitasvir/paritaprevir/ritonavir had an SVR of 97% in all treatment groups [11].

In phase 2 and 3 studies of sofosbuvir plus daclatasvir with or without ribavirin in patients infected with HCV genotype 1, both treatment naïve and experienced, an SVR of 100% was seen in patients with baseline RASs. In patients with genotype 3 infections treated with sofosbuvir plus daclatasvir without ribavirin for 12 weeks, SVR in noncirrhotics was 97% for treatment naïve patients and 94% for treatment-experienced patients, and for patients with cirrhosis, 58% for treatment-naive patients and 69% for treatment-experienced patients. In patients with baseline NS5A RASs with cirrhosis treated for only 12 weeks, a reduced rate of SVR was seen [11, 14]. Although the sample size was small, and the treatment lacked ribavi-rin, this may suggest a benefit of prolonging treatment in genotype 3 patients with baseline NS5A RRASs and cirrhosis.

In patients treated with sofosbuvir plus simeprevir without ribavirin for 12 weeks, a phase 2 study showed an SVR rate of 95% for genotype 1b, 88% for genotype 1a with Q80K present, and 94% for genotype 1a without the Q80K variant [15]. In a phase 3 study, SVR rates were studied in patients who were either treatment naïve or had been treated with pegylated-INF-based regimens with or without cirrhosis. In patients without cirrhosis, SVR rates of 97% in genotype 1b, 96% genotype 1a with Q80K, and 97% in genotype 1a without Q80K were seen. In patients with cirrhosis, the SVR was 84% in genotype 1b, 74% genotype 1a with Q80K, and 92% genotype 1a without Q80K [16]. This suggested a decreased rate of SVR in genotype 1a in cirrhotic patients who had the Q80K RAS [11].

In phase 2 and 3 trials on patients treated with grazoprevir/elbasvir, the NS3 protease RAS was found not to affect SVR. However, the presence of NS5A RASs did affect the SVR in patients with genotype 1a. Patients without the elbasvir-specific NS5A RAS had an SVR of 98% compared to 58% in those with the RAS. NS5A RASs did not affect SVR in patients with genotype 1b. This effect was not observed with the addition of ribavirin and prolonging treatment to 16–18 weeks. The SVR was 94 and 100% with and without the NS5A RAS in genotype 1b, respectively. [11]

The combination of sofosbuvir/velpatasvir was studied in three phase 3 trials and the presence of NS5A RAS at baseline did not affect SVR in patients with genotypes 1a, 1b, 2, 4, 5 or 6. In patients with genotype 3 without the NS5A RAS at baseline, SVR was 97% compared to 88% in those with the RAS. Another phase 3 trial studied sofosbuvir/velpatasvir treatment in patients with decompensated cirrhosis (Child-Pugh B) and genotypes 1 to 6 HCV infections. Patients were treated for 12 weeks with ribavirin or 24 weeks without ribavirin. In patients with genotype 1 infection with and without baseline NS5A RAS, SVRs were 80% versus 96% for 12 weeks without ribavirin, 100% versus 98% for 12 weeks with ribavirin, and 90% versus 98% for 24 weeks without ribavirin. [11, 17] This suggests that adding ribavirin reduced the effect of NS5A RAS more than extending the duration of treatment [17–19]. Although asunaprevir plus daclatasvir has not been approved in the United Stated or Europe, it is used in Asia and the Middle East. Studies have suggested that patients with HCV genotype 1b with a NS5A RASs at positions 31 or 93 should not use this treatment regimen [11, 20].

In compliant patients, most treatment failures are relapses. The relapse rate has been described in several trials. One phase 3 trial studied treatment with sofosbuvir plus simeprevir in patients without cirrhosis and found a relapse rate of 17% and 3% at 8 and 12 weeks, respectively. In patients treated with grazoprevir/elbasvir, the relapse rate was 2.3% in HIV co-infected patients. A phase 3 trial studied sofosbuvir/velpatasvir and found that 20 patients with Child-Pugh B had relapse and 19 of these patients had NS5A RASs. Alternatively, 2 of 625 patients with genotype 1a, 1b, 4, 5, 6 without cirrhosis or with compensated cirrhosis experienced relapse and they both were found to have the NS5A substitution. In patients with genotype 3 and NS5A RASs, 10/277 had a relapse [11].

4.1. Retreatment studies

Retreatment strategies with DAAs in patients who have failed an interferon-free regimen can lead to SVR in the majority of patients including patients with known RASs. Studies suggested that sofosbuvir in combination with 1–3 other DAAs can be considered for retreatment. In addition, prolonging treatment to 24 weeks and/or adding ribavirin may also be considered [11]. These recommendations were based mainly on small scale studies. One study investigated 15 patients who failed a daclatasvir-based regimen. They were retreated with sofosbuvir and simeprevir without ribavirin for 12 weeks and achieved an SVR of 87%. In a study on retreatment with sofosbuvir, ombitasvir/paritaprevir/ritonavir and dasabuvir with or without ribavirin, 92% of noncirrhotic patients with genotype 1a achieved SVR after 12 weeks with ribavirin and 100% achieved SVR after 24 weeks with ribavirin in patients with cirrhosis. In cirrhotics with genotype 1b, SVR without ribavirin achieved 100% after 12 weeks. Variants resistant to sofosbuvir were rarely selected and appeared not to affect retreatment with sofosbuvir possibly because sofosbuvir-resistant variants tend to be poorly fit and to disappear rapidly after treatment is stopped. In contrast, variants associated with NS5A RASs tend to persist which can affect re-treatment. [11].

5. Conclusions

In the era of DAAs, about 90–95% of persons treated for HCV to achieve SVR. While these new treatment regimens have significantly and dramatically improved SVR rates, about 5–10% of patients fail to achieve SVR [1]. Factors that influence SVR rates include the absorption and metabolism of the DAA, the immune response of the patient, the presence or absence of cirrhosis, and the severity and resistance of HCV to DAAs. [11] HCV resistance plays an important role in treatment failure. Most of the treatment failures on DAA treatment regimens are not due to on-treatment failures, but due to relapses. The persistence and development of resistant variants post treatment depend on the DAA class used [7].

There are several possible mechanisms of mutation-associated relapse. It seems most likely that relapse involves persistent intrahepatocytic viral replication. Treatment with DAAs is known to be biphasic with a rapid initial response followed by a slower second phase. The first phase is dependent on drug potency, exposure, and susceptibility. The second phase, which can be accelerated by ribavirin, is dependent on drug potency, host genetic features, and the severity of immune response [11]. During treatment, drug-sensitive HCV is suppressed in the blood, and the virus remains undetectable. Due to differences in host-specific hepatocyte factors or aggressiveness of the host immune system, the level of resistant variants in the hepatocytes may be higher in relapsers compared to responders.

Acknowledgements

The support of a grant from Alexion Corporation, and the Herman Lopata Chair in hepatitis Research are gratefully acknowledged.

Abbreviations

DAAs   direct acting antivirals

HCV   hepatitis C virus

SVR   sustained virological response

HIV   human immunodeficiency virus

HBV   hepatitis B virus

RdRp   RNA-dependent RNA polymerase

SNP   single nucleotide polymorphism

RASs   resistance-associated substitutions

RAVs   resistance-associated variants

NMR   nucleic magnetic resonance

Author details

Shaina M. Lynch[1]* and George Y. Wu[2]

*Address all correspondence to: slynch@mcw.edu

1 Medical College of Wisconsin, Division of Gastroenterology and Hepatology, Milwaukee, USA

2 University of Connecticut, Division of Gastroenterology and Hepatology, Farmington, USA

References

[1] Kim S, Han KH, Ahn SH. Hepatitis C virus and antiviral drug resistance. Gut and Liver. 2016;**10**(6):890-895

[2] Esteban R, Nyberg L, Lalezari J, Ni L, Doehle B, Kanwar B, Brainard D, Subramanian M, Symonds WT, McHutchinson JG, Rodriguez-Torres M, Zeuzem S. Successful retreatment with sofosbuvir-containing regimens for HCV genotype 2 or 3 infected patients who failed prior sofosbuvir plus ribavirin therapy. Elsevier Science: Journal of Hepatology. 2014;**60**(1): Supplement, S4-S5

[3] Bartenschlager R, Lohmann V, Penin F. The molecular and structural basis of advanced antiviral therapy for hepatitis C virus infection. Nature Reviews. Microbiology. 2013;**11**(7):482-496

[4] Panel AIHG. Hepatitis C guidance: AASLD-IDSA recommendations for testing, managing, and treating adults infected with hepatitis C virus. Hepatology. 2015;**62**(3):932-954

[5] Romano KP, et al. The molecular basis of drug resistance against hepatitis C virus NS3/4A protease inhibitors. PLoS Pathogens. 2012;**8**(7):e1002832

[6] Perales C, et al. Resistance of hepatitis C virus to inhibitors: Complexity and clinical implications. Virus. 2015;**7**(11):5746-5766

[7] Fourati S, Pawlotsky JM. Virologic tools for HCV drug resistance testing. Virus. 2015;**7**(12): 6346-6359

[8] Ghany MG, et al. Diagnosis, management, and treatment of hepatitis C: An update. Hepatology. 2009;**49**(4):1335-1374

[9] Dienstag J. Chronic hepatitis C. In: Longo DL, Kasper DL, Jameson JL, Fauci AS, Hauser SL, Loscalzo J, editors. Harrison's Principles of Internal Medicine. McGraw Hill; New York, 2012. p. 2579-2585

[10] Rong L, et al. Rapid emergence of protease inhibitor resistance in hepatitis C virus. Science Translational Medicine. 2010;**2**(30):30ra32

[11] Pawlotsky JM. Hepatitis C virus resistance to direct-acting antiviral drugs in interferon-free regimens. Gastroenterology. 2016;**151**(1):70-86

[12] Sarrazin C. The importance of resistance to direct antiviral drugs in HCV infection in clinical practice. Journal of Hepatology. 2016;**64**(2):486-504

[13] Krishnan P, et al. Resistance analysis of baseline and treatment-emergent variants in hepatitis C virus genotype 1 in the AVIATOR study with paritaprevir-ritonavir, ombitasvir, and dasabuvir. Antimicrobial Agents and Chemotherapy. 2015;**59**(9):5445-5454

[14] Nelson DR, et al. All-oral 12-week treatment with daclatasvir plus sofosbuvir in patients with hepatitis C virus genotype 3 infection: ALLY-3 phase III study. Hepatology. 2015;**61**(4): 1127-1135

[15] Lawitz E, et al. Simeprevir plus sofosbuvir, with or without ribavirin, to treat chronic infection with hepatitis C virus genotype 1 in non-responders to pegylated interferon and ribavirin and treatment-naive patients: The COSMOS randomised study. Lancet. 2014;**384**(9956):1756-1765

[16] Kwo P, et al. Simeprevir plus sofosbuvir (12 and 8 weeks) in hepatitis C virus genotype 1-infected patients without cirrhosis: OPTIMIST-1, a phase 3, randomized study. Hepatology. 2016;**64**(2):370-380

[17] Curry MP, et al. Sofosbuvir and velpatasvir for HCV in patients with decompensated cirrhosis. The New England Journal of Medicine. 2015;**373**(27):2618-2628

[18] Feld JJ, et al. Sofosbuvir and velpatasvir for HCV genotype 1, 2, 4, 5, and 6 infection. The New England Journal of Medicine. 2015;**373**(27):2599-2607

[19] Foster GR, et al. Sofosbuvir and velpatasvir for HCV genotype 2 and 3 infection. The New England Journal of Medicine. 2015;**373**(27):2608-2617

[20] McPhee F, et al. High sustained virologic response to daclatasvir plus asunaprevir in elderly and cirrhotic patients with hepatitis C virus genotype 1b without baseline NS5A polymorphisms. Advances in Therapy. 2015;**32**(7):637-649

13

Current Therapeutic Options for HCV-HIV Coinfection

Ljiljana Perić and Dario Sabadi

Abstract

Due to shared risk factors for transmission, coinfection with human immunodeficiency virus (HIV) and hepatitis C virus (HCV) is a very common event. The prevalence of HCV infection among HIV-positive patients averages about 35%. In HIV/HCV co-infected patients, liver-related morbidity and mortality is a prominent non-AIDS-defining complication: up to 90% of liver-related deaths in HIV-infected patients are attributable to HCV. The progression of liver fibrosis is accelerated in HIV/HCV-coinfected patients, particularly in individuals with low CD4 counts ($\leq$350 cells/mm^3). Antiretroviral therapy may slow liver disease progression in HIV/HCV-coinfected patients and should, therefore, be considered for all coinfected patients regardless of CD4 cell count. Most patients with HIV/HCV coinfection are taking multi-drug antiretroviral therapy, which may pose a problem with drug–drug interactions when initiating therapy with HCV medications. Rapid advances in HCV drug development led to the discovery of new classes of direct-acting antiviral (DAA) agents that target the HCV replication cycle. Several studies demonstrated comparable rates of sustained virological response (SVR) in coinfected and monoinfected patients with new DAA-based therapy.

Keywords: HCV/HIV-coinfection, liver cirrhosis, CD4 T lymphocytes, antiretroviral therapy (ART), direct-acting antiviral (DAA) agents, drug–drug interaction

1. Introduction

By the Global AIDS Update: 2016, around 36.7 million people are living with human immunodeficiency virus (HIV) in the world today [1]. Five million of them are also infected with hepatitis C virus (HCV) [1]. HIV accelerate the progression of hepatitis C, inducing increased morbidity and mortality [2]. HIV-infected people are on average six times more likely than HIV-uninfected people to have HCV infection [3].

HIV and HCV share modes of transmission: often occurring by exposure to blood, sexual intercourse or by mother-to-child transmission.

2. Epidemiology

The prevalence of HCV antibodies varies widely among HIV transmission groups, ranging from 7–8% in men who have sex with men to 60–70% in hemophiliacs and 80–90% in intravenous drug users (IDUs), the most important group (**Figure 1**) [4].

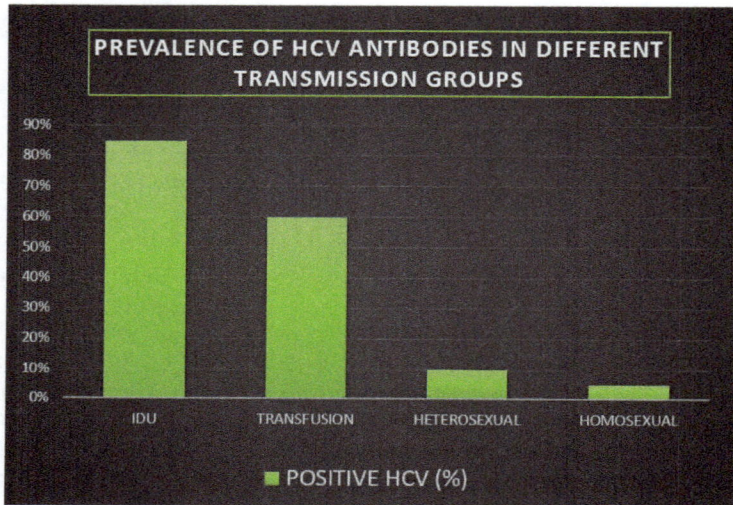

Figure 1. Prevalence of HCV antibodies in different transmission groups. IDU, intravenous drug users; HCV, hepatitis C virus. Inspired by Management of Hepatitis C and HIV coinfection, Clinical Protocol for the WHO European Region. Available at: http://www.euro.who.int/data/assets/pdf_file/0008/78146/E90840Chapter6.pdf, Version September 1th, 2015.

For HIV-infected patients with HCV coinfection, liver-related morbidity and mortality is a prominent non-AIDS-defining complication [5]. Up to 90% of liver-related deaths in HIV-infected patients are attributable to HCV [5].

Among patients with chronic HCV infection, approximately one-third progress to cirrhosis, at a median time of 20 years [6–8]. The risk of progression is even greater in HCV/HIV-coinfected patients with low CD4 T lymphocyte (CD4) cell counts ($\leq$350 cells/mm^3) [6, 9, 10]. Cirrhosis has been observed to occur 12–16 years earlier in HIV/HCV-coinfected patients compared with those who have HCV monoinfection [11].

3. Antiretroviral therapy (ART) in HIV/HCV-coinfected patients

Antiretroviral therapy (ART) may slow liver disease progression in HIV/HCV-coinfected patients and should, therefore, be considered for all coinfected patients regardless of CD4

NRTIs	NNRTIs	Protease inhibitors	Entry inhibitors	Integrase inhibitors
Abacavir	Efavirenz	Atazanavir, atazanavir/ritonavir	Enfuvirtide	Dolutegravir
Didanosine	Etravirine	Darunavir/ritonavir Darunavir/cobicistat	Maraviroc	Raltegravir
Emtricitabine	Nevirapine	Fosamprenavir		
Lamivudine	Rilpivirine	Lopinavir		
Stavudine		Saquinavir		
Tenofovir				
Zidovudine				

Table 1. Standard recommended treatments for naive patients with HIV-1 infection.

cell count [12]. This recommendation is supported by observational studies that suggest that antiretroviral therapy may reduce the risk of liver-related morbidity. The key issues in the clinical management of HIV/HCV-coinfected patients are which treatment for each condition and when to initiate it [12].

Classes of antiretroviral agents are nucleoside reverse transcriptase inhibitors (NRTIs), non-nucleoside reverse transcriptase inhibitors (NNRTIs), protease inhibitors (PIs), integrase inhibitors (INSTIs), entry/fusion inhibitors (FIs) and chemokine receptor antagonists (CCR5 antagonists).

Standard recommended treatments for naive patients with HIV-1 infection (**Table 1**) generally consist of two nucleoside reverse transcriptase inhibitors (NRTIs) in combination with a third active antiretroviral drug from one of three drug classes: an integrase strand transfer inhibitor (INSTI), a non-nucleoside reverse transcriptase inhibitor (NNRTI) or a protease inhibitor (PI) with a pharmacokinetic (PK) enhancer (booster) (cobicistat or ritonavir) [12].

Antiretroviral therapy (ART) associated with liver injury is more common in HIV/HCV-coinfected patients than in those with HIV monoinfection [6, 13]. Some older ART have been associated with higher rates of liver injury in patients with chronic HCV infection, but newer ART drugs currently in use appear to be less hepatotoxic [6, 13]. Patients with significant alanine aminotransferase (ALT) and/or aspartate aminotransferase (AST) elevation should be carefully evaluated for signs and symptoms of liver insufficiency and for alternative causes of liver injury (e.g., acute HAV or HBV infection, hepatobiliary disease, or alcoholic hepatitis) [6, 14]. Short-term interruption of the ART regimen or of the specific drug suspected of causing the liver injury may be required [6, 14].

4. Concurrent treatment of HIV and HCV by the Office of AIDS Research advisory council (OARAC 2016)

If the decision is made to treat HCV, the antiretroviral regimen may need to be modified before HCV treatment is initiated to reduce the potential drug–drug interactions and/or toxicities that may develop during the period of concurrent HIV and HCV treatment [6].

In patients with suppressed plasma HIV RNA and modified antiretroviral therapy, HIV RNA should be measured within 4–8 weeks after changing antiretroviral therapy to confirm the effectiveness of the new regimen [6]. After completion of HCV treatment, the modified ART regimen should be continued for at least 2 weeks before reinitiating the original regimen [6]. This is necessary because of the prolonged half-life of some HCV drugs and the potential risk of drug–drug interactions if a prior HIV regimen is resumed soon after HCV treatment is completed [6].

5. HCV therapy in HIV/HCV-coinfected patients by EASL recommendations on treatment of hepatitis C, 2016

With direct-acting antivirals (DAAs), HCV cure rates of both HCV mono and HIV/HCV-coinfected persons are greater than 95% [15]. Current treatment guidelines no longer separate these two groups. Indications for HCV treatment and choice of direct-acting antiviral (DAA) agents combination are now the same for all HCV patients. In HIV/HCV co-infection, drug interactions between HIV and HCV agents need be checked prior to starting HCV therapy [15]. The higher risk of hepatic decompensation in HIV/HCV-coinfected patients, including those receiving successful antiretroviral therapy, continues to make these patients a high priority group for receiving access to direct-acting antiviral (DAA) agents as combination therapy [15].

6. Key studies for treatment of HCV with HIV coinfection

Using DAA therapy, several studies demonstrated comparable rates of sustained virological response (SVR) in coinfected and monoinfected patients.

These trials, however, have primarily included individuals with CD4 counts >200 cells/mm^3, and most patients in these trials did not have cirrhosis.

6.1. Sofosbuvir for genotype 1–4 in HIV coinfection by Rodriguez-Torres et al.

In an open-label trial, 23 HCV/HIV-coinfected treatment-naive patients with genotype 1–4 received the 12-week triple therapy of peginterferon alfa-2a, ribavirin (weight-based) and sofosbuvir [16]. Mean CD4 count was 562 cells/mm^3, and all were on antiretroviral therapy (tenofovir-emtricitabine plus one of the following: efavirenz, atazanavir plus ritonavir, darunavir plus ritonavir, rilpivirine or raltegravir) [16]. The overall SVR12 rate was 91%; of the 19 patients with genotype 1, 89% achieved an SVR12 (**Figure 2**) [16].

6.2. TURQUOISE-I by Wyles et al.

This open-label study randomized treatment-naive and experienced patients with chronic HCV genotype 1 and HIV coinfection to receive a 12- or 24-week course of ombitasvir-paritaprevir-ritonavir and dasabuvir plus ribavirin [17]. Patients were required to have

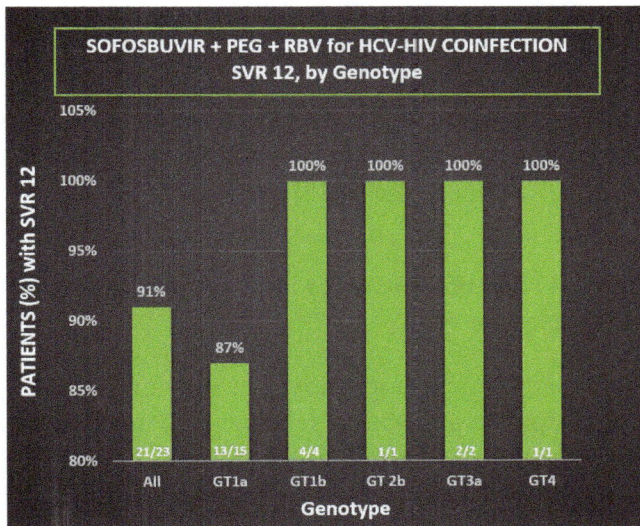

Figure 2. Sofosbuvir for genotype 1-4 in HIV coinfection. PEG, peginterferon alfa-2a; RBV, ribavirin; SVR12, sustained viral response 12 weeks after the end of treatment; GT, genotype. Inspired by http://slides.hcvonline.org/uploads/151/sofosbuvir_for_genotype_14_in_hiv_coinfection.pdf

a CD4 > 200 cells/mm^3 and an HIV RNA level < 40 copies while receiving an atazanavir- or raltegravir-based regimen [17]. The sustained virological response (SVR) 12 rates were 93.5% (29 of 31) in the 12-week group and 90.6% (29 of 32) in the 24-week group (**Figure 3**) [17].

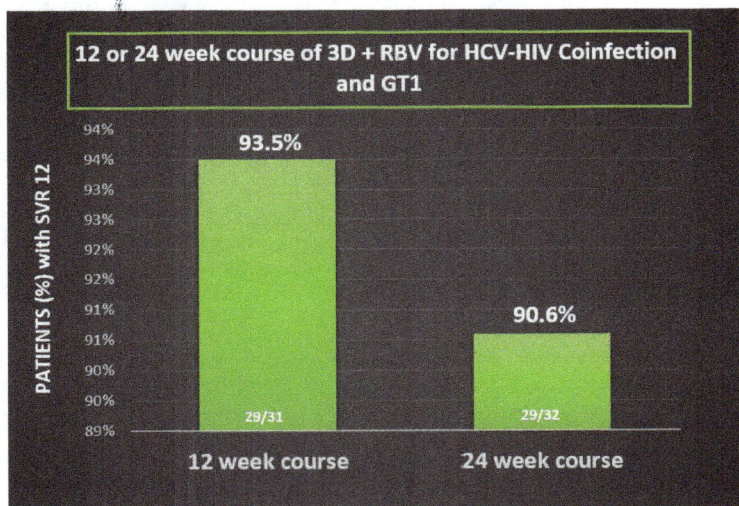

Figure 3. TURQUOISE-I. 3 D, Ombitasvir-Paritaprevir-Ritonavir and Dasabuvir; RBV, ribavirin; GT, genotype; SVR, sustained viral response. Inspired by https://depts.washington.edu/hepstudy/presentations/uploads/137/turquoise13d.pdf

6.3. ALLY-2 study (daclatasvir + sofosbuvir in HCV GT 1–4 and HIV coinfection) by Wyles et al.

Among HIV/HCV-coinfected patients who received 12 weeks of daclatasvir plus sofosbuvir, sustained virologic response across all genotypes was 97.0% (including black patients and those with cirrhosis) and 76.0% after 8 weeks [18].

6.4. ION-4 study (ledipasvir and sofosbuvir for HCV genotype 1 or 4 in patients coinfected with HIV-1) by Naggie et al.

In this multicenter, open-label, single-group study, 12 weeks of treatment with the once-daily, single-tablet regimen of ledipasvir-sofosbuvir resulted in a sustained virologic response in 96% of patients [19]. In exploratory subgroup analyses, rates of sustained virologic response 12 weeks after the end of therapy (the primary efficacy end point) were similar across all subgroups except that black patients, who made up 34% of the study population, had lower rates of sustained virologic response (**Figure 4**) [19].

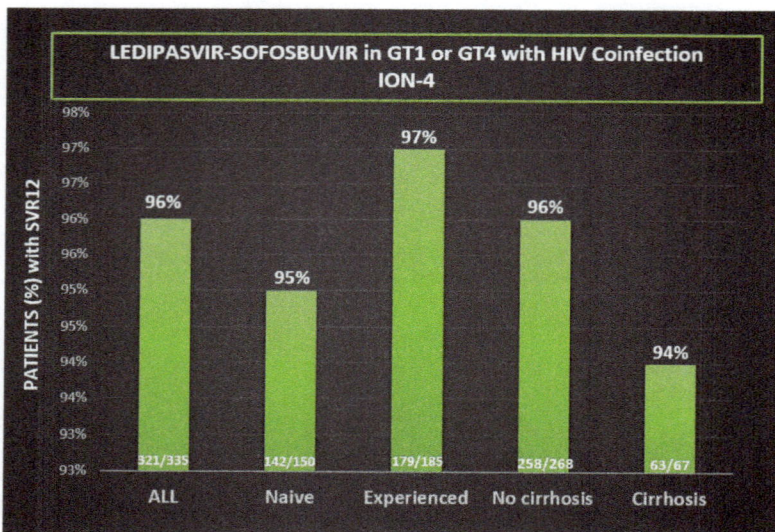

Figure 4. Ledipasvir and sofosbuvir for HCV genotype 1 or 4 in patients coinfected with HIV-1. GT 1 or 4, genotype 1 or 4; SVR 12, sustained viral response 12 weeks after the end of treatment. Inspired by http://slides.hcvonline.org/uploads/149/ion4_ls.pdf

7. Conclusions

Due to shared risk factors for transmission, HIV/HCV coinfection is a very common event, the prevalence averages about 35% in the United States and Europe [20, 21].

The progression of liver fibrosis is accelerated in HIV/HCV-coinfected patients. HCV guidance recommends using the same HCV treatment approach for patients coinfected with HIV as those with HCV monoinfection.

DAAs and interferon-free combination therapy has changed the landscape of therapy for HIV/HCV-coinfected patients.

Multiple studies demonstrating comparable rates of SVR in coinfected and monoinfected patients.

Author details

Ljiljana Perić[1,2]* and Dario Sabadi[1,2]

*Address all correspondence to: ljiljana.peric@mefos.hr

1 Department of Infectious Diseases and Dermatology, Faculty of Medicine Osijek, University of Osijek, Osijek, Croatia

2 Clinic for Infectious Diseases, University Hospital Center Osijek, Osijek, Croatia

References

[1] Global AIDS Response Progress Reporting (GARPR) 2016. Geneva, Switzerland: UNAIDS 2016 Estimates; 2016

[2] Operskalski EA, Kovacs A. HIV/HCV co-infection: Pathogenesis, clinical complications, treatment, and new therapeutic technologies. Current HIV/AIDS Reports. 2011;8(1):12-22

[3] Platt L, Easterbrook P, Gower E, McDonald B, Sabin K, McGowan C, Yanny I, Razavi H, Vickerman P. Prevalence and burden of HCV co-infection in people living with HIV: A global systematic review and meta-analysis. 2016.

[4] Management of hepatitis C and HIV coinfection, Clinical Protocol for the WHO European Region, Chapter6.pdf, Version 1 September 2015. Available from: http://www.euro.who.int/data/assets/pdf_file/0008/78146/ E90840

[5] Spach DH, Nina Kim H. Treatment of Chronic Hepatitis C Infection Overview. Available from: http://www.hepatitisc.uw.edu/go/treatment-infection

[6] Guidelines for the Use of Antiretroviral Agents in HIV-1-Infected Adults and Adolescents, Developed by the DHHS Panel on Antiretroviral Guidelines for Adults and Adolescents – A Working Group of the Office of AIDS Research Advisory Council (OARAC), 8/25/2017. Available from: https://aidsinfo.nih.gov/contentfiles/lvguidelines/AdultandAdolescentGL.pdf

[7] Alter MJ, Margolis HS, Krawczynski K, et al. The natural history of community-acquired hepatitis C in the United States. The Sentinel Counties Chronic non-A, non-B Hepatitis

Study Team. The New England Journal of Medicine 1992;**327** (27):1899-1905. Available at: http://www.ncbi.nlm.nih.gov/entrez/query.fcgi?cmd=Retrieve&db=PubMed&dopt=Citation&list_uids=1280771

[8]   Thomas DL, Astemborski J, Rai RM, et al. The natural history of hepatitis C virus infection: Host, viral, and environmental factors. Journal of the American Medical Association. 2000;**284**(4):450-456 Available from: http://www.ncbi.nlm.nih.gov/entrez/query.fcgi?cmd=Retrieve&db=PubMed&dopt=Citation&list_uids=10904508

[9]   Considerations for Antiretroviral Use in Patients with Coinfections, Hepatitis C (HCV)/HIV Coinfection, Last Updated: July 14, 2016; Last Reviewed: July 14, 2016. Developed by the DHHS Panel on Antiretroviral Guidelines for Adults and Adolescents – A Working Group of the Office of AIDS Research Advisory Council (OARAC), Available at: https://aidsinfo.nih.gov/guidelines/html/1/adult-and-adolescent-arv-guidelines/26/hcv-hiv

[10] Graham CS, Baden LR, Yu E, et al. Influence of human immunodeficiency virus infection on the course of hepatitis C virus infection: A meta-analysis. Clinical Infectious Diseases. 2001;**33**(4):562-569 Available from: http://www.ncbi.nlm.nih.gov/entrez/query.fcgi?cmd=Retrieve&db=PubMed&dopt=Citation&list_uids=11462196

[11] Benhamou Y, Bochet M, Di Martino V, Charlotte F, Azria F, Coutellier A, Vidaud M, Bricaire F, Opolon P, Katlama C, Poynard T. Liver fibrosis progression in human immunodeficiency virus and hepatitis C virus coinfected patients. Hepatology. 1999;**30**:1054-1058

[12] Considerations for Antiretroviral Use in Patients with Coinfections, Hepatitis C (HCV)/HIV Coinfection, Last Updated: 14 July 2016; Last Reviewed: 14 July 2016. Available from: https://aidsinfo.nih.gov/guidelines/html/1/adult-and-adolescent-arv-guidelines/26/hcv-hiv

[13] Aranzabal L, Casado JL, Moya J, et al. Influence of liver fibrosis on highly active antiretroviral therapy-associated hepatotoxicity in patients with HIV and hepatitis C virus coinfection. Clinical Infectious Diseases. 2005;**40**(4):588-593 Available from: http://www.ncbi.nlm.nih.gov/entrez/query.fcgi?cmd=Retrieve&db=PubMed&dopt=Citation&list_uids=15712082

[14] Sulkowski MS, Thomas DL. Hepatitis C in the HIV-infected patient. Clinics in Liver Disease. 2003;**7**(1):179-194 Available from: http://www.ncbi.nlm.nih.gov/entrez/query.fcgi?cmd=Retrieve&db=PubMed&dopt=Citation&list_uids=12691466

[15] Rockstroh JK, Hardy WD. Current treatment options for hepatitis C patients co-infected with HIV, Expert Rev Gastroenterol Hepatol. 2016;**10**:689-695. Available from: https://www.ncbi.nlm.nih.gov/pubmed/26799571

[16] Rodriguez-Torres M et al. Sofosbuvir for chronic hepatitis C virus infection genotype 1-4 in patients coinfected with HIV. Journal of Acquired Immune Deficiency Syndrome. 2015;**68**:543-549 Available from: https://www.ncbi.nlm.nih.gov/pubmed/25622055, http://slides.hcvonline.org/uploads/151/sofosbuvir_for_genotype_14_in_hiv_coinfection.pdf

[17] Wyles D et al. TURQUOISE-I Part 1b: Ombitasvir/Paritaprevir/Ritonavir and Dasabuvir with Ribavirin for Hepatitis C Virus Infection in HIV-1 Coinfected Patients on Darunavir. The Journal of Infectious Disease. 2017;**215**(4):599-605. doi: 10.1093/infdis/jiw597. Available from: https://www.ncbi.nlm.nih.gov/pubmed/28329334 and https://depts.washington.edu/hepstudy/presentations/uploads/137/turquoise13d.pdf

[18] Wyles DL et al. Daclatasvir in combination with sofosbuvir for HIV/HCV coinfection: ALLY-2 Study. The New England Journal of Medicine. 2015;**373**:714-725 Available from: http://slides.hcvonline.org/uploads/163/ally2_daclatasvir.pdf and http://www.nejm.org/doi/full/10.1056/NEJMoa1503153#t=article

[19] Naggie S et al. Ledipasvir and sofosbuvir for HCV in patients coinfected with HIV-1-ION-4 Study. The New England Journal of Medicine. 2015;**378**:705-713 Available at http://www.nejm.org/doi/full/10.1056/NEJMoa1501315?rss=searchAndBrowse#t=article and http://slides.hcvonline.org/uploads/149/ion4_ls.pdf

[20] Nina Kim H, Spach DH. Treatment of Hepatitis C in Patients with HIV Coinfection. Available from: http://www.hepatitisc.uw.edu/go/special-populations-situations/treatment-hiv-coinfection/core-concept/all#drug-drug-interactions-hiv-hcv-coinfection-treatment

[21] Verucchi G et al. Human immunodeficiency virus and hepatitis C virus coinfection: Epidemiology, natural history, therapeutic options and clinical management. Infection. 2004;**32**(1):33-46 Available from: https://www.ncbi.nlm.nih.gov/pubmed/15007741

14

Progress in Vaccine Development for HCV Infection

Ashraf Tabll, Reem El-Shenawy and Yasmine El Abd

Abstract

Hepatitis C virus (HCV) is a blood-transmitted disease that spreads among 3% of the world's population causing seriously increasing mortality rates. The HCV prevalence in Egypt in October 2008 was 14.7% and declined to 6.3% in the survey carried out in October 2015. Nowadays, the new direct-acting antivirals (DAAs) show amazing results especially with regard to HCV genotype 1, but there is still a great necessity to produce a vaccine to avoid this viral infection. Additionally, neutralizing anti-HCV antibodies could be utilized in combination with DAAs empowering their effect. A powerful candidate HCV vaccine should create comprehensively cross-receptive T cells CD4 and CD8 and effectively neutralizing antibodies to successfully clear the virus. The current clinical trials for HCV vaccines comprise synthetic peptides, DNA-based vaccines, or recombinant protein vaccines. Several preclinical vaccine studies are under research including cell culture-derived HCV (HCVcc), HCV-like particles, and recombinant adenoviral vaccines. This mini-review will discuss the prevalence of HCV worldwide and in Egypt. We will present the recent progress in basic research and preclinical and clinical studies for HCV vaccine. Finally, it will present the phenomena of spontaneous clearance of HCV without treatment as a model for study of HCV vaccine development.

Keywords: HCV vaccine, cell culture-derived HCV, HCV-like particles, spontaneous clearance, neutralizing antibodies

1. Introduction

Hepatitis C virus (HCV) infection is the main health problem worldwide and in Egypt. Until now there is no prophylactic or therapeutic vaccine for HCV. The development of a protective vaccine is essential in combating the global HCV epidemic. Understanding the immune response in those who spontaneously resolve HCV infections versus those who develop chronic

infection is the key to the development of prophylactic or therapeutic vaccine. In this mini review, we will discuss the recent and more promising progress in the HCV vaccine development.

2. Prevalence of HCV in the world

HCV is a worldwide predominant pathogen with very high mortality rates [1]. Sub-Saharan Africa accounts for almost one-fifth of worldwide infections; in Southeast Asia, approximately 32.2 million people have chronic HCV infection, and over 6 million infected people are in Latin America [2]. In [3], it is reported that 2.8% people equating more than 185 million are infected by HCV worldwide. Egypt was from the countries with the high prevalence rates (14.7%), followed by Pakistan (4.8%) and China (3.2%). Constant HCV disease is connected with the advancement of liver fibrosis, liver cirrhosis, hepatocellular malignancy, and death [3]. Although the HCV occurrence rate is clearly diminishing in the developing countries, Razavi et al. [4] reported that over the next 20 years the mortality from liver diseases secondary to HCV will keep on rising.

3. Prevalence of HCV in Egypt

The 2015 Egypt Health Issues Survey conducted on behalf of the Ministry of Health and Population by El-Zanaty and Associates (http://www.dhsprogram.com) showed that the prevalence of HCV antibodies was 6.3% of the tested individuals ($n = 26{,}027$) in cases with ages 1–59 years, while prevalence of HCV RNA was 4.4%. In 2008, according to the health survey carried out, the prevalence of HCV antibodies was 14.7% (number of examined individuals was 11,126) and that of HCV RNA was 9.8% (as shown in **Figure 1**). Interestingly, a

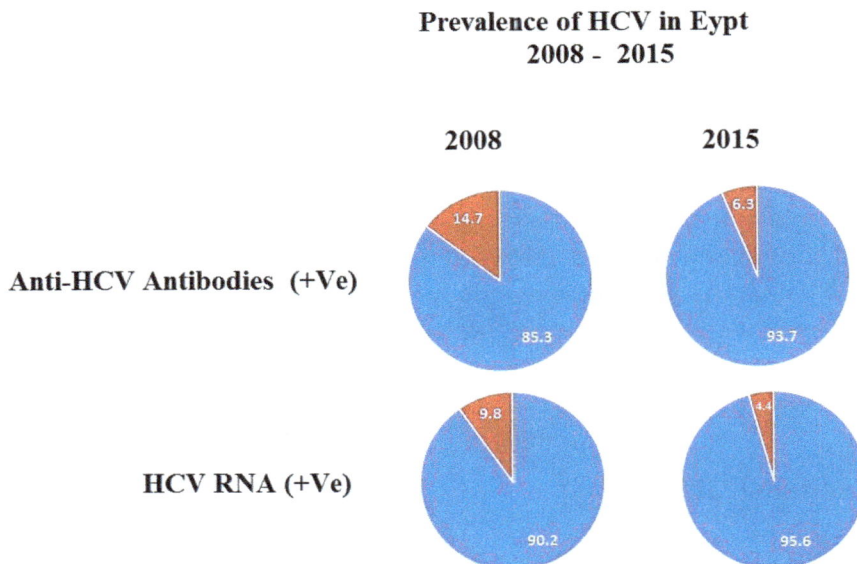

Figure 1. Prevalence of HCV in Egypt according to health survey carried out at 2008 and 2015 in cases aged from 1 to 59 years (male and females).

promising finding of the 2015 survey is that the prevalence of HCV antibodies was 0.7 and HCV RNA was 0.3 among cases with age 10–14, while the percentage of HCV antibodies in cases with ages 50–59 years ($n = 627$) was 30.5–41.9%, and that of HCV RNA was 23.7–27.8%. This means that low prevalence of HCV infection is expected among the future generation. The decline of prevalence of HCV antibodies and HCV RNA is due to single usage of syringes and needles, sterilization of medical, dental and dialysis instruments, regular check-up, testing of blood donors, and also activity of Egyptian National Control Strategy for viral hepatitis.

4. Barriers that limit HCV vaccine development

HCV is the world's most common blood-borne viral infection for which there is no vaccine [5, 6]. Most acute HCV infections are asymptomatic, and viral persistence is established in the majority of infected subjects. Vaccine development is fundamental to globally eliminate HCV infection through prevention, representing a public health priority. Generally, a good vaccine must induce cellular and humoral immunity, during early phase of viral infection, before the virus gets the opportunity to trigger its numerous immune escape mechanisms [7]. Also a new vaccine should be affordable, safe, not inducing autoimmunity or hypersensitivity, and finally providing long-lasting immunity. Progress in HCV vaccine development is hampered due to the high level of genetic diversity among different HCV strains resulting from the absence of proofreading activity for the NS5B RNA-dependent polymerase [8], which led to the production of genetically distinct but closely related variants within the same genotype designated quasi species [9]. Also, the high viral mutation rate enabled the viral persistence by evading the cellular and humoral immune control [10], either by binding low-density lipoproteins or infecting surrounding cells through cell-to-cell contact mediated by CD81 and Claudin-1 and inducing interfering antibodies by continuous mutation [11]. Also the barriers that challenges vaccine research against HCV is the lack of small and suitable animal models for studying HCV pathogenesis and protective specific immunity. Nowadays, the chimpanzee is the only suitable infectious animal model with lots of ethical and financial obstacles to acquire [12]. Progression to chronic liver disease results from the ineffective weak immune response against the virus. In summary, many barriers occur for HCV vaccine development such as the presence of several HCV genotypes, restricted accessibility of animal models, and the complicated nature of the immunological response to HCV. Neutralizing antibody (Nab) and cellular immune responses to CD4$^+$ and CD8$^+$ T cells are essential for HCV clearance [13]. Some reports suggest that the highly changeable, quasi-species' nature of HCV and the continuous emergence of resistant strains are reasons for the HCV resistance attitude. However, the HCV resistance in the presence of circulating antibodies cannot be completely explained by the continuous and rapid acquired viral genetic variability alone.

5. HCV vaccine strategies

The target of all strategies is to activate a long-lasting T-cell response involving both helper CD4$^+$ and CD8$^+$ rather than only adaptive immune response. HCV is vastly mutable, thus developing an effective vaccine is very challenging. In 2013 [14], scientists from Scripps Research Institute reported that the virus uses HCV E2 envelope glycoprotein as the key protein to invade liver cells. Discovering that E2 binds to the CD81 receptor on the liver cells through a relatively conserved binding region will empower designing of a vaccine which triggers effective antibody responses to various HCV genotypes. Previous studies focused on certain peptide sequences from envelope regions 1 and 2 of HCV as a candidate vaccine. They found that peptide region E1 (aa 315–323) and peptide regions from HCV E2 (aa 412–219) and HCV E2 (aa 517–531) had capability to introduce neutralizing antibodies in mice, rabbits, and goats, while peptide sequence from HCV E2 (aa 430–447) produced nonneutralizing antibodies, which are known interference antibodies [15–22]. Another strategy is to use viral vectors inducing T-cell responses against HCV-infected cells, e.g., adenoviral vectors that have big areas of the HCV genome itself. Early vaccines targeted only genotypes 1a and 1b, accounting for more than 60% of chronic HCV infections worldwide, while subsequent vaccines might target other genotypes by prevalence [23].

Various HCV candidate vaccines were described, comprising synthetic peptides [24], recombinant E1 and E2 proteins [25, 26], recombinant adenoviral and prime-boost strategies with modified vaccinia Ankara (MVA) vaccines or recombinant E1 and E2 glycoproteins [27–30]. However, only few proceeded to phases I and II using recombinant poxvirus [31], DNA vaccines [29, 32], synthetic peptide-based vaccines [33], and MVA vaccines and adenoviral [34, 35]. Recently, Teimourpour et al. [36] successfully cloned structural viral genes in pCDNA3.1 (+) vector and expressed them in eukaryotic expression system facilitating the development of new DNA vaccines against HCV. These candidate vaccines produced robust cross-reactive HCV-specific cellular responses, and HCV viral load was reduced.

On the other hand, plant-based vaccine is a new approach for making an inexpensive and easily producible HCV vaccine. Infecting plants with a genetically engineered tobacco mosaic virus (TMV) produced the hyper variable region 1 (HVR1) peptide fused to the B subunit of cholera toxin CTB. The plant-derived HVR1/CTB reacted with specific antibodies acquired from HCV-infected individuals [37].

6. HCV-like particles and cell culture-derived HCV (HCVcc)

Special focus will be drawn on candidate vaccine HCV-like particles and HCVcc, which is expected to boom in the next years. Virus-like particle consists of some of the structural viral proteins. These proteins self-assemble into particles which resemble the virus but lack viral nucleic acid; thus, they are not infectious. Viral-like particles (VLP) are typically more immunogenic because of their highly repetitive and multivalent structure.

6.1. HCV-viral like particles (VLP)

HCV VLP vaccine is very promising for the development of a prophylactic vaccine. VLP are vectors for gene delivery that closely resemble the mature HCV. Hence, using a single VLP-based vaccine, neutralizing antibodies and T-cell responses against many epitopes can be induced. Hepatitis B virus (HBV) and human papillomavirus (HPV) have licensed VLP vaccines [38]. Baumert et al. [39] generated HCV-LPs using a recombinant baculovirus containing the complementary DNA for HCV structural proteins in insect cells.

Recently, results of Kumar et al. [40] suggested that the combined regimen of HCV viral-like particles followed by recombinant adenovirus could more effectively inhibit HCV infection, endorsing the novel vaccine strategy.

HCV-LPs were used to immunize four chimpanzees, and all developed HCV-specific T-cell and proliferative lymphocyte responses against core, E1, and E2 proteins. Challenging with infectious HCV, one chimpanzee developed transitory viremia, and the other three displayed higher levels of viremia, but after 10 weeks, their viral levels became immeasurable as reported by Elmowalid et al. [41]. Technique for high-capacity purification of HCV VLPs was defined by Earnest-Silveira et al. [42]. The structural HCV protein coding sequences of genotypes 1a, 1b, 2a, or 3a were coexpressed using a recombinant adenoviral expression system in Huh7 cell line. Using iodixanol ultracentrifugation and Stirred cell ultrafiltration, the structural proteins self-assembled into VLPs which were purified from Huh7 cell lysates. VLPs of the different genotypes are morphologically similar as revealed by electron microscopy. Results showed that it is feasible to produce big quantities of individual HCV genotype VLPs, making this approach an alternative for the manufacture of a quadrivalent mammalian cell-derived HCV VLP vaccine. HCV-specific neutralizing antibodies (Nabs) recognize quaternary structures [43, 44]. The particulate structure of HCV VLPs makes them an attractive vaccine candidate [45–47].

6.2. Cell culture-derived HCV (HCVcc)

Kato and Wakita [48] introduced the HCV infection system in cell culture using clone JFH-1, taken from a fulminant HCV-infected Japanese patient. JFH-1 replicates well in hepatic cancer cells and releases infectious virion in the cells' media. Understanding how hosts react to HCV infection and how the viruses escape from host immune reactions was studied using HCVcc systems. Although it is difficult to understand the mechanisms underlying the HCV infection outcomes, innate immune responses seem to have a crucial effect on HCV infection outcomes. Later, robust production of HCVcc particles was obtained by introducing a few specific mutations in JFH-1 structural proteins [49].

Also, Akazawa et al. [50] showed that a protective vaccine can be developed from inactivated HCV particles derived from cultured cells that protected chimeric liver uPA(+/+)-SCID mice against HCV infection. Also, Gottwein and Bukh [51] cultured virus particles constituting the antigen in most antiviral vaccines.

Recently, Yokokawa evaluated neutralizing antibody induction and cellular immune responses following the immunization of a nonhuman primate model with (HCVcc) in [52]. This preclinical study demonstrated that the vaccine included both HCVcc and K3-SPG-induced humoral and cellular immunity in marmosets. Vaccination with this combination resulted in the production of antibodies exhibiting cross-neutralizing activity against multiple HCV genotypes. Based on these findings, the vaccine created in this study represents a promising, potent, and safe prophylactic option against HCV.

Generally, we can conclude the comparison between the two strategies of candidate vaccines of HCVcc and HCV VLP in **Table 1**.

C virus induce humoral and cellular responses in goats. Virology Journal. 2009;6(1):66. DOI: 10.1186/1743-422X-6-66

[22] El-Shenawy R, Tabll A, Bader El Din NG, El Abd Y, Mashaly M, Abdel Malak CA, Dawood R, El-Awady M. Antiviral activity of virocidal peptide derived from NS5A against two different HCV genotypes: An in vitro study. Journal of Immunoassay and Immunochemistry. 2015;36:63-79. DOI: 10.1080/15321819.2014.896264

[23] Kong L, Giang E, Nieusma T, Kadam RU, Cogburn KE, Hua Y, Dai X, Stanfield RL, Burton DR, Ward AB, Wilson IA, Law M. Hepatitis C virus E2 envelope glycoprotein core structure. Science. 2013;342:1090-1094. DOI: 10.1126/science.1243876

[24] Kong L, Lee DE, Kadam RU, Liu T, Giang E, Nieusma T, Garces F, Tzarum N, Woods Jr. VL, Ward AB, Li S, Wilson IA, Law M. Structural flexibility at a major conserved antibody target on hepatitis C virus E2 antigen. Proceedings of the National Academy of Sciences of the United States of America. October 2016. pii: 201609780. PMID: 27791120

[25] Colombatto P, Brunetto MR, Maina AM, Romagnoli V, Almasio P, Rumi MG, Ascione A, Pinzello G, Mondelli M, Muratori L, Rappuoli R, Rosa D, Houghton M, Abrignani S, Bonino F. *HCV E1E2-MF59* vaccine in chronic hepatitis C patients treated with PEG-IFNα2a and Ribavirin: A randomized controlled trial. Journal of Viral Hepatitis. 2014;21:458-465. DOI: 10.1111/jvh.12163

[26] Houghton M. Prospects for prophylactic and therapeutic vaccines against the hepatitis C viruses. Immunological Reviews. 2011;239:99-108. DOI: 10.1111/j.1600-065X.2010.00977

[27] Grubor-Bauk B, Yu W, Wijesundara D, Gummow J, Garrod T, Brennan AJ, Voskoboinik I, Gowans EJ. Intradermal delivery of DNA encoding HCV NS3 and perforin elicits robust cell-mediated immunity in mice and pigs. Gene Therapy. 2016;23:26-37. DOI: 10.1038/gt.2015.86

[28] Gummow J, Li Y, Yu W, Garrod T, Wijesundara D, Brennan AJ, Mullick R, Voskoboinik I, Grubor-Bauk B, Gowans EJ. A multiantigenic DNA vaccine that induces broad hepatitis C virus-specific T-cell responses in mice. Journal of Virology. 2015;89:7991-8002. DOI: 10.1128/JVI.00803-15

[29] Sällberg M, Frelin L, Weiland O. DNA vaccine therapy for chronic hepatitis C virus (HCV) infection: Immune control of a moving target. Expert Opinion on Biological Therapy. 2009;9:805-815. DOI: 10.1517/14712590902988444

[30] Chmielewska AM, Naddeo M, Capone S, Ammendola V, Hu K, Meredith L, Verhoye L, Rychlowska M, Rappuoli R, Ulmer JB, Colloca S, Nicosia A, Cortese R, Leroux-Roels G, Balfe P, Bienkowska-Szewczyk K, Meuleman P, McKeating JA, Folgori A. Combined adenovirus vector and hepatitis C virus envelope protein prime-boost regimen elicits T cell and neutralizing antibody immune responses. Journal of Virology. 2014;88:5502-5510. DOI: 10.1128/JVI.03574-13

[31] Habersetzer F, Honnet G, Bain C, Maynard-Muet M, Leroy V, Zarski JP, Feray C, Baumert TF, Bronowicki JP, Doffoël M, Trépo C, Agathon D, Toh ML, Baudin M, Bonnefoy JY,

Limacher JM, Inchauspé G. A poxvirus vaccine is safe, induces T-cell responses, and decreases viral load in patients with chronic hepatitis C. Gastroenterology. 2011;**141**(3):890-899.e1-4. DOI: 10.1053/j.gastro.2011.06.009 PMID: 21699798

[32] Levander S, Sällberg M, Ahlén G, Frelin L. A non-human hepadnaviral adjuvant for hepatitis C virus-based genetic vaccines. Vaccine. 2016;**34**(25):2821-2833. DOI: 10.1016/j.vaccine.2016.04.030

[33] Klade CS, Schuller E, Boehm T, von Gabain A, Manns MP. Sustained viral load reduction in treatment-naive HCV genotype 1 infected patients after therapeutic peptide vaccination. Vaccine 2012;30:2943-2950. DOI: 10.1016/j.vaccine.2012.02.070

[34] Swadling L, Halliday J, Kelly C, Brown A, Capone S, Ansari MA, Bonsall D, Richardson R, Hartnell F, Collier J, Ammendola V, Del Sorbo M, Von Delft A, Traboni C, Hill AV, Colloca S, Nicosia A, Cortese R, Klenerman P, Folgori A, Barnes E. Highly-immunogenic virally-vectored T-cell vaccines cannot overcome subversion of the T-cell response by HCV during chronic infection. Vaccines (Basel). 2016;**4**(3). pii: E27). DOI: 10.3390/vaccines4030027 PMID: 27490575

[35] Swadling L, Capone S, Antrobus RD, Brown A, Richardson R, Newell EW, Halliday J, Kelly C, Bowen D, Fergusson J, Kurioka A, Ammendola V, Del Sorbo M, Grazioli F, Esposito ML, Siani L, Traboni C, Hill A, Colloca S, Davis M, Nicosia A, Cortese R, Folgori A, Klenerman P, Barnes E. A human vaccine strategy based on chimpanzee adenoviral and MVA vectors that primes, boosts, and sustains functional HCV-specific T cell memory. Science Translational Medicine. 2014;**5**(6):261ra153. DOI: 10.1126/scitranslmed.3009185

[36] Teimourpour R, Tajani AS, Askari VR, Rostami S, Meshkat Z. Designing and development of a DNA vaccine based on structural proteins of hepatitis C virus. Iranian Journal of Pathology. 2016;**11**:222-230 PMC5079455

[37] Nemchinov LG, Liang TJ, Rifaat MM, Mazyad HM, Hadidi A, Keith JM. Development of a plant-derived subunit vaccine candidate against hepatitis C virus. Archives of Virology. 2000;**145**:2557-2573 11205105

[38] Roldão A, Mellado MC, Castilho LR, Carrondo MJ, Alves PM. Virus-like particles in vaccine development. Expert Review of Vaccines. 2010;**9**:1149-1176. DOI: 10.1586/erv.10.115

[39] Baumert TF, Vergalla J, Satoi J, Thomson M, Lechmann M, Herion D, Greenberg HB, Ito S, Liang TJ. Hepatitis C virus-like particles synthesized in insect cells as a potential vaccine candidate. Gastroenterology. 1999;**117**:1397-1407 10579981

[40] Kumar A, Das S, Mullick R, Lahiri P, Tatineni R, Goswami D, Bhat P, Torresi J, Gowans EJ, Karande AA, Das S. Immune responses against hepatitis C virus genotype 3a virus-like particles in mice: A novel VLP prime-adenovirus boost strategy. Vaccine. 2016;**34**:1115-1125. DOI: 10.1016/j.vaccine.2015.11.061

[41] Elmowalid GA, Qiao M, Jeong SH, Borg BB, Baumert TF, Sapp RK, Hu Z, Murthy K, Liang TJ. Immunization with hepatitis C virus-like particles results in control of hepatitis

C virus infection in chimpanzees. Proceedings of the National Academy of Sciences of the United States of America. 2007;**104**:8427-8432. DOI: 10.1073/pnas.0702162104

[42] Earnest-Silveira L, Chua B, Chin R, Christiansen D, Johnson D, Herrmann S, Ralph SA, Vercauteren K, Mesalam A, Meuleman P, Das S, Boo I, Drummer H, Bock CT, Gowans EJ, Jackson DC, Torresi J. Characterization of a hepatitis C virus-like particle vaccine produced in a human hepatocyte-derived cell line. Journal of General Virology. 2016;**97**:1865-1876. DOI: 10.1099/jgv.0.000493

[43] Keck ZY, Saha A, Xia J, Wang Y, Lau P, Krey T, Rey FA, Foung SK. Mapping a region of hepatitis C virus E2 that is responsible for escape from neutralizing antibodies and a core CD81-binding region that does not tolerate neutralization escape mutations. Journal of Virology. 2011;**85**:10451-10463. DOI: 10.1128/JVI.05259-11

[44] Giang E, Dorner M, Prentoe JC, Dreux M, Evans MJ, Bukh J, Rice CM, Ploss A, Burton DR, Law M.Human broadly neutralizing antibodies to the envelope glycoprotein complex of hepatitis C virus. Proceedings of the National Academy of Sciences of the United States of America. 2012;109:6205-6210. DOI:10.1073/pnas.1114927109

[45] Elmowalid GA, Qiao M, Jeong SH, Borg BB, Baumert TF, Sapp RK, Hu Z, Murthy K, Liang TJ. Immunization with hepatitis C virus-like particles results in control of hepatitis C virus infection in chimpanzees. Proceedings of the National Academy of Sciences of the United States of America. 2007;104:8427-8432. DOI: 10.1073/pnas.0702162104

[46] Chua BY, Johnson D, Tan A, Earnest-Silveira L, Sekiya T, Chin R, Torresi J, Jackson DC. Hepatitis C VLPs delivered to dendritic cells by a TLR2 targeting lipopeptide results in enhanced antibody and cell-mediated responses. PloS One. 2012;7(10):e47492. DOI: 10.1371/journal.pone.0047492

[47] Kumar A, Gupta V, Sharma P, Bansal N, Singla V, Arora A. Association of overt diabetes mellitus with the Non-CC but not the CC genotype of Interleukin-28B in hepatitis C virus infected patients. Journal of Clinical and Translational Hepatology 2016;4:26-31. DOI: 10.14218/JCTH.00040

[48] Kato T, Wakita T. Production of infectious hepatitis C virus in cell culture. Uirusu. 2005;**55**:287-295 16557015

[49] Delgrange D, Pillez A, Castelain S, Cocquerel L, Rouillé Y, Dubuisson J, Wakita T, Duverlie G, Wychowski C. Robust production of infectious viral particles in Huh-7 cells by introducing mutations in hepatitis C virus structural proteins. Journal of General Virology 2007;88:2495-2503. DOI: 10.1099/vir.0.82872-0 DOI:10.1099/vir.0.82872-0

[50] Akazawa D, Moriyama M, Yokokawa H, Omi N, Watanabe N, Date T, Morikawa K, Aizaki H, Ishii K, Kato T, Mochizuki H, Nakamura N, Wakita T. Neutralizing antibodies induced by cell culture-derived hepatitis C virus protect against infection in mice. Gastroenterology. 2013;**145**:447-455. DOI: 10.1053/j.gastro.2013.05.007

[51] Gottwein JM, Bukh J. Viral hepatitis: Cell-culture-derived HCV--a promising vaccine antigen. Nature Reviews Gastroenterology & Hepatology. 2013;10(9):508-509. DOI: 10.1038/nrgastro.2013.136. PMID: 23897287

[52] Yokokawa H, Higashino A, Suzuki S, Moriyama M, Nakamura N, Suzuki T, Suzuki R, Ishii K, Kobiyama K, Ishii KJ, Wakita T, Akari H, Kato T. Induction of humoural and cellular immunity by immunisation with HCV particle vaccine in a non-human primate model. Gut. 2016;26. pii: gutjnl-2016-312208. DOI: 10.1136/gutjnl-2016-312208

[53] Kelly C, Swadling L, Capone S, Brown A, Richardson R, Halliday J, von Delft A, Oo Y, Mutimer D, Kurioka A, Hartnell F, Collier J, Ammendola V, Del Sorbo M, Grazioli F, Esposito ML, Di Marco S, Siani L, Traboni C, Hill AV, Colloca S, Nicosia A, Cortese R, Folgori A, Klenerman P, Barnes E. Chronic hepatitis C viral infection subverts vaccine-induced T-cell immunity in humans. Hepatology 2016;63:1455-1470. DOI: 10.1002/hep.28294

[54] Ogholikhan S, Schwarz KB. Hepatitis vaccines. Vaccines (Basel). 2016;4(1). DOI: 10.3390/vaccines4010006

[55] Schulze ZJ, Ciuffreda D, Lewis-Ximenez L, Kasprowicz V, Nolan BE, Streeck H, Aneja J, Reyor LL, Allen TM, Lohse AW, McGovern B, Chung RT, Kwok WW, Kim AY, Lauer GM. Broadly directed virus-specific CD4+ T cell responses are primed during acute hepatitis C infection, but rapidly disappear from human blood with viral persistence. Journal of Experimental Medicine. 2012;209:61-75. DOI: 10.1084/jem.201003

[56] Razvi S, Schneider L, Jonas MM, Cunningham-Rundles C. Outcome of intravenous immunoglobulin-transmitted hepatitis C virus infection in primary immunodeficiency. Journal of Clinical Immunology. 2001;101:284-288. DOI: 10.1006/clim.2001.5132

15

Hepatitis C: Host and Viral Factors Associated with Response to Therapy and Progression of Liver Fibrosis

Snezana Jovanovic-Cupic, Ana Bozovic,
Milena Krajnovic and Nina Petrovic

Abstract

The goal of this study was to identify the baseline host and viral factors of response to antiviral therapy in patients with chronic hepatitis C. Compared with interferon/ribavirin therapy, new current direct-acting antiviral (DAA) combination regimens significantly increased rate of sustained virologic response (SVR) and shorter treatment durations, but is still limited by viral resistance, adverse effects, and high cost especially in developing countries. Human genetic factors and heterogeneity within the HCV genome may be associated with virologic treatment failure before and after antiviral therapy. Further, HCV infection may contribute to the development of HCV-related liver disease and hepatocarcinogenesis, through modulating genetic and epigenetic state of certain genes implicated in control of critical cellular pathways. Previous results confirm the importance of host and viral factors and virus-induced genetic and epigenetic changes in predicting outcome and treatment response.

Keywords: hepatitis C virus, response to therapy, IFN-based antiviral therapies, direct-acting antiviral (DAA) agents, genetic variability, liver fibrosis, hepatocarcinogenesis, epigenetic changes

1. Introduction

Chronic hepatitis C virus (HCV) infection with the estimated worldwide prevalence of 1.1% is a global health problem, affecting 170 million people worldwide [1, 2]. About 15–45% of infected persons spontaneously clear the virus without any treatment, but remaining 60–80% will develop chronic HCV infection leading to fibrosis, cirrhosis and/or hepatocellular carcinoma (HCC) [1, 3]. Previous results suggest that, worldwide, there were 1.75 million new HCV infections and annually an estimated 700,000 persons with chronic HCV die untreated [1]. Until 2014, the standard of care to treat HCV infection was pegylated interferon and ribavirin (PEG-IFN and RBV). However, first generation of (DAAs) NSA3/4A protease inhibitors (PI) were boceprevir and telaprevir, administrated with PEG-IFN and RBV [1]. These protease inhibitors were limited by viral resistance, adverse effect and long treatment duration and high cost especially in development countries [4]. The standard care of therapy is changing rapidly and new (DAAs) therapy such as sofosbuvir, daclatasvir, and the sofosbuvir/ledipasvir combination are part of the preferred regimens in the WHO guidelines with achieve cure rates above 95%. In comparison with older therapies, new therapy is more effective, safer, and better-tolerated with shorter treatment (usually 12 weeks), but high prices of the medicines limit the expansion of HCV in many countries [1]. However, challenges remain in optimizing current drug regimens, limiting the problem of resistance mutations and promote individual therapy [5–7]. Treatment predictors are important factors for management of therapy in patients with chronic hepatitis C infection.

1.1. Host and virus-related factors associated with response to therapy

Previous studies indicated that baseline host and virus related factors such genotype, viral load, age, gender, stage of liver fibrosis, and *IL28B* (interleukin-28B) polymorphisms were associated with therapy outcome [8–16]. Among viral factors, HCV genotype and baseline level of HCV-RNA are significant determinants of treatment outcome. Sustained virologic response (SVR) was defined as undetectable levels of HCV RNA, 24 weeks after cessation of treatment. Rapid virologic response (RVR) was defined as undetectable levels of HCV RNA at 4 weeks. Early virologic response (EVR) was defined as undetectable levels of HCV-RNA at week 12 (complete EVR) or ≥2 log reduction in HCV viral load from baseline (partial EVR), while non-response NR was defined as detection of serum HCV RNA 6 months after cessation of treatment. Thus, RVR is a strong predictor of SVR, but absence of an EVR is significant predictor for non-response (NR) to antiviral treatment. Moreover, viral kinetics during therapy provides information on how to individualize treatment [16, 17]. It is known that stages of liver fibrosis may be associated with response rates to PEG-IFN/RBV therapy. Further, patients with advanced liver fibrosis (METAVIR score F3-F4) were more frequently in non-responders (NR) than in patients with minimal or mild fibrosis (F0-F2), especially in patients with genotype 1 [8, 12, 18]. According to the previous results, infection with genotypes 2 or 3, younger ages, lower baseline viral load, and absence of advanced fibrosis were all strong predictors of SVR. Since 2011, therapeutic regimens for HCV genotype 1 patients were modified. Combination of NS3/4a protease inhibitors and pegylated interferon and ribavirin improved the SVR rates [19]. However, boceprevir- and telaprevir-based regimens are associated with side effect and lower efficacy than the newer DAA therapies. Also, this therapy is effective only in patients with genotype 1 [1, 20]. With respect to host and viral factors and first generation DAAs, viral kinetics is the most important predictive factor of SVR. The IL28B was associated with greater chances to shorten therapy but there is no correlation with SVR [8]. Second-generation DAAs have higher rates of SVR, are safer and can be used in combinations that obviate the need for interferon and ribavirin [1]. However, failure to new DAAs combinations is in association with patients with poor response, genotypes 1a or 3, advanced liver cirrhosis, elevated level of viral load and the presence of human immunodeficiency virus (HIV) coinfection [21]. In contrast, some authors suggest that therapy outcomes are not significantly influenced by *IL28B* polymorphisms, HCV genotype, high baseline viral load, or prior interferon failure [22]. In the era of DAAs, surveillance of HCC after eradication of HCV by antivirus therapy is particularly important. Current new therapies with DAAs are associated with high rates of SVR, generally exceeding 90% even among patients with cirrhosis or prior treatment failure. Therefore, understanding of various host and viral factors associated with disease progression and development of HCC in chronic hepatitis C infection is important for implementing personalized treatment. One of the most interesting current questions concerns the impact of DAAs on HCC incidence [23].

1.2. HCV-host interactions and host genetic alterations

In the specific environment of every host, the outcomes of the HCV infection will be different. There are many factors which influence the therapy outcome and progression of liver disease. These factors include baseline clinical and pathohistological parameters. Also, host genetic landscape has effects on therapy outcomes and development of liver disease phenotypes. Genome-wide association studies (GWAS) have been created to track genetic polymorphisms in the human genome which associate with, virus clearance, therapy outcomes, and different stages of liver disease. Thus, this kind of the genome screening could be a useful tool in the diagnostics and the therapy of hepatitis C, and could lead to a personalized therapy.

1.2.1. Role of interferons (IFN) in HCV infection

HCV infection induces production of interferons λ (IFN-λ). IFN-λs bind to IFNL receptors (IFNLR) activating JAK-STAT signaling pathway which induces expression of *ISGs* (interferon-stimulated genes). The IFNLR is a heterodimer, consisting of two subunits, IL10R2 and IL28RA. There are four IFN-λs described so far: IFNL 1–4. The gene loci for these proteins are located on the chromosome 19. Study of GWAS has revealed polymorphisms in IFNL gene loci, which are in association with HCV clearance, either spontaneous or therapy-induced. Previously it was shown that single nucleotide polymorphisms (SNPs) near *IL28B* (rs12979869 and rs8099917) were strongly associated with response to PEG-IFN/RBV therapy in patients with genotype 1 and with spontaneous virus clearance [24–27]. In the neighborhood of *ILR3*, a novel dinucleotide polymorphism, ss469415590 (TT/ΔG), has recently been discovered which is in high linkage disequilibrium with rs12979869 and participate in formation of a novel gene *IFNL4*. The *IFNL4* gene creates IFNL4 protein, but TT variant of ss469415590 does not form the protein [28]. The TT variant has been shown to be beneficial to its carriers because it influences the spontaneous and therapy-induced virus clearance [26]. Among people of African ancestry, the polymorphism ss469415590 is in stronger association with virus clearance than the rs12979869 [28]. There are two variants of IFNL4 protein with impact on antiviral activity, which differ in only one amino acid at the place 70. The carriers of the variant with serine (P70S) have better therapy response and higher spontaneous virus clearance rate compared to carriers of the variant with proline. However, the expression of *ISGs* in the variant P70S is decreased, which is in discrepancy with its better antiviral activity. The researchers have speculated this is probably due to decreased adaptive immunity as the consequence of high expression of *ISGs* in carriers of IFNL4-P70 variant [28]. The genes of human leukocyte antigen (HLA) family located on the chromosome 6 are associated with clearance of HCV infection. Some authors found that this connection is inconsistent, because of different systems of HLA typing, clinical phenotypes, and ethnic backgrounds. The only polymorphisms of *HLA* genes which are confirmed so far to have an association with virus clearance are HLA-DQB1*03 and HLA-DRB1*11 [29–32]. The receptors of natural killer (NK) cells Killer-cell immunoglobulin-like receptors (KIR) and their corresponding ligands, HLA class 1 proteins, also have a role in the immune response. Studies of the association of the polymorphisms of KIR and HLA-C and virus clearance have given controversial results. In some studies, the carriers of a KIR2DS3 (killer cell immunoglobulin like receptor, two Ig domains and short cytoplasmic tail 3) and homozygosity for *HLA-C1* were associated with spontaneous virus clearance [33, 34]. Polymorphisms of some other genes coding for the proteins which have a role in the immune response have also been shown to correlate with spontaneous/therapy-induced virus clearance. One of these genes is the gene for osteopontin which initiates T helper cells type 1 response, and has been shown to associate with the sustained viral response after the IFN therapy [35, 36]. Today, the role of the host genetic variability has been reduced due to high efficacy of new era interferon-free antiviral therapy. However, the high cost of this therapy limits its availability to the developed parts of the world.

1.2.2. The influence of host genetic alterations on the progression of liver fibrosis in chronic HCV infection

On the other hand, the host genetic variability has a significant role in the formation of different liver phenotypes. The phenotypes, such as fibrosis, steatosis, cirrhosis, or hepatocellular carcinoma (HCC) are the consequence of virus infection and disease progression. The polymorphisms of the immune response genes have effect on disease progression or inhibition. For example, the patients with chronic hepatitis C, which carry rs12979860CC variant, have higher fibrosis progression rate. This effect is even more pronounced in the younger females and in the carriers of the HCV type 3 [37]. The polymorphisms of apoptosis-related genes *MERTK* (MER proto-oncogene, tyrosine kinase), *TULP1* (tubby like protein 1) and *RNF* (ring finger proteins) gene family have association with the progression of the HCV-related fibrosis [38] and the genes of the major histocompatibility complex (MHC) with cirrhosis [39] and HCC [40]. However, these results need confirmation in the further research. Although having some potential, GWAS studies have many flaws. One of them is the impossibility of the screening of more extensive genetic changes, e.g., *copy number variation* (CNV) and epigenetic events, which also take part in the disease progression and the therapy response. Methodological failure is that these studies use conservative significance thresholds to eliminate false positive signals and many significant polymorphisms of low frequency could be unregistered, as reviewed in [41]. All discovered polymorphisms so far are currently not applicable to the clinical classification of the liver disease, because of their low predictive value. One of the possible solutions is the formation of the polygenic scores. For example, there is an earlier study which resulted in the formation of cirrhosis risk scores (CRS) based on the gene signature of seven genes [42]. In another study, a prediction model for liver fibrosis was based on gene polymorphisms. This model includes polymorphisms of *IFNL* and clinical risk factors, which taken together give a risk for liver fibrosis [43]. Based on the fibrosis/cirrhosis risk score, therapy decisions can be made. Chronic inflammation and cirrhosis of hepatic cells lead to HCC. Hepatocellular carcinoma is the one of the deadliest type of cancer in the world. It represents a heterogeneous disease consisting of many tumor subpopulations with different frequencies of mutated genes. There are several genes which are affected, during the HCC progression, either by genetic or epigenetic alterations. In recent studies, the alterations of the *TERT* (telomerase reverse transcriptase), *CTNNB1* (catenin beta 1), *TP53* (tumor protein p53), and *AXIN1* (axin 1) genes are shown to correlate with tumor progression [44, 45]. *TERT* promoter mutations have been present in 64% of HCV-related HCC [44]. TERT is a subunit of the telomerase enzyme, whose mutations lead to telomere shortening and uncapping of chromosomes, which then leads to chromosome fusion and general chromosomal instability. *TERT* mutations and silencing of *CDKN2A* (cyclin dependent kinase inhibitor 2A) gene by promoter hypermethylation are the events that coincided [46]. It seems that *TERT* mutation is an early event in the cancerogenesis [45]. Frequent *CTNNB1* mutations have also been observed in HCV-related HCC [46]. There were attempts to classify HCC based on genetic signatures. The genetic signature represents one gene or a collection of genes, with characteristic expression profile, which is confirmed to be specific for the diagnosis, prognosis, and treatment response prediction [47]. Genetic signatures could be the means of classifying HCC in the groups which would facilitate diagnosis and therapy decisions. In the first attempt to make a molecular model for a diagnosis of an early HCC in the HCV patients, the best accuracy was achieved using the signature of three genes *LYVE1* (lymphatic vessel endothelial hyaluronan receptor 1), *GPC3* (glypican 3), and *BIRC5* (baculoviral IAP repeat containing 5). The *TERT* gene and *E-cadherin* were also shown to be informative in that model [48]. One European study revealed molecular signatures of 243 HCCs, based on fibrosis and cirrhosis score, and various risk factors, among which HCV was present in 26% of the cases. However, this study did not find any associations of these molecular signatures with HCV infection [45]. Cancer Genome Atlas Research found 26 frequently mutated genes in HCC. They identified *ALB* (albumin), *APOB* (apolipoprotein B), *LZTR1* (leucine zipper like transcription regulator 1), *EEF1A1* (eukaryotic translation elongation factor 1 alpha 1), *SMARCA4* (SWI/SNF related, matrix associated, actin dependent regulator of chromatin, subfamily a, member 4), *AZIN1* (antizyme inhibitor 1), *RP1L1* (retinitis pigmentosa 1 like 1), *GPATCH4* (G-patch domain containing 4), *CREB3L3* (cAMP responsive element binding protein 3 like 3), *AHCTF1* (AT-hook containing transcription factor 1) and *HIST1H1c* (histone cluster 1 H1 family member c) gene mutations. Additionally, this study used methylation profiles, based on which the HCC were divided into four methylation clusters. The fourth cluster was characterized by high frequency of *CTNNB1* and *TERT* mutations, *CDKN2A* promoter hypermethylation and presence of HCV infection [46]. Besides smaller genetic changes, the changes which encompass bigger regions of DNA such as deletions, insertions, copy number variations, loss of heterozygosity also have a role in the HCC progression. All of these changes alongside hyper and hypomethylation lead to general chromosomal instability, which is prerequisite for tumor progression. There are examples of the direct influence of HCV on host genomic instability. HCV protein NS5A interacts with host gene *ASPM* (abnormal spindle microtubule assembly), which regulates mitotic spindle formation, causing interruption of the cell cycle, eventually leading to chromosomal instability and HCC [49]. HCV Core protein induces polyploidy by decreasing of retinoblastoma-associated protein expression, thereby influencing mitotic cycle checkpoint, which also leads to chromosomal instability [50]. In addition, interaction of NS3/4A with serine protein kinase, which has a role in the cell cycle, leads to disabling cell repair system [51]. The polymorphisms in the host genome have effect on therapy response, virus clearance, and differentiation of HCV-induced liver phenotypes. The genetic signatures in the host genomes could be the means of therapy decisions making, and a way to personalize therapy. However, some other factors, such as epigenetic events and alterations of larger DNA regions, should also be taken into an account.

1.3. Impact of hepatitis C virus heterogeneity on therapy outcomes

The persistence of hepatitis C virus (HCV) infection and its poor susceptibility to treatment have been attributed, at least in part, to the high rate of genetic variability exhibited by the virus.

The persistence of HCV infection and its poor susceptibility to treatment is the consequence of high rate of virus genetic variability. Variability of virus is due to the low fidelity of viral RNA-dependent RNA-polymerase, which lacks proof-reading capacity, thus allowing the generation of quasispecies. Genetic variability is segregated within particular segments of the HCV genome, resulting in a number of highly variable regions [52]. These quasispecies play an important role in the escape from selective pressures by immune responses and antiviral therapies. A decrease or no change in the number of nucleotides substitutions in the protein kinase (PKR) binding domain (PKRBD) and the interferon-sensitivity-determining region (ISDR) were associated with failed to respond to PEG-IFN/RBV treatment [53]. It was reported that the presence of >4 mutations in the PKRBD region of NS5A protein was correlated with SVR to peg-IFN/RBV therapy [54]. Moreover, PKRBD sequences might be used as a prognostic guide for treating HCV-1-infected patients [54, 55]. Absence of substitutions at positions 70 and 91 in Core protein is a significant predictor for the success of IFN-based therapy [54]. On the other side, amino acid substitutions in the Core protein play an important role in early dynamics of viral replication during IFN-based therapy in chronic HCV infection and more frequent occurrence HCC. With respect to new DAAs therapy, efficacy of NS5A inhibitors can be blocked by presence of NS5A resistance-associated substitutions (RASs), but choice of DAA regimen and duration of therapy depends on multiple viral and host factors.

2. Epigenetic changes in HCV-induced liver diseases

Persistent infection with HCV is associated with the development of chronic liver diseases: fibrosis, cirrhosis and ultimately, HCC [56, 57]. Prevention of chronic hepatitis C and its complications is based on antiviral therapy and early detection of reliable molecular markers in persons under the risk [57, 58]. However, current antiviral therapies are not effective in many patients with chronic hepatitis C, so there is a need for a greater understanding of the factors leading to progression to HCC in order to design novel approaches to prevention of HCV-associated complications [59]. Here, we discuss the current knowledge about the inter-relationship between HCV and pathophysiology of HCV-associated chronic liver diseases, with particular focus on the virus-induced host epigenetic changes leading to hepatocarcinogenesis.

2.1. Hepatocellular carcinoma

According to epidemiological evaluation, HCC is the fifth most common cancer and the second most common cause for cancer death in the world [60]. Although the prognosis of patients with HCC has marginally improved over the last few decades, the five-year survival rate remains poor as a result of late diagnosis. Consequently, the majority of patients with advanced HCC do not survive for longer than 6 months from the time of diagnosis [61]. It has been shown that in chronically infected patients, the risk of developing HCC is strictly correlated to fibrosis stage, and the incidence of HCC is more frequent in patients with liver cirrhosis than in those with mild fibrosis [62]. SVR to IFN-based therapies decreases HCC incidence in a large number of HCV patients, indicating the importance of eradicating the virus to prevent carcinogenesis [63, 64]. However, despite a successful virus clearance, the risk of HCC still exists in individuals with severe fibrosis and continuous HCC monitoring is recommended [65]. So, it is of great importance to determine molecular markers of progressive fibrosis, that could indicate the chronically HCV infected persons under the risk of developing HCC [66, 67]. HCV-induced hepatocarcinogenesis is a multifactorial process which results from a complex interaction among host, environmental, and viral factors [67]. It is considered that at least three host cellular pathways are affected in this process: cell cycle, proliferation, and apoptosis [68]. As HCV is an RNA virus with limited integration of its genetic material into the host's genome, it was first assumed that its ability to transform hepatocytes is linked to indirect mechanisms. Chronic inflammation induced by viral infection results in a permanent degenerative and regenerative processes and occurrence of progressive fibrosis and cirrhosis [69–71]. In addition, chronic inflammation leads to increased levels of reactive oxygen species (ROS), which damage hepatocytes and can lead to accumulation of genetic and epigenetic alterations in hepatic cells [67, 72]. All these events can promote neoplastic transformation of hepatocytes and the progression of malignant clones [73]. Later studies have shown that HCV is directly involved in hepatocarcinogenesis, through direct action of viral proteins on host tumor suppressors and proto-oncogenes [74, 75]. Several viral proteins have been shown *in vitro* to possess functions that could favor hepatocarcinogenesis, through inducing genetic and epigenetic alterations. In particular, the Core protein, NS3, NS4B and NS5A can transform various cell lines, either alone or in cooperation with oncogenes [76–80]. These proteins interact with a number of host factors and signaling pathways leading to the progression from chronic hepatitis C to liver cirrhosis and HCC [68].

2.1.1. Epigenetic changes in HCV-induced HCC

Many lines of evidence suggest that aberrant epigenetic changes associated with viral infection may trigger events that promote the neoplastic transformation of hepatocytes [59, 73]. Epigenetics is defined as heritable state of gene expression without altering DNA sequences. Epigenetic mechanisms include genomic DNA methylation, chemical modifications of histone tails, and non-coding miRNA regulation [81]. Epigenetic changes play a critical role in control of cellular processes through switching genes on and off, thus leading to differential expression of proteins [82]. HCV infection has been shown to induce or correlate with some epigenetic changes that may contribute to HCV-related liver diseases, including hepatocarcinogenesis [68]. It has been proven that certain HCV-encoded proteins induce promoter methylation of multiple genes, thereby affecting their expression [83, 84].

2.1.2. Host genes promoter methylation induced by HCV

DNA methylation represents the addition of methyl group (CH_3) to a fifth carbon of cytosine residues within a CG dinucleotide, frequently referred to as cytosine-guanine dinucleotide (CpG). DNA methylation is an essential component of epigenetic machinery that regulates transcriptional state of many genes. Methylated promoters often lack transcriptional activity, which could result in gene inactivation. As a transcriptional regulator, DNA methylation has a considerable impact on the development of many cancers, including HCC [81, 85]. Aberrant promoter hypermethylation of tumor suppressor genes involved in the cell proliferation, apoptosis, cell adhesion, DNA repair, and detoxification is frequently detected in HCC, resulting in loss of the corresponding gene function [86, 87]. It is believed that changes in DNA methylation patterns are early events in hepatocarcinogenesis and they can even occur at the early stages of HCV induced liver fibrosis [88]. This is supported by the results of the study conducted by Zekri et al., in which they demonstrated that methylation of certain host genes increase with liver disease progression, from fibrosis to HCC [89]. Moreover, the same group of authors has been shown that methylation of certain tumor suppressor genes affect the response to the antiviral therapy [90]. Considering this, a better understanding of methylation changes and how they correlate with disease progression will help in finding novel biomarkers for early detection of HCC and its prevention.

2.1.3. HCV-encoded proteins inducing host genes methylation

It has been demonstrated that HCV Core protein up-regulates levels of DNA methyltransferase (DNMT) 1 and 3b and induces promoter hypermethylation of tumor suppressor genes like *p16* (*CDKN2A*) and *E-cadherin* [91, 92]. Consequent inhibition of p16 expression results in inactivation of pRb (retinoblastoma protein) and subsequent activation of E2F transcription factor 1 (E2F1), which lead to growth stimulation of hepatocytes. Inactivation of *p16* tumor suppressor gene, that regulates cell cycle, appears to play an important role in the pathogenesis of HCC. It has been demonstrated that reactivation of p16 by transferring the *p16* gene can inhibit the proliferation and reduce the invasive ability of HCC cells [93]. Down-regulation of *E-cadherin* by Core-induced hypermethylation leads to epithelial-mesenchymal transition, cell detachment from the surrounding matrix, and migration outside of the primary tumor site, which is known to be a critical event during the late stage of carcinogenesis [94]. Besides these, methylation of some other tumor suppressor genes, like suppressor of *SOCS-1* (cytokine signaling 1), *GSTP1* (glutathione S-transferase pi 1), *APC* (adenomatous polyposis coli), and *RASSF1A* (Ras association domain family member 1), has been detected in HCV-associated HCC compared normal liver [95, 96]. Abnormal promoter methylation of most of these genes was detected in the plasma/serum DNA as well as in the tissue DNA of HCC patients, which gives opportunity for designing noninvasive blood tests for detection of methylation markers and to distinguish HCV patients who will eventually progress to advanced stages of fibrosis [97]. Zhang et al. reported that the analysis of methylation status of *RASSF1A*, *p16*, and *p15* (cyclin-dependent kinase inhibitor 2B, *CDKN2B*) in serum DNA of infected people could be a valuable biomarker for early detection of HCC in the populations at high risk, including chronic HCV infection [98]. Iyer et al. recorded high frequencies of *p15*, *p16*, *APC*, *FHIT* (fragile histidine triad), and *E-cadherin* promoter methylation in the plasma and liver tissue of HCV-associated HCC patients, with high concordance for all examined genes [99]. Zekri et al. have shown that methylation of *MGMT* (O-6-methylguanine-DNA methyltransferase) gene can be used as a predictor of response to the antiviral therapy, while *RASSF1A* methylation status could be a marker of fibrosis severity [90]. As authors reported, promoter methylation of *MGMT* gene appeared at higher frequencies in the NR than in the responders, which was explained by the fact that MGMT has an important role in protecting cells against DNA damage, via triggering DNA repair mechanisms [100]. On the other hand, the same group of authors has shown that *RASSF1A* methylation was significantly higher in HCV patients with mild fibrosis, which support the role of an intact *RASSF1A* gene in inducing the fibrogenesis in chronic HCV patients [90]. Another study by Hayashi et al. reported that HCC patients with SVR have different molecular alterations compared to NR with continuous HCV infection [101]. This group of authors observed lower frequencies of *v16*, *RB1* (RB transcriptional corepressor 1) and *PTEN* (phosphatase and tensin homolog) genes promoter hypermethylation in patients with SVR, while methylation of *p15* and *p14* (ARF tumor suppressor) genes was not detected in this group of patients, compared to those with the present HCV infection. Interestingly, *p16* methylation was detected with the highest frequency in the both groups, suggesting important role of p16 gene in the development of SVR-HCC. Authors speculated that *p16* in hepatic stem cells might be methylated in the continuous presence of HCV. These cells with methylated *p16* gene might survive and grow after eradication of HCV by IFN therapy. In addition, despite an improved understanding of mechanisms leading to HCV-induced HCC and development of highly potent antiviral therapy, HCV-related HCC remains a global health problem. The development of valuable molecular biomarkers will be of a great importance to distinguish a group of HCV infected people with a high risk for hepatocarcinogenesis. Based on the studies conducted so far, genomic DNA methylation could function as a non-invasive, sensitive, and specific biomarker for prediction the response to the antiviral therapy and early detection of HCC.

2.2. MicroRNA biogenesis and function

MicroRNA (miRNA) are non-coding genetic elements participating in the regulation of gene expression by RNA interference in plants and animals, while in human cells, are associated with viral infection, as well. According to The Encyclopedia of DNA Elements (ENCODE), approximately 75% of the human genome transcribes into a various types of RNA molecules, coding and non-coding [102, 103]. Among non-coding RNA (ncRNA), miRNAs emerged as biologically, physiologically, and clinically significant, considering the fact that they silence translation of partially complementary target messenger (mRNA) molecules. MicroRNAs participate in the regulation of gene expression by RNA interference. In the last 15 years,

miRNAs were linked with various types of diseases and disorders, and majority of investigations were based on the changes in their expression levels. MicroRNAs are encoded by a
miRNA gene, which transcribes into an immature-primary microRNA (pri-miRNA) molecule, a double stranded, hairpin-like genetic structure. Then, two enzymes-RNase endonucle-
ase III Drosha, and DGCR8 (molecular anchor part of a microprocessor complex), transform
pri-miRNA into a 70 nucleotides (nt) long precursor microRNA (pre-miRNA) in the nucleus
[104]. The process of miRNA maturation occurs in the cytoplasm, where Dicer or Argonaute
(Ago), and other protein-partners, cooperators cleave pri-miRNA into a 22 nt long miRNA,
ready to be recognized by RNA-induced silencing complex-RISC [105, 106]. The recognition
and binding of miRNA "seed" sequence to 3' untranslated region (3'UTR) of target mRNA
incompletely complementary with "seed" region at miRNA molecule results in either translational repression, or mRNA degradation. Translational repression and degradation result
in the decrease of protein levels, thus changing genetic, biological, and physiological processes, activity of various signaling pathways. So, main characteristic of miRNAs is to regulate amounts of synthesized proteins [107]. miRNAs are present in every human cell, and
in body fluids (as circulating), such as serum, plasma, urine, saliva, and even gingival liq-
uid. MicroRNA circulates through the body via body fluids as free-circulating miRNAs, and
packed into the exosomes and vesicles, as exosomal miRNAs. Extracellular, exosomal circulating miRNAs may carry over the information about disease progression, infection status,
and other clinic pathological parameters of HCV infection and HCC formation and progression, but it is still not completely clear. Liver-specific miRNAs such as miR-122 and miR-192,
may be released from damaged liver cells, providing the information about liver. Exosomal
and circulating miRNAs, as well as miRNAs extracted from tissue may be involved in inter-
cellular communication. Besides the fact that nearly 300 miRNAs are expressed in normal,
healthy liver, miR-122 represents the major fraction of liver-specific miRNAS, together with
miR-192, miR-199a/b-3p, miR-101/99a, and members of oncogenic let-7 family [108].

2.2.1. MicroRNA in HCV infection and HCC

MicroRNAs are described as onco miRNAs, some of them as tumor suppressive, and several
of them even have dual role in cancer pathogenesis and presumably in other physiological
processes and pathological condition [109]. During the HCV infection, onco miRNAs such
as miR-21/155/221 activate and might cause formation and facilitate progression of HCC. On
the other hand, the decrease of some tumor suppressive miRNAs during the HCV infection
might also cause hepatocarcinogenesis, such as miR-198 [110]. Firstly, some miRNAs directly
interact with the genome of HCV. Secondly, several miRNAs are potential biomarkers of the
presence or progression of the HCV infection. Thirdly, several miRNAs are indicators of HCC
formation and/or progression. Fourthly, there are miRNAs associated with HCC genotype and
clinicopathological characteristics of infected patients and histopathological characteristics of
tumors, while some miRNAs such as miR-134/320c/483-5p may be used as early biomarkers
for HCV infection in the future. Finally, some miRNAs, such as miR-122 represent potentially
great targets for future therapeutics in the aspects of treatment of HCV-associated liver diseases and HCC. Large numbers of different studies have recently been focused on miRNAs in
a different points related to different points of HCV infection, i.e., replication of the virus, viral

genotype, response to HCV therapy, lipid status, liver function indicators, stage of liver fibrosis, HCC grading, and response to chemotherapy. Changes in the expression levels of miRNA several micro RNAs such as miR-21/122/134/141/155/192/199/221/320c/373/483-5p/491/758, let-7b, etc., are associated with different stages of the viral life cycle and the progression of infection [111]. Circulating miRNAs, miR-122, and miR-222 have been shown to be valuable as potential future diagnostic tool for HCV infection within the Egyptian patients [112]. Upregulated miR-10a/15a/17-5p were associated with HCV-related HCC, miR-122 was characterized as potential diagnostic tool for HCC within HCV-infected individuals, while overexpression of miR-221/222-3p was characteristic exclusively for HCV-related HCC [108]. MicroRNA 122 is a liver-specific miRNA, a regulator of HCV tendency to infect hepatic cells. miR-122 is crucial for efficient HCV infection and viral spread and speed up the replication of the virus in hepatocytes, and facilitates viral protein synthesis [113]. Besides miR-122, as the mostly studied miRNA in HCV-HCC patients that recognizes two different sites at HCV 5'UTR, increased levels of miR-448 and miR-196 attenuate HCV replication by binding to the Core and NS5A sequences of the HCV genome [114]. Secondly, some miRNAs, such as miR-199a have opposing characteristics during the HCV infection. Namely, miR-199 targets sequences of HCV genome and blocks the transcription of HCV RNA [115]. Thirdly, during the HCV infection, miR-155 is usually up-regulated. Higher levels of the well-known onco-miRNA, miR-155 induce proliferation of hepatocytes, increasing the chance of HCC formation [116]. For example, changes in the expression levels of miRNAs such as miR-134/320c/483-5p were shown to be significantly higher within the HCV-infected individuals, compared with healthy controls. In our previous article, we described heterogeneity in behavior of microRNA in cancer studies [109, 117]. Another evidence is supporting our observation on the importance to notice how level changes of the particular miRNA can be important for one event, while having no significance for another similar event, related to the same type of the disease or pathological condition, showing high specificity of some miRNA molecules. Namely, miR-20a/92a levels investigated in the sera of the patients having HCV-related liver disease were associated with the disease severity, and the higher grade of liver fibrosis, while levels of the same miRNAs have not shown any association with grade of liver fibrosis and other pathological characteristics examined within the patients with non-HCV-related liver diseases. Another example of involvement of miRNAs in various segments of HCV-HCC pathology, HCV proteins change levels of miR-193a that results in reduction of sensitivity to chemotherapy of HCC patients [118]. Furthermore, in our article related to the heterogeneity of miRNAs. According to several researches, it has been shown that miR-122 may be anti-tumorigenic properties in mice knockdown studies [119].

2.2.2. MicroRNA as future therapeutics for HCV and HCC

Considering the fact that several miRNAs can modulate expression of up to a dozens or even hundreds of target genes, it is not surprising that miRNA-based therapy is still challenging. Nevertheless, this multi-targeting ability also represents an advantage for future miRNA-based therapeutics. There are two major approaches for future miRNA-related therapeutics miRNA inhibition (Lock nucleic acid (LNA) anti miRNAs, antago miRNAs, miRNA zippers, small molecules inhibitors of miRNAs, and miRNA sponges) and miRNA substitution strategies (miRNA mimics and miRNA vectors), with the purpose to either silence miRNA activity or to replace absent miRNA molecules [109, 110]. Several studies proposing that miRNA panels could be used in near future as biomarkers for screening of the HCV-related liver diseases. The changes in their expression levels were associated with staging of liver disease progression and anti-HCV therapeutics [108]. Probably, manipulation with several miRNAs at the same time might be crucial in treatment of HCV-HCC. For example, inhibition of upregulated miRNAs involved in viral replication, such as miR-122, simultaneously with miRNAs, in combination with inhibition of miRNA such as miR-155 which promotes cancerogenesis, or mimicking miRNA whose under expression helps HCV replication, and mimicking downregulated miRNA with tumor suppressive function in HCC.

3. Nomenclature

The Family: Flaviviridae, Genus: Hepacivirus, species: Hepacivirus C.

(Guidelines of the International Committee on Virus Taxonomy (ICTV) https://talk.ictvonline.org/)

4. Conclusions

Chronic HCV infection ultimately leading to HCC will remain a global health problem in the coming decades. Despite increasing knowledge regarding mechanisms of HCV-induced HCC, prevention of HCV-induced HCC is not yet fully established. So, it is important to define both viral- and host genetic and epigenetic patterns on the onset of infection and in early and advanced stages of inflammation and fibrosis in order to predict response to the antiviral therapy, and thus avoid potential complications of persistent HCV infection. Further, for screening a population and making a correct diagnosis about the presence of infection, it is necessary to use standardized commercial tests with universal values and analyze homogenous group of patients. Despite new DAAs therapy, this virus remains unbeatable. When the heterogeneity of the HCV virus, the host genetic and epigenetic variability, and the differences in the therapy outcomes are taken into account, the only right way to fight this disease is personalized therapy.

Acknowledgements

This study supported by the Ministry of Education, Science and Technological Development of the Republic of Serbia, Grants OI 173049 and TR 3702.

Author details

Snezana Jovanovic-Cupic*, Ana Bozovic, Milena Krajnovic and Nina Petrovic

*Address all correspondence to: cupic@vinca.rs

University of Belgrade - Vinča Institute of Nuclear Sciences, Laboratory for Radiobiology and Molecular Genetics, Belgrade, Serbia

References

[1] World Health Organization. Guidelines for the Screening, Care and Treatment of Persons with Chronic Hepatitis C Infection. 2016. Available from: http://apps.who.int/iris/bitstr eam/10665/205035/1/9789241549615_eng.pdf (Accessed March 6, 2018)

[2] Poynard T, Yuen M-F, Ratziu V, Lai CL. Viral hepatitis C. Lancet. 2003;**362**:2095-2100

[3] Perz JF, Alter MJ. The coming wave of HCV-related liver disease: Dilemmas and challenges. Journal of Hepatology. 2006;**44**(3):441. DOI: 10.1016/j.jhep.2005.12.007

[4] Vo KP, Vutien P, Akiyama MJ, Vu VD, Ha NB, Piotrowski JI, et al. Poor sustained virological response in a Multicenter real-life cohort of chronic hepatitis C patients treated with Pegylated interferon and ribavirin plus telaprevir or boceprevir. Digestive Diseases and Sciences. 2015;**60**:1045-1051. DOI: 10.1007/s10620-015-3621-0

[5] Bukh J. The history of hepatitis C virus (HCV): Basic research reveals unique features in phylogeny, evolution and the viral life cycle with new perspectives for epidemic control. Journal of Hepatology. 2016;**65**:S2-S21. DOI: 10.1016/j.jhep.2016.07.035

[6] Pawlotsky J. New hepatitis C therapies: The toolbox, strategies, and challenges. Gastroenterology. 2014;**146**:1176-1192. DOI: 10.1053/j.gastro.2014.03.003

[7] Pawlotsky J-M. Hepatitis C virus resistance to direct-acting antiviral drugs in interferon-free regimens. Gastroenterology. 2016;**151**:70-86. DOI: 10.1053/j.gastro.2016.04.003

[8] Cavalcante LN, Lyra AC. Predictive factors associated with hepatitis C antiviral therapy response. World Journal of Hepatology. 2015;**7**:1617. DOI: 10.4254/wjh.v7.i12.1617

[9] Promrat K, McDermott DH, Gonzalez CM, Kleiner DE, Koziol DE, Lessie M, et al. Associations of chemokine system polymorphisms with clinical outcomes and treatment responses of chronic hepatitis C. Gastroenterology. 2003;**124**:352-360. DOI: 10.1053/gast.2003.50061

[10] Asselah T, Bièche I, Paradis V, Bedossa P, Vidaud M, Marcellin P. Genetics, genomics, and proteomics: Implications for the diagnosis and the treatment of chronic hepatitis C. Seminars in Liver Disease. 2007;**27**:013-027. DOI: 10.1055/s-2006-960168

[11] Saludes V, Bracho MA, Valero O, Ardèvol M, Planas R, González-Candelas F, et al. Baseline prediction of combination therapy outcome in hepatitis C virus 1b infected

patients by discriminant analysis using viral and host factors. PLoS One. 2010;**5**:e14132. DOI: 10.1371/journal.pone.0014132

[12] Jovanovic-Cupic S, Glisic S, Stanojevic M, Nozic D, Petrovic N, Mandusic V, et al. The influence of host factors and sequence variability of the p7 region on the response to pegylated interferon/ribavirin therapy for chronic hepatitis C genotype 1b in patients from Serbia. Archives of Virology. 2016;**161**:1189-1198. DOI: 10.1007/s00705-016-2777-z

[13] Jovanović-Ćupić S, Glisić S, Stanojević M, Vasiljević N, Bojić-Milinović T, Božović A, et al. Response factors to pegylated interferon-alfa/ribavirin treatment in chronic hepatitis c patients genotype 1b. Archives of Biological Sciences. 2014;**66**. DOI: 10.2298/ABS1401193J

[14] Antonucci G, Longo MA, Angeletti C, Vairo F, Oliva A, Comandini UV, et al. The effect of age on response to therapy with peginterferon ? Plus ribavirin in a cohort of patients with chronic HCV hepatitis including subjects older than 65 yr. The American Journal of Gastroenterology. 2007;**102**:1383-1391. DOI: 10.1111/j.1572-0241.2007.01201.x

[15] Manns MP, McHutchison JG, Gordon SC, Rustgi VK, Shiffman M, Reindollar R, et al. Peginterferon alfa-2b plus ribavirin compared with interferon alfa-2b plus ribavirin for initial treatment of chronic hepatitis C: A randomised trial. Lancet (London, England). 2001;**358**:958-965

[16] Fried MW, Hadziyannis SJ, Shiffman ML, Messinger D, Zeuzem S. Rapid virological response is the most important predictor of sustained virological response across genotypes in patients with chronic hepatitis C virus infection. Journal of Hepatology. 2011;**55**:69-75. DOI: 10.1016/j.jhep.2010.10.032

[17] Davis GL. Monitoring of viral levels during therapy of hepatitis C. Hepatology. 2002;**36**:S145-S151. DOI: 10.1002/hep.1840360719

[18] Poynard T, McHutchison J, Manns M, Trepo C, Lindsay K, Goodman Z, et al. Impact of pegylated interferon alfa-2b and ribavirin on liver fibrosis in patients with chronic hepatitis C. Gastroenterology. 2002;**122**:1303-1313

[19] Manns MP, Markova AA, Serrano BC, Cornberg M. Phase III results of Boceprevir in treatment naïve patients with chronic hepatitis C genotype 1. Liver International. 2012;**32**:27-31. DOI: 10.1111/j.1478-3231.2011.02725.x

[20] Parekh PJ, Shiffman ML. The role of interferon in the new era of hepatitis C treatments. Expert Review of Gastroenterology & Hepatology. 2014;**8**:649-656. DOI: 10.1586/17474124.2014.910453

[21] Benítez-Gutiérrez L, Barreiro P, Labarga P, de Mendoza C, Fernandez-Montero JV, Arias A, et al. Prevention and management of treatment failure to new oral hepatitis C drugs. Expert Opinion on Pharmacotherapy. 2016;**17**:1215-1223. DOI: 10.1080/14656566.2016.1182156

[22] Arias A, Aguilera A, Soriano V, Benítez-Gutiérrez L, Lledó G, Navarro D, et al. Rate and predictors of treatment failure to all-oral HCV regimens outside clinical trials. Antiviral Therapy. 2017;**22**:307-312. DOI: 10.3851/IMP3061

[23] Finkelmeier F, Dultz G, Peiffer K-H, Kronenberger B, Krauss F, Zeuzem S, et al. Risk of de novo hepatocellular carcinoma after HCV treatment with direct-acting antivirals. Liver Cancer. 2018. DOI: 10.1159/000486812

[24] Jovanović-Ćupić S, Kokanov N, Petrović N, Krajnović M, Kožik B, Kojić M SG. The influence of baseline viral and host factors on therapy response in patients with chronic hepatitis C genotype 1b from Serbia. First Congr. Mol. Biol. Serbia with Int. Particip., Belgrade, Serbia: n.d. p. 135

[25] Tanaka Y, Nishida N, Sugiyama M, Kurosaki M, Matsuura K, Sakamoto N, et al. Genome-wide association of IL28B with response to pegylated interferon-α and ribavirin therapy for chronic hepatitis C. Nature Genetics. 2009;**41**:1105-1109. DOI: 10.1038/ng.449

[26] Thomas DL, Thio CL, Martin MP, Qi Y, Ge D, O'hUigin C, et al. Genetic variation in IL28B and spontaneous clearance of hepatitis C virus. Nature. 2009;**461**:798-801. DOI: 10.1038/nature08463

[27] Prokunina-Olsson L, Muchmore B, Tang W, Pfeiffer RM, Park H, Dickensheets H, et al. A variant upstream of IFNL3 (IL28B) creating a new interferon gene IFNL4 is associated with impaired clearance of hepatitis C virus. Nature Genetics. 2013;**45**:164-171. DOI: 10.1038/ng.2521

[28] Terczyńska-Dyla E, Bibert S, Duong FHT, Krol I, Jørgensen S, Collinet E, et al. Reduced IFNλ4 activity is associated with improved HCV clearance and reduced expression of interferon-stimulated genes. Nature Communications. 2014;**5**:5699. DOI: 10.1038/ncomms6699

[29] Miki D, Ochi H, Takahashi A, Hayes CN, Urabe Y, Abe H, et al. HLA-DQB1*03 confers susceptibility to chronic hepatitis C in Japanese: A genome-wide association study. PLoS One. 2013;**8**:e84226. DOI: 10.1371/journal.pone.0084226

[30] Duggal P, Thio CL, Wojcik GL, Goedert JJ, Mangia A, Latanich R, et al. Genome-wide association study of spontaneous resolution of hepatitis C virus infection: Data from multiple cohorts. Annals of Internal Medicine. 2013;**158**:235. DOI: 10.7326/0003-4819-158-4-201302190-00003

[31] Kuniholm MH, Kovacs A, Gao X, Xue X, Marti D, Thio CL, et al. Specific human leukocyte antigen class I and II alleles associated with hepatitis C virus viremia. Hepatology. 2010;**51**:1514-1522. DOI: 10.1002/hep.23515

[32] Singh R, Kaul R, Kaul A, Khan K. A comparative review of HLA associations with hepatitis B and C viral infections across global populations. World Journal of Gastroenterology. 2007;**13**:1770-1787. DOI: 10.3748/WJG.V13.I12.1770

[33] Knapp S, Warshow U, Hegazy D, Brackenbury L, Guha IN, Fowell A, et al. Consistent beneficial effects of killer cell immunoglobulin-like receptor 2DL3 and group 1 human leukocyte antigen-C following exposure to hepatitis C virus. Hepatology. 2010;**51**:1168-1175. DOI: 10.1002/hep.23477

[34] Khakoo SI, Thio CL, Martin MP, Brooks CR, Gao X, Astemborski J, et al. HLA and NK cell inhibitory receptor genes in resolving hepatitis C virus infection. Science. 2004;**305**:872-874. DOI: 10.1126/science.1097670

[35] Shaker O, El-Shehaby A, Fayez S, Zahra A, Marzouk S, Raziky M El. Osteopontin gene polymorphisms as predictors for the efficacy of interferon therapy in chronic hepatitis C Egyptian patients with genotype 4. Cell Biochemistry and Function. 2013:n/a-n/a. DOI:10.1002/cbf.2954

[36] Angelo ALD, Cavalcante LN, Abe-Sandes K, Machado TB, Lemaire DC, Malta F, et al. Myxovirus resistance, osteopontin and suppressor of cytokine signaling 3 polymorphisms predict hepatitis C virus therapy response in an admixed patient population: Comparison with IL28B. Clinics (São Paulo, Brazil). 2013;68:1325-1332. DOI: 10.6061/clinics/2013(10)06

[37] Eslam M, Hashem AM, Leung R, Romero-Gomez M, Berg T, Dore GJ, et al. Interferon-λ rs12979860 genotype and liver fibrosis in viral and non-viral chronic liver disease. Nature Communications. 2015;6:6422. DOI: 10.1038/ncomms7422

[38] Patin E, Kutalik Z, Guergnon J, Bibert S, Nalpas B, Jouanguy E, et al. Genome-wide association study identifies variants associated with progression of liver fibrosis from HCV infection. Gastroenterology. 2012;143:1244-1252.e12. DOI: 10.1053/j.gastro.2012.07.097

[39] Urabe Y, Ochi H, Kato N, Kumar V, Takahashi A, Muroyama R, et al. A genome-wide association study of HCV-induced liver cirrhosis in the Japanese population identifies novel susceptibility loci at the MHC region. Journal of Hepatology. 2013;58:875-882. DOI: 10.1016/j.jhep.2012.12.024

[40] Kumar V, Kato N, Urabe Y, Takahashi A, Muroyama R, Hosono N, et al. Genome-wide association study identifies a susceptibility locus for HCV-induced hepatocellular carcinoma. Nature Genetics. 2011;43:455-458. DOI: 10.1038/ng.809

[41] Heim MH, Bochud P-Y, George J. Host - hepatitis C viral interactions: The role of genetics. Journal of Hepatology. 2016;65:S22-S32. DOI: 10.1016/j.jhep.2016.07.037

[42] Huang H, Shiffman ML, Friedman S, Venkatesh R, Bzowej N, Abar OT, et al. A 7 gene signature identifies the risk of developing cirrhosis in patients with chronic hepatitis C. Hepatology. 2007;46:297-306. DOI: 10.1002/hep.21695

[43] Eslam M, Hashem AM, Romero-Gomez M, Berg T, Dore GJ, Mangia A, et al. FibroGENE: A gene-based model for staging liver fibrosis. Journal of Hepatology. 2016;64:390-398. DOI: 10.1016/j.jhep.2015.11.008

[44] Totoki Y, Tatsuno K, Covington KR, Ueda H, Creighton CJ, Kato M, et al. Trans-ancestry mutational landscape of hepatocellular carcinoma genomes. Nature Genetics. 2014; 46:1267-1273. DOI: 10.1038/ng.3126

[45] Schulze K, Imbeaud S, Letouzé E, Alexandrov LB, Calderaro J, Rebouissou S, et al. Exome sequencing of hepatocellular carcinomas identifies new mutational signatures and potential therapeutic targets. Nature Genetics. 2015;47:505-511. DOI: 10.1038/ng.3252

[46] Ally A, Balasundaram M, Carlsen R, Chuah E, Clarke A, Dhalla N, et al. Comprehensive and integrative genomic characterization of hepatocellular carcinoma. Cell. 2017;169: 1327-1341.e23. DOI: 10.1016/j.cell.2017.05.046

[47] Chibon F. Cancer gene expression signatures—The rise and fall? European Journal of Cancer. 2013;**49**:2000-2009. DOI: 10.1016/j.ejca.2013.02.021

[48] Llovet JM, Chen Y, Wurmbach E, Roayaie S, Fiel MI, Schwartz M, et al. A molecular signature to discriminate dysplastic nodules from early hepatocellular carcinoma in HCV cirrhosis. Gastroenterology. 2006;**131**:1758-1767. DOI: 10.1053/j.gastro.2006.09.014

[49] Wu S-C, Chang SC, Wu H-Y, Liao P-J, Chang M-F. Hepatitis C virus NS5A protein down-regulates the expression of spindle gene Aspm through PKR-p38 signaling pathway. The Journal of Biological Chemistry. 2008;**283**:29396-29404. DOI: 10.1074/jbc.M802821200

[50] Machida K, Liu J-C, McNamara G, Levine A, Duan L, Lai MMC. Hepatitis C virus causes uncoupling of mitotic checkpoint and chromosomal polyploidy through the Rb pathway. Journal of Virology. 2009;**83**:12590-12600. DOI: 10.1128/JVI.02643-08

[51] Lai C-K, Jeng K-S, Machida K, Cheng Y-S, Lai MMC. Hepatitis C virus NS3/4A protein interacts with ATM, impairs DNA repair and enhances sensitivity to ionizing radiation. Virology. 2008;**370**:295-309. DOI: 10.1016/J.VIROL.2007.08.037

[52] Martell M, Esteban JI, Quer J, Genescà J, Weiner A, Esteban R, et al. Hepatitis C virus (HCV) circulates as a population of different but closely related genomes: Quasispecies nature of HCV genome distribution. Journal of Virology. 1992;**66**:3225-3229

[53] Figlerowicz M, Alejska M, Kurzyńska-Kokorniak A, Figlerowicz M. Genetic variability: The key problem in the prevention and therapy of RNA-based virus infections. Medicinal Research Reviews. 2003;**23**:488-518. DOI: 10.1002/med.10045

[54] Muñoz de Rueda P, Fuentes Rodríguez JM, Quiles Pérez R, Gila Medina A, Martín Álvarez AB, Casado Ruíz J, et al. Hepatitis C virus NS5A region mutation in chronic hepatitis C genotype 1 patients who are non-responders to two or more treatments and its relationship with response to a new treatment. World Journal of Gastroenterology. 2017;**23**:4538. DOI: 10.3748/wjg.v23.i25.4538

[55] Munoz de Rueda P, Casado J, Paton R, Quintero D, Palacios A, Gila A, et al. Mutations in E2-PePHD, NS5A-PKRBD, NS5A-ISDR, and NS5A-V3 of hepatitis C virus genotype 1 and their relationships to pegylated interferon-ribavirin treatment responses. Journal of Virology. 2008;**82**:6644-6653. DOI: 10.1128/JVI.02231-07

[56] Saito I, Miyamura T, Ohbayashi A, Harada H, Katayama T, Kikuchi S, et al. Hepatitis C virus infection is associated with the development of hepatocellular carcinoma. Proceedings of the National Academy of Sciences of the United States of America. 1990;**87**:6547-6549

[57] Pawlotsky J-M. Pathophysiology of hepatitis C virus infection and related liver disease. n.d. DOI:10.1016/j.tim.2003.12.005

[58] NIH Consensus Statement on Management of Hepatitis C: 2002. NIH Consens State Sci Statements. n.d.;**19**:1-46

[59] McGivern DR, Lemon SM. Virus-specific mechanisms of carcinogenesis in hepatitis C virus associated liver cancer. Oncogene. 2011;**30**:1969-1983. DOI: 10.1038/onc.2010.594

[60] International Agency for Research on Cancer WHO. Liver Cancer Estimated Incidence, Mortality and Prevalence Worldwide in 2012. Globocan 2012 Estim Cancer Incid Mortal Preval Worldw 2012. http://globocan.iarc.fr/Pages/fact_sheets_cancer.aspx (Accessed March 6, 2018)

[61] Nagai H, Sumino Y. Therapeutic strategy of advanced hepatocellular carcinoma by using combined intra-arterial chemotherapy. Recent Patents on Anti-Cancer Drug Discovery. 2008;3:220-226

[62] Yang JD, Roberts LR. Hepatocellular carcinoma: A global view. Nature Reviews. Gastroenterology & Hepatology. 2010;7:448-458. DOI: 10.1038/nrgastro.2010.100

[63] Yoshida H, Tateishi R, Arakawa Y, Sata M, Fujiyama S, Nishiguchi S, et al. Benefit of interferon therapy in hepatocellular carcinoma prevention for individual patients with chronic hepatitis C. Gut. 2004;53:425-430. DOI: 10.1136/GUT.2003.030353

[64] Shiratori Y, Ito Y, Yokosuka O, Imazeki F, Nakata R, Tanaka N, et al. Antiviral therapy for cirrhotic hepatitis C: Association with reduced hepatocellular carcinoma development and improved survival. Annals of Internal Medicine. 2005;142:105-114

[65] D'Ambrosio R, Colombo M. Should surveillance for liver cancer be modified in hepatitis C patients after treatment-related cirrhosis regression? Liver International. 2016;36:783-790. DOI: 10.1111/liv.13106

[66] de Oliveria Andrade LJ, D'Oliveira A, Melo RC, De Souza EC, Costa Silva CA, Paraná R. Association between hepatitis C and hepatocellular carcinoma. Journal of Global Infectious Diseases. 2009;1:33-37. DOI: 10.4103/0974-777X.52979

[67] Vescovo T, Refolo G, Vitagliano G, Fimia GM, Piacentini M. Molecular mechanisms of hepatitis C virus-induced hepatocellular carcinoma. Clinical Microbiology and Infection. 2016;22:853-861. DOI: 10.1016/j.cmi.2016.07.019

[68] Bartosch B, Thimme R, Blum HE, Zoulim F. Hepatitis C virus-induced hepatocarcinogenesis. Journal of Hepatology. 2009;51:810-820. DOI: 10.1016/j.jhep.2009.05.008

[69] Nakamoto Y, Guidotti LG, Kuhlen CV, Fowler P, Chisari FV. Immune pathogenesis of hepatocellular carcinoma. The Journal of Experimental Medicine. 1998;188:341-350

[70] Mitochondrial injury, oxidative stress, and antioxidant gene expression are induced by hepatitis C virus core protein. Gastroenterology. 2002;122:366-375. DOI: 10.1053/GAST.2002.30983

[71] Helmut Bartsch JN. Oxidative stress and lipid peroxidation-derived DNA-lesions in inflammation driven carcinogenesis. Cancer Detection and Prevention. 2004;28:385-391. DOI: 10.1016/J.CDP.2004.07.004

[72] Gurtsevitch VE. Human oncogenic viruses: Hepatitis B and hepatitis C viruses and their role in hepatocarcinogenesis. The Biochemist. 2008;73:504-513. DOI: 10.1134/S0006297908050039

[73] Hoshida Y, Fuchs BC, Bardeesy N, Baumert TF, Chung RT. Pathogenesis and prevention of hepatitis C virus-induced hepatocellular carcinoma. Journal of Hepatology. 2014;**61**:S79-S90. DOI: 10.1016/j.jhep.2014.07.010

[74] Koike K. Hepatitis C virus contributes to hepatocarcinogenesis by modulating metabolic and intracellular signaling pathways. Journal of Gastroenterology and Hepatology. 2007;**22**:S108-S111. DOI: 10.1111/j.1440-1746.2006.04669.x

[75] Mesri EA, Feitelson MA, Munger K. Human viral oncogenesis: A cancer hallmarks analysis. Cell Host & Microbe. 2014;**15**:266-282. DOI: 10.1016/j.chom.2014.02.011

[76] Sakamuro D, Furukawa T, Takegami T. Hepatitis C virus nonstructural protein NS3 transforms NIH 3T3 cells. Journal of Virology. 1995;**69**:3893-3896

[77] Ray RB, Lagging LM, Meyer K, Ray R. Hepatitis C virus core protein cooperates with ras and transforms primary rat embryo fibroblasts to tumorigenic phenotype. Journal of Virology. 1996;**70**:4438-4443

[78] Ghosh AK, Majumder M, Steele R, Meyer K, Ray R, Ray RB. Hepatitis C virus NS5A protein protects against TNF-α mediated apoptotic cell death. Virus Research. 2000;**67**:173-178. DOI: 10.1016/S0168-1702(00)00141-6

[79] Ray RB, Meyer K, Ray R. Hepatitis C virus Core protein promotes immortalization of primary human hepatocytes. Virology. 2000;**271**:197-204. DOI: 10.1006/VIRO.2000.0295

[80] Park JS, Yang JM, Min MK. Hepatitis C virus nonstructural protein NS4B transforms NIH3T3 cells in cooperation with the ha-ras oncogene. Biochemical and Biophysical Research Communications. 2000;**267**:581-587. DOI: 10.1006/bbrc.1999.1999

[81] Egger G, Liang G, Aparicio A, Jones PA. Epigenetics in human disease and prospects for epigenetic therapy. Nature. 2004;**429**:457-463. DOI: 10.1038/nature02625

[82] Robertson KD. DNA methylation and human disease. Nature Reviews. Genetics. 2005;**6**:597-610. DOI: 10.1038/nrg1655

[83] Kaneto H, Sasaki S, Yamamoto H, Itoh F, Toyota M, Suzuki H, et al. Detection of hypermethylation of the p16 INK4A gene promoter in chronic hepatitis and cirrhosis associated with hepatitis B or C virus n.d

[84] Roncalli M, Bianchi P, Bruni B, Laghi L, Destro A, Di Gioia S, et al. Methylation framework of cell cycle gene inhibitors in cirrhosis and associated hepatocellular carcinoma. Hepatology. 2002;**36**:427-432. DOI: 10.1053/jhep.2002.34852

[85] Feinberg AP. Epigenetics at the epicenter of modern medicine. Journal of the American Medical Association. 2008;**299**:1345. DOI: 10.1001/jama.299.11.1345

[86] Feitelson M. Parallel epigenetic and genetic changes in the pathogenesis of hepatitis virus-associated hepatocellular carcinoma. Cancer Letters. 2006;**239**:10-20. DOI: 10.1016/j.canlet.2005.07.009

[87] Nishida N, Nagasaka T, Nishimura T, Ikai I, Boland CR, Goel A. Aberrant methylation of multiple tumor suppressor genes in aging liver, chronic hepatitis, and hepatocellular carcinoma. Hepatology. 2008;**47**:908-918. DOI: 10.1002/hep.22110

[88] Zekri AE-RN, Nassar AA-M, El-Din El-Rouby MN, Shousha HI, Barakat AB, El-Desouky ED, et al. Disease progression from chronic hepatitis C to cirrhosis and hepatocellular carcinoma is associated with increasing DNA promoter methylation. Asian Pacific Journal of Cancer Prevention. 2014;**14**:6721-6726

[89] Zekri A-RN, Bahnasy AA, Shoeab FEM, Mohamed WS, El-Dahshan DH, Ali FT, et al. Methylation of multiple genes in hepatitis C virus associated hepatocellular carcinoma. Journal of Advanced Research. 2014;**5**:27-40. DOI: 10.1016/j.jare.2012.11.002

[90] N Zekri A-R, Raafat AM, Elmasry S, Bahnassy AA, Saad Y, Dabaon HA, et al. Promotor methylation: Does it affect response to therapy in chronic hepatitis C (G4) or fibrosis? Annals of Hepatology. n.d.;**13**:518-524

[91] Arora P, Kim E-O, Jung JK, Jang KL. Hepatitis C virus core protein downregulates E-cadherin expression via activation of DNA methyltransferase 1 and 3b. Cancer Letters. 2008;**261**:244-252. DOI: 10.1016/j.canlet.2007.11.033

[92] Park S-H, Lim JS, Lim S-Y, Tiwari I, Jang KL. Hepatitis C virus Core protein stimulates cell growth by down-regulating p16 expression via DNA methylation. Cancer Letters. 2011;**310**:61-68. DOI: 10.1016/j.canlet.2011.06.012

[93] Huang J-Z, Xia S-S, Ye Q-F, Jiang H-Y, Chen Z-H. Effects of p16 gene on biological behaviours in hepatocellular carcinoma cells. World Journal of Gastroenterology. 2003;**9**:84-88

[94] Park J, Jang KL. Hepatitis C virus represses E-cadherin expression via DNA methylation to induce epithelial to mesenchymal transition in human hepatocytes. Biochemical and Biophysical Research Communications. 2014;**446**:561-567. DOI: 10.1016/j.bbrc.2014.03.009

[95] Lee S, Lee HJ, Kim J-H, Lee H-S, Jang JJ, Kang GH. Aberrant CpG island hypermethylation along multistep hepatocarcinogenesis. The American Journal of Pathology. 2003;**163**:1371-1378. DOI: 10.1016/S0002-9440(10)63495-5

[96] Feng Q, Stern JE, Hawes SE, Lu H, Jiang M, Kiviat NB. DNA methylation changes in normal liver tissues and hepatocellular carcinoma with different viral infection. Experimental and Molecular Pathology. 2010;**88**:287-292. DOI: 10.1016/j.yexmp.2010.01.002

[97] Chan KCA, Lai PBS, Mok TSK, Chan HLY, Ding C, Yeung SW, et al. Quantitative analysis of circulating methylated DNA as a biomarker for hepatocellular carcinoma. Clinical Chemistry. 2008;**54**:1528-1536. DOI: 10.1373/clinchem.2008.104653

[98] Zhang Y-J, Wu H-C, Shen J, Ahsan H, Tsai WY, Yang H-I, et al. Predicting hepatocellular carcinoma by detection of aberrant promoter methylation in serum DNA. Clinical Cancer Research. 2007;**13**:2378-2384. DOI: 10.1158/1078-0432.CCR-06-1900

[99] Iyer P, Zekri A-R, Hung C-W, Schiefelbein E, Ismail K, Hablas A, et al. Concordance of DNA methylation pattern in plasma and tumor DNA of Egyptian hepatocellular carcinoma patients. Experimental and Molecular Pathology. 2010;**88**:107-111. DOI: 10.1016/j.yexmp.2009.09.012

[100] Li Z, Zhang H, Yang J, Hao T, Li S. Promoter hypermethylation of DNA damage response genes in hepatocellular carcinoma. Cell Biology International. 2012;36:427-432. DOI: 10.1042/CBI20100851

[101] Hayashi T, Tamori A, Nishikawa M, Morikawa H, Enomoto M, Sakaguchi H, et al. Differences in molecular alterations of hepatocellular carcinoma between patients with a sustained virological response and those with hepatitis C virus infection. Liver International. 2009;29:126-132. DOI: 10.1111/j.1478-3231.2008.01772.x

[102] Djebali S, Davis CA, Merkel A, Dobin A, Lassmann T, Mortazavi A, et al. Landscape of transcription in human cells. Nature. 2012;489:101-108. DOI: 10.1038/nature11233

[103] Ling H, Vincent K, Pichler M, Fodde R, Berindan-Neagoe I, Slack FJ, et al. Junk DNA and the long non-coding RNA twist in cancer genetics. Oncogene. 2015;34:5003-5011. DOI: 10.1038/onc.2014.456

[104] Lee Y, Ahn C, Han J, Choi H, Kim J, Yim J, et al. The nuclear RNase III Drosha initiates microRNA processing. Nature. 2003;425:415-419. DOI: 10.1038/nature01957

[105] Koscianska E, Starega-Roslan J, Krzyzosiak WJ. The role of dicer protein partners in the processing of MicroRNA precursors. PLoS One. 2011;6:e28548. DOI: 10.1371/journal.pone.0028548

[106] Cheloufi S, Dos Santos CO, Chong MMW, Hannon GJ. A dicer-independent miRNA biogenesis pathway that requires ago catalysis. Nature. 2010;465:584-589. DOI: 10.1038/nature09092

[107] Monroig P del C, Chen L, Zhang S, Calin GA. Small molecule compounds targeting miRNAs for cancer therapy. Advanced Drug Delivery Reviews. 2015;81:104-116. DOI: 10.1016/j.addr.2014.09.002

[108] Jelen MM, Glavač D. Importance of MicroRNAs in hepatitis B and C diagnostics and treatment. In: Allam N, editor. Adv. Treat. Hepat. C B. Vol. 3. InTech; 2017. DOI: 10.5772/62815

[109] Petrovic N, Ergün S, Isenovic ER. Levels of MicroRNA heterogeneity in cancer biology. Molecular Diagnosis & Therapy. 2017;21:511-523. DOI: 10.1007/s40291-017-0285-9

[110] Varnholt H. The role of microRNAs in primary liver cancer. Annals of Hepatology. 2008;7:104-113

[111] Shrivastava S, Steele R, Ray R, Ray RB. MicroRNAs: Role in hepatitis C virus pathogenesis. Genes and Diseases. 2015;2:35-45. DOI: 10.1016/j.gendis.2015.01.001

[112] Motawi TMK, Sadik NAH, Shaker OG, Ghaleb MH. Elevated serum microRNA-122/222 levels are potential diagnostic biomarkers in Egyptian patients with chronic hepatitis C but not hepatic cancer. Tumor Biology. 2016;37:9865-9874. DOI: 10.1007/s13277-016-4884-6

[113] Ono C, Fukuhara T, Motooka D, Nakamura S, Okuzaki D, Yamamoto S, et al. Characterization of miR-122-independent propagation of HCV. PLoS Pathogens. 2017;13:e1006374. DOI: 10.1371/journal.ppat.1006374

[114] Pang PS, Pham EA, Elazar M, Patel SG, Eckart MR, Glenn JS. Structural map of a MicroRNA-122: Hepatitis C virus complex. Journal of Virology. 2012;**86**:1250-1254. DOI: 10.1128/JVI.06367-11

[115] Murakami Y, Aly HH, Tajima A, Inoue I, Shimotohno K. Regulation of the hepatitis C virus genome replication by miR-199a. Journal of Hepatology. 2009;**50**:453-460. DOI: 10.1016/j.jhep.2008.06.010

[116] Zhang Y, Wei W, Cheng N, Wang K, Li B, Jiang X, et al. Hepatitis C virus-induced up-regulation of microRNA-155 promotes hepatocarcinogenesis by activating Wnt signaling. Hepatology. 2012;**56**:1631-1640. DOI: 10.1002/hep.25849

[117] Petrovic N, Davidovic R, Jovanovic-Cupic S, Krajnovic M, Lukic S, Petrovic M, et al. Changes in miR-221/222 levels in invasive and in situ carcinomas of the breast: Differences in association with Estrogen receptor and TIMP3 expression levels. Molecular Diagnosis & Therapy. 2016;**20**:603-615. DOI: 10.1007/s40291-016-0230-3

[118] Braconi C, Valeri N, Gasparini P, Huang N, Taccioli C, Nuovo G, et al. Hepatitis C virus proteins modulate MicroRNA expression and Chemosensitivity in malignant hepatocytes. Clinical Cancer Research. 2010;**16**:957-966. DOI: 10.1158/1078-0432.CCR-09-2123

[119] Hsu S, Wang B, Kota J, Yu J, Costinean S, Kutay H, et al. Essential metabolic, anti-inflammatory, and anti-tumorigenic functions of miR-122 in liver. The Journal of Clinical Investigation. 2012;**122**:2871-2883. DOI: 10.1172/JCI63539

16

Health-Related Quality of Life in Antiviral-Treated Chronic Hepatitis C Patients

Aleksandar Včev, Jelena Jakab, Lucija Kuna and Martina Smolić

Abstract

Chronic hepatitis C has a profound negative impact on both physical and mental well-being, thus decreasing health-related quality of life (HRQL). The most common complaints include symptoms such as fatigue, depression, and neurocognitive deficits. The burden of chronic HCV infections is multiplied by emotional and psychological issues that affect patients' functional health and work ability. Treatment of chronic HCV infection may at the beginning cause worse HRQL rates, as a result of common adverse effects like fatigue, muscle aches, and depression. However, the relationship between sustained virologic response (SVR) and improvement in HRQL is well known. Treatment-related adverse effects may discourage patients from starting therapy and reduce their adherence to treatment. Novel agents, with improved adverse effect profiles and SVR rates, allow more patients the opportunity to achieve improvements in HRQL during and after treatment.

Keywords: chronic hepatitis C, HCV treatment, adverse effects, health-related quality of life

1. Introduction

Life expectancy and causes of death have been used as key indicators of population health. Although these indicators provide information about the health status of populations, they do not offer any evidence about the quality of the physical, mental, or social functioning. To date, health is systematically included as a significant aspect of quality of life. Health-related quality of life (HRQL) measures have been developed to evaluate numerous aspects of an individual's subjective experience that cover health, disease, and different disabilities [1]. Despite the huge interest in quality of life, agreement is lacking on the definition and measurement of quality of life. Therefore, quality of life is used as a generic designation to describe a range of different physical and psychosocial variables [2].

2. Health-related quality of life (HRQL)

At the beginning of the 1990s, the World Health Organization (WHO) accepted the importance of evaluating and improving people's quality of life and developed a project in order to create a cross-cultural instrument of quality of life assessment: the World Health Organization Quality of Life (WHOQOL) [3]. WHO started its own project for several reasons. One of the reasons was to develop an international quality of life evaluation. Also, it was important to include a consideration of patients' quality of life in treatment decisions, approval of new pharmaceuticals, and policy research. Hence, having an international quality of life assessment as WHOQOL makes it possible to follow up quality of life research in different cultural settings and to directly compare results obtained in these different placements [4].

Likewise, clinicians and public health professionals have used health-related quality of life (HRQL) to evaluate the effects of the chronic diseases, treatments, and different disabilities. Institutes at the National Institutes of Health (NIH): for instance, the National Cancer Institute (NCI) and centers within the Centers for Disease Control and Prevention (CDC) have involved the evaluation and improvement of HRQL as a public health preference [5].

There are two potential explanations for the increasing interest in the assessment of quality of life in health care. The first explanation is an increased life expectancy as a result of improved medical care. Diagnostic and therapeutic treatments have increasingly advanced prognoses and management of many diseases, also increasing the life expectancy of individuals affected by these diseases. Consequently, many more patients are diagnosed with chronic, clinically manageable diseases than terminal diseases [2]. This evolution has led to the conclusion that health care interventions can no longer be evaluated solely on the basis of mortality or morbidity. Indeed, the impact of a disorder on a patient's life must also be observed [6]. The second explanation is referred to as the proliferation of improved medical and surgical technologies. Quality of life is included in the evaluation of the benefits of different treatment options.

HRQL aims at measuring disabilities related to specific diseases and also on effectiveness of treatment. Studies on HRQL focus on quality of life components that can be impacted by specific diseases. For example, measures of well-being typically evaluate the positive aspects of a person's life such as positive emotions. Therefore, numerous studies evaluate the quality and outcome of provided health care [2, 5].

It is important to emphasize that in HRQL, the experience of patients is most important. However, not only patient's estimation of their level of functioning is significant, for instance, cognitive process, but also the level of satisfaction in the different scopes, for instance, emotional process [7]. Investigators focused on HRQL may overestimate the impact of health-related factors. In addition, they could seriously underestimate the importance of nonmedical phenomena [8]. Some analyses of quality of life that have been undertaken have recognized this idea. Therefore, the majority of analyses have demonstrated that quality of life is most properly defined in patient satisfaction [9]. Finally, health should be observed as significant indicator as well as an important contributor to better quality of life.

3. HRQL measurements

Assessment of HRQL is related to functioning and well being in physical, mental, and social parts of life. Moreover, it shows importance in screening for disability and in improving communication between patients and clinicians [10, 11].

Common HRQL profile measures use multiple points to evaluate each of multiple parts of health and to decrease response burden. For that purpose, short-form HRQL measures, such as short-form 36 (SF-36), are widely used. Their briefness makes short-form measures practical for use as only 7 to 10 minutes are required to complete the form [12]. To provide the briefest possible measure of HRQL, the Dartmouth Cooperative Functional Assessment Charts (COOP) were designed. They consist of global items representing every single domain of health. These items are managed using five response choices: *Excellent, Very good, Good, Fair, Poor*, and COOP charts are original examples of global health items to evaluate multiple HRQL domains [13]. The NIH Patient-Reported Outcomes Measurement Information System (PROMIS) assesses global physical, mental, and social HRQL. It also designs, develops, validates, and standardizes item banks to measure patient-reported outcomes (PROs) relevant across common medical conditions. PRO is a 10-question measure which was developed through PROMIS, a NIH Roadmap electronic system designed to collect self-reported HRQL data from different populations with different types of chronic diseases [14]. The PROMIS global measure includes questions that evaluate self-rated health, physical HRQL, mental HRQL and evaluate for fatigue, pain, emotional distress, and their effects on different types of social activities. Recent investigations showed that psychometric evaluation of the PROMIS global health questions identified global physical and mental health summary scales but also separate scoring for global health, social activities, and numerous roles. Since it has been demonstrated, individual questions can be used to assess physical and mental HRQL, and social questions are included to assess social HRQL [14]. The PROMIS global health measure is scheduled to be managed on the National Health Interview Survey (NHIS) every 5 years. Analysis of summary scores and individual questions are expected to provide useful results and information. Their results are also expected to be reported every 5 years.

Well-being measures evaluate the positive aspects of people's lives. These measures have an association with their health and satisfaction, the quality of their relationships, positive emotions, their resiliency, and also with the realization of their potential. Well-being indicators measure when people feel very healthy and satisfied with life. Therefore, these characteristics representing well-being are associated with different benefits related to health, work, family, and economics. For instance, positive emotions are associated with decreased risk of disease and injury, as well as better immune functioning, which includes faster recovery time and

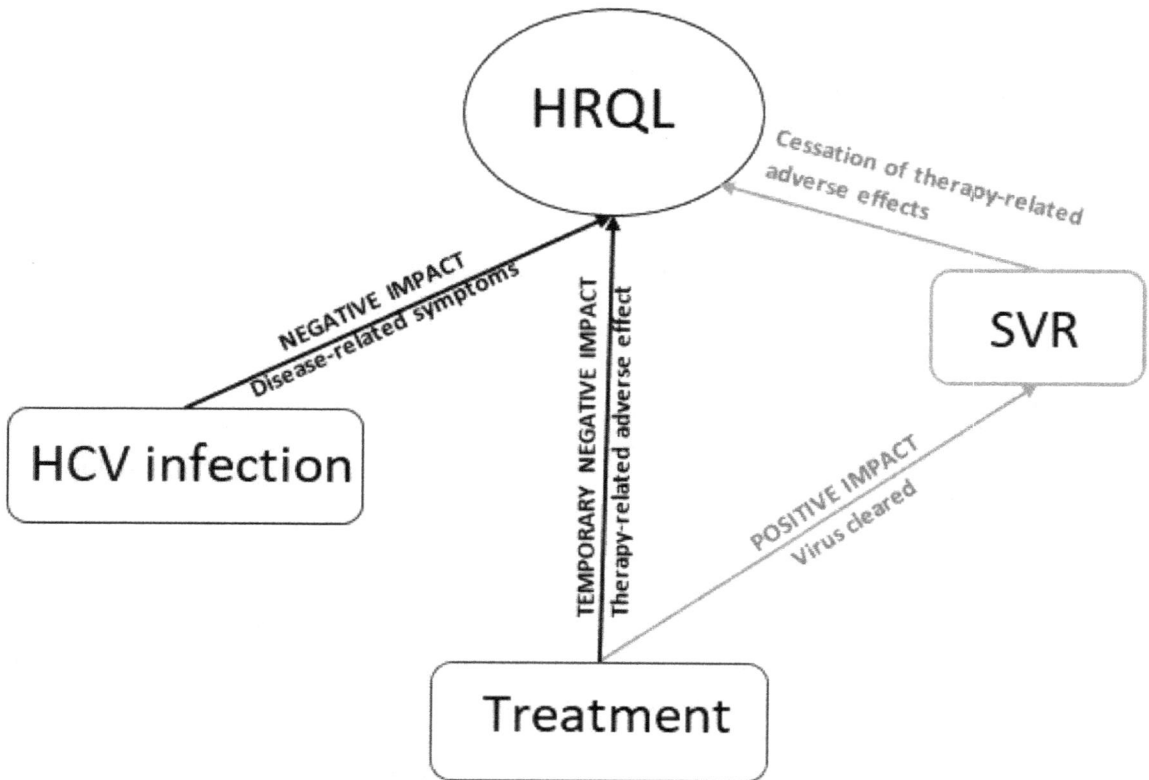

Figure 1. Chronic infection with hepatitis C compromises HRQL due to disease-related symptoms. Antiviral therapy affects HRQL negatively through side effects, but successful treatment of CHC improves HRQL because of cessation of treatment-related adverse effects and also due to disease eradication and virus clearance.

hepatitis C, and it serves as an independent predictor of low HRQL. Neuropsychological symptoms and hepatic encephalopathy can be found among patients with chronic hepatitis C, as well as mild cognitive deficits. Those symptoms may be the result of released inflammatory cytokines and altered neurotransmission [35]. Depression is another common feature of chronic hepatitis C which has been shown to be associated with lower work and social adjustment, lower acceptance of illness, and higher rates of subjective physical symptoms [36]. It is possible that mood-related aspects of HRQL are mediated by HCV colonization of brain microglia.

Poor baseline HRQL is partly psychosocial in origin, relating to the psychiatric comorbidity associated with acquisition of HCV, stigma of illness, and history of illicit drug use [37]. Patients with HCV infection are stigmatized in society which affects their HRQL but may also be a barrier to treatment, resulting in decreased social support [36]. Chronic hepatitis C as a disease with uncertain outcome raises serious concerns about future health status and presents significant emotional and psychological burden. Patients with chronic HCV infection aware of their diagnosis had worse HRQL scores as compared with unaware seropositive patients, suggesting the psychological impact of diagnosis awareness.

HCV patients who experience greater physical and psychiatric symptoms and have poorer HRQL are more likely to discontinue treatment prematurely. These issues highlight the importance of investigating the physical and psychosocial experiences and HRQL of patients chronically infected with HCV [38].

6. HCV treatment impact on HRQL

Patient-reported outcome (PRO) measures are important to evaluate the impact of chronic infection, willingness for treatment and assessment of HRQL during and post treatment. These measures ensure that patient preferences are taken into consideration when deciding between treatment options. While antiviral treatment can eradicate the virus and prevent liver-related death, associated toxicity can have effect on HRQL by decreasing physical, social, and emotional functioning [39].

In recent years, treatment options for HCV infection have moved from the use of interferon with low efficacy and significant toxicity to first-generation direct antiviral agents (DAAs) which were more efficient but still toxic to interferon-free regimens with high efficacy and minimal toxicity [40].

Besides HRQL burden of HCV infection, the previous anti-HCV treatment with interferon and ribavirin had further negative impact on patients' HRQL due to substantial side effects. Well documented side effects of interferon include fever, myalgias, and headache, often described as influenza-like illness. IFN-mediated myelosuppression may lead to decreases in erythrocyte, leukocyte, and platelet counts. Neuropsychiatric side effects include irritability, depression, anxiety, and fatigue. Fatigue is the most commonly reported adverse effect which occurs as a part of neurovegetative symptoms during the first 3 months of treatment [41]. Anorexia, nausea, vomiting, and diarrhea are gastrointestinal adverse effect [36]. Adding RBV to interferon improves SVR, but it substantially impairs physical functioning, which may be the result of hemolytic anemia, occasional rash, and additional fatigue [42]. The use of peg-IFN and RBV is associated with less fatigue and bodily pain than standard IFN and RBV, but it is also characterized by considerable toxicity, neuropsychiatric side-effects, lethargy, and influenza-like symptoms [43]. The side effects of HCV therapy increase the likelihood that patients will discontinue treatment, and because of that, adjunctive therapy must be considered to treat those side effects. Fatigue, depression, and anemia are more difficult to control so addressing those symptoms is of major importance for patients' adherence to therapy [36].

However, successful clearance of the virus after treatment results in certain HRQL improvement in patients who respond well to therapy. Patient-reported outcomes, including HRQL, fatigue, and work productivity improved in patients after achieving sustained virologic response (SVR) with interferon and ribavirin-containing regimens [44]. Therefore, reaching SVR is crucial in achieving long-term HRQL in patients with chronic HCV infection.

The first-generation direct antiviral agents (DAA) shifted the treatment focus to protease inhibitors (PI). A triple combination therapy (PEG-IFN + ribavirin + a protease inhibitor) increased SVR rates but decreased HRQL. Along with the pegylated interferon and RBV side effects, PIs carried plenty of additional side effects. Telaprevir treatment causes nausea, rectal burning, diarrhea, and recently, it has been connected to decrease renal function. Lower glomerular filtration rate led to decreased renal elimination of RBV. Boceprevir has been associated with nausea, headache, and anemia. Furthermore, these regimens had significant drug–drug interactions (DDIs) [41]. However, symptom alleviation after successful treatment can improve HRQL, having economic and social benefits and resulting in removal of social stigma [39].

The next generation of DAAs focused on different targets: HCV viral replication in the cytoplasm. These new drugs, given without concomitant interferon, can result in SVR in over 90% of cases. Additionally, toxicity is reduced in comparison with second generation triple combinations, although response is influenced by genotype, stage of hepatic fibrosis, and drug-resistant mutations [39]. Shortly after initiation of treatment, there is an improvement in PRO scores which correlates with viral suppression. Furthermore, therapy with the new generation of DAAs maximizes PRO rates during treatment as well as after achieving SVR [40]. Most of the data about HRQL come from sofosbuvir (SOF)-based treatment options. Analysis showed that the PRO profile of interferon-free regimens (SOF/RBV) was significantly better compared to peg-IFN/RBV regimens. However, RBV-containing regimens still carry important HRQL impairment, possibly due to hemolytic anemia and mental health side effects of RBV. When both RBV and interferon are removed from the regimen, improvements in HRQL, work productivity, and other PROs were noted 2 weeks after starting treatment (**Figure 1**) [41].

7. The road to success: future directions to improve HCV HRQL

Regardless of the regimen, there are significant improvements in PRO scores after achieving SVR. Still, these improvements are more noticeable in patients who achieve SVR with DAAs. It is shown in multivariate analysis that receiving a regimen that contained IFN and RBV was the strongest negative predictor of HRQL during treatment [45]. On the other hand, IFN- and RBV-free was the only regimen independently associated with improved HRQL during treatment. Moreover, DAAs remained the only independent predictor of HRQL improvement after achieving SVR [46]. However, there are still unanswered questions in terms of DAA safety, and we require data from real-world settings. For example, postauthorization studies would be useful to identify and characterize safety profiles of the new DAAs [47].

8. Conclusions

Chronic HCV infection causes a decline in HRQL measures through a broad spectrum of clinical complaints. The impact on HRQL affects physical, social, and mental health domains. SVR is associated with improvement in HRQL, thereby indicating that treatment of HCV may improve PRO rates in patients who respond well to therapy. Considering low efficacy and significant toxicity of IFN/RBV regimens, treatment options are shifting to the new DAAs which offer improved SVR rates with less toxicity, leading to improvements in HRQL in patients with chronic hepatitis C.

Author details

Aleksandar Včev[1,2]*, Jelena Jakab[2], Lucija Kuna[2] and Martina Smolić[2,3]

*Address all correspondence to: aleksandar.vcev@mefos.hr

1 Department of Medicine, Faculty of Medicine Osijek, University of Osijek, Osijek, Croatia

2 Department of Integrative Medicine, Faculty of Medicine Osijek, University of Osijek, Osijek, Croatia

3 Department of Pharmacology, Faculty of Medicine Osijek, University of Osijek, Osijek, Croatia

References

[1] Coletta SL. Adults with congenital heart disease: Utilizing quality of life and Husted's nursing theory as a conceptual framework. Critical Care Nursering Quarterly. 1999;**22**(3): 1-11

[2] Moons P. Why call it health-related quality of life when you mean perceived health status? European Journal of Cardiovascular Nursing. 2004;**3**(4):275-277

[3] Canavarro MC, Serra AV, Simões MR, Rijo D, Pereira M, Gameiro S, et al. Development and psychometric properties of the World Health Organization quality of life assessment instrument (WHOQOL-100) in Portugal. International Journal of Behavioral Medicine. 2009;**16**(2):116-124

[4] Diener Ed, Seligman M.E.P. Beyond money: toward an economy of well-being. Psychological Science in the Public Interest. 2004;**5**(1):1-31

[5] The WHOQOL Group. The World Health Organization Quality of Life assessment (WHOQOL): position paper from the World Health Organization. Soc Sci Med. 1995; **41**(10):1403-9

[6] Colin M. Respondent-generated quality of life measures: Useful tools for nursing or more fool's gold? Journal of Advanced Nursing. 2000;**32**(2):375-382

[7] Kamphuis M, Zwinderman KH, Vogels T, Vliegen HW, Kamphuis RP, Ottenkamp J, et al. A cardiac-specific health-related quality of life module for young adults with congenital heart disease: Development and validation. Quality of Life Research. 2004;**13**(4):735-745

[8]   Gill TM, Feinstein AR. A critical appraisal of the quality of quality-of-life measurements. Journal of the American Medical Association. 1994;**272**(8):619-626

[9]   Ferrans CE. Development of a conceptual model of quality of life. Scholarly Inquiry for Nursing Practice. 1996;**10**(3):293-304

[10] McHorney CA. Health status assessment methods for adults: Past accomplishments and future challenges. Annual Review of Public Health. 1999;**20**:309-335

[11] Velikova G, Booth L, Smith AB, Brown PM, Lynch P, Brown JM, et al. Measuring quality of life in routine oncology practice improves communication and patient well-being: A randomized controlled trial. Journal of Clinical Oncology. 2004;**22**(4):714-724

[12] Coons SJ, Rao S, Keininger DL, Hays RD. A comparative review of generic quality-of-life instruments. PharmacoEconomics. 2000;**17**(1):13-35

[13] Nelson EC, Wasson JH, Johnson DJ, Hays RD. Dartmouth COOP Functional Health Assessment Charts: Brief measures for clinical practice. in: B Spilker (Ed.) Quality of Life and Pharmacoeconomics in Clinical Trials. ed 2. Lippincott-Raven, Philadelphia, PA; 1996

[14] Cella D, Yount S, Rothrock N, Gershon R, Cook K, Reeve B, et al. The patient-reported outcomes measurement information system (PROMIS): Progress of an NIH roadmap cooperative group during its first two years. Medical Care. 2007;**45**(5 Suppl 1):S3-S11

[15] Lyubomirsky S, King L, Diener E. The benefits of frequent positive affect: Does happiness lead to success? Psychological Bulletin. 2005;**131**(6):803-855

[16] Ed D. Well-Being for Public Policy. New York: Oxford University Press. Oxford Scholarship Online; 2010

[17] Albrecht GL, Devlieger PJ. The disability paradox: High quality of life against all odds. Social Science & Medicine. 1999;**48**(8):977-988

[18] Ronald DM. Healthy People 2010: national health objectives for United States. BMJ. 1998;**317**(7171):1513-1517

[19] Smith-Palmer J, Cerri K, Valentine W. Achieving sustained virologic response in hepatitis C: A systematic review of the clinical, economic and quality of life benefits. BMC Infectious Diseases. 2015;**15**:19

[20] Webster K, Cella D, Yost K. The functional assessment of chronic illness therapy (FACIT) measurement system: Properties, applications, and interpretation. Health and Quality of Life Outcomes. 2003;**1**:79

[21] Younossi ZM, Stepanova M, Henry L, Gane E, Jacobson IM, Lawitz E, et al. Effects of sofosbuvir-based treatment, with and without interferon, on outcome and productivity of patients with chronic hepatitis C. Clinical Gastroenterology and Hepatology. 2014;**12**(8): 1349-1359 e13

[22] Younossi ZM, Guyatt G, Kiwi M, Boparai N, King D. Development of a disease specific questionnaire to measure health related quality of life in patients with chronic liver disease. Gut. 1999;**45**(2):295-300

[23] Luciana S. The societal burden of chronic liver diseases: results from the COME study. BMJ Open Gastroenterol. 2015;**2**(1):e000025. Published online 2015 Mar 30. DOI:10.1136/bmjgast-2014-000025

[24] Lavanchy D. Evolving epidemiology of hepatitis C virus. Clinical Microbiology and Infection. 2011;**17**(2):107-115

[25] Van Herck K, Vorsters A, Van Damme P. Prevention of viral hepatitis (B and C) reassessed. Best Practice & Research. Clinical Gastroenterology. 2008;**22**(6):1009-1029

[26] NIH Consensus Statement on management of hepatitis C: 2002. NIH Consensus and State-of-The-Science Statements. 2002;**19**(3):1-46

[27] Edlin BR, Kresina TF, Raymond DB, Carden MR, Gourevitch MN, Rich JD, et al. Overcoming barriers to prevention, care, and treatment of hepatitis C in illicit drug users. Clinical Infectious Diseases. 2005;**40**(Suppl 5):S276-S285

[28] McHutchison JG, Bacon BR, Owens GS. Making it happen: Managed care considerations in vanquishing hepatitis C. The American Journal of Managed Care. 2007;**13**(Suppl 12):S327-S336 quiz S37-40

[29] Chong CA, Gulamhussein A, Heathcote EJ, Lilly L, Sherman M, Naglie G, et al. Health-state utilities and quality of life in hepatitis C patients. The American Journal of Gastroenterology. 2003;**98**(3):630-638

[30] Seeff LB, Hoofnagle JH. National Institutes of Health consensus development conference: Management of hepatitis C: 2002. Hepatology. 2002;**36**(5 Suppl 1):S1-S2

[31] Spiegel BMR. Impact of hepatitis C on health related quality of Life: A systematic review and quantitative assessment. Hepatology. 2005;**41**:790-800

[32] El Khoury AC, Vietri J, Prajapati G. Health-related quality of life in patients with hepatitis C virus infection in Brazil. Revista Panamericana de Salud Pública. 2014;**35**(3):200-206

[33] Bezemer G, Van Gool AR, Verheij-Hart E, Hansen BE, Lurie Y, Esteban JI, et al. Long-term effects of treatment and response in patients with chronic hepatitis C on quality of life. An international, multicenter, randomized, controlled study. BMC Gastroenterology. 2012;**12**:11

[34] Kallman J, O'Neil MM, Larive B, Boparai N, Calabrese L, Younossi ZM. Fatigue and health-related quality of life (HRQL) in chronic hepatitis C virus infection. Digestive Diseases and Sciences. 2007;**52**(10):2531-2539

[35] Vera-Llonch M, Martin M, Aggarwal J, Donepudi M, Bayliss M, Goss T, et al. Health-related quality of life in genotype 1 treatment-naïve chronic hepatitis C patients receiving telaprevir combination treatment in the ADVANCE study. Alimentary Pharmacology & Therapeutics. 2013;**38**(2):124-133

[36] Younossi ZM, Kallman J, Kincaid J. The effects of HCV infection and management on health-related quality of life. Hepatology. 2007;**45**(3):806-816

List of Contributors

Tomasz I. Michalak
Molecular Virology and Hepatology Research Group, Division of BioMedical Science, Faculty of Medicine, Health Sciences Center, Memorial University, St. John's, NL, Canada

Vanja Vojnović
Faculty of Medicine, Josip Juraj Strossmayer University, Osijek, Croatia
Department of Neurology, University Hospital Dubrava, Zagreb, Croatia

Philip Aston, Katie Cranfield and Haley O'Farrell
University of Surrey, Guildford, United Kingdom

Alex Cassenote, Cassia J. Mendes-Correa and Aluisio Segurado
University of Sao Paulo, Sao Paulo, Brazil

Phuong Hoang, George Lankford and Hien Tran
North Carolina State University, Raleigh, United States

Takashi Honda, Masatoshi Ishigami, Kazuhiko Hayashi, Teiji Kuzuya, Yoji Ishizu, Yoshiki Hirooka and Hidemi Goto
Department of Gastroenterology and Hepatology, Nagoya University Graduate School of Medicine, Nagoya, Japan

Binod Kumar, Akshaya Ramachandran and Gulam Waris
Department of Microbiology and Immunology, H.M. Bligh Cancer Research Laboratories, Chicago Medical School, Rosalind Franklin University of Medicine and Science, North Chicago, IL, USA

Milan Milošević
University of Zagreb, School of Medicine, Andrija Stampar School of Public Health, WHO Collaborative Centre for Occupational Health, Zagreb, Croatia

Jelena Jakab, Lucija Kuna and Martina Smolić
Josip Juraj Strossmayer University of Osijek, Faculty of Medicine, Osijek, Croatia

Moustafa Nouh Elemeery
Center for Systemic Biotechnology, Korea Institute of Science and Technology, Gangneung, Gwang-do, Republic of Korea
Division of Biomedical Science and Technology, Korea University of Science and Technology, Daejeon, Republic of Korea
Microbial Biotechnology Department, Genetic Engineering and Biotechnology Research Division, National Research Centre, Dokki-Giza, Egypt

Kazuhiko Hayashi, Masatoshi Ishigami, Yoji Ishizu, Teiji Kuzuya, Takashi Honda, Tetsuya Ishikawa, Hidemi Goto and Yoshiki Hirooka
Department of Gastroenterology and Hepatology, Nagoya University Graduate School of Medicine, Nagoya, Japan

Yoshihiko Tachi
Department of Gastroenterology, Komaki City Hospital, Komaki, Japan

Yoshiaki Katano
Department of Internal Medicine, Banbuntane Hotokukai Hospital, Fujita Health University, School of Medicine, Nagoya, Japan

Kentaro Yoshioka
Division of Liver and Biliary Diseases, Department of Internal Medicine, Fujita Health University, Toyoake, Japan

Hidenori Toyoda and Takashi Kumada
Department of Gastroenterology, Ogaki Municipal Hospital, Ogaki, Japan

Robert Smolić and Aleksandar Včev
University Hospital Center Osijek, Osijek, Croatia

Faculty of Medicine, Josip Juraj Strossmayer University of Osijek, Osijek, Croatia

Jelena Jakab, Lucija Kuna, Martina Smolić and Marinko Žulj
Faculty of Medicine, Josip Juraj Strossmayer University of Osijek, Osijek, Croatia

Martina Kajić
Pharmaceutical Company Pliva, Zagreb, Croatia

Nina Blažević
Division of Gastroenterology and Hepatology, Department of Internal Medicine, Sestre Milosrdnice University Hospital Center, Zagreb, Croatia

Marko Duvnjak and Lucija Virović Jukić
Division of Gastroenterology and Hepatology, Department of Internal Medicine, Sestre Milosrdnice University Hospital Center, Zagreb, Croatia
University of Zagreb School of Medicine, Zagreb, Croatia

Livia M Villar, Allan P da Silva and Letícia P Scalioni
Viral Hepatitis Laboratory, Oswaldo Cruz Institute, FIOCRUZ, Rio de Janeiro, Brazil

Cristiane A Villela-Nogueira
University Hospital Clementino Fraga Filho, School of Medicine, Federal University of Rio de Janeiro, Rio de Janeiro, RJ, Brazil

Shaina M. Lynch
Medical College of Wisconsin, Division of Gastroenterology and Hepatology, Milwaukee, USA

George Y. Wu
University of Connecticut, Division of Gastroenterology and Hepatology, Farmington, USA

Ljiljana Perić and Dario Sabadi
Department of Infectious Diseases and Dermatology, Faculty of Medicine Osijek, University of Osijek, Osijek, Croatia
Clinic for Infectious Diseases, University Hospital Center Osijek, Osijek, Croatia

Ashraf Tabll, Reem El-Shenawy and Yasmine El Abd
Microbial Biotechnology Department, Genetic Engineering and Biotechnology Research Division, National Research Center, Dokki, Giza, Egypt

Snezana Jovanovic-Cupic, Ana Bozovic, Milena Krajnovic and Nina Petrovic
University of Belgrade - Vinča Institute of Nuclear Sciences, Laboratory for Radiobiology and Molecular Genetics, Belgrade, Serbia

Aleksandar Včev
Department of Medicine, Faculty of Medicine Osijek, University of Osijek, Osijek, Croatia

Jelena Jakab and Lucija Kuna
Department of Integrative Medicine, Faculty of Medicine Osijek, University of Osijek, Osijek, Croatia

Martina Smolić
Department of Integrative Medicine, Faculty of Medicine Osijek, University of Osijek, Osijek, Croatia
Department of Pharmacology, Faculty of Medicine Osijek, University of Osijek, Osijek, Croatia

Index

www.ingramcontent.com/pod-product-compliance
Lightning Source LLC
Chambersburg PA
CBHW061952190326
41458CB00009B/2852